Health and Illness in Close Relationships

Health and Illness in Close Relationships provides an integrated theoretical framework for understanding the complexities of health trajectories and relationship processes. It is the first volume to review and synthesize current empirical evidence and associated theoretical constructs from the literature on health and illness in close relationships across the social and behavioral sciences. In doing so, it provides a unique cross-disciplinary understanding of how health and illness redefine relationships. The volume also maps out an explanatory framework of how the pathways and processes of close relationships pose considerations for resilience and flourishing or, on the contrary, for relational and health decline. It will appeal to researchers and students across psychology, communication, and relationship studies, as well as to health professionals who are interested in understanding how health conditions can shape or be shaped by patients' close relationships.

ASHLEY P. DUGGAN is an associate professor in the Communication Department and the Medical Humanities Program at Boston College, USA. She is also the co-director of the Communication and Family Medicine Research Division, a collaboration between Tufts University School of Medicine and Boston College, USA.

T0371364

Advances in Personal Relationships

Christopher R. Agnew
Purdue University

John P. Caughlin
University of Illinois at Urbana–Champaign

C. Raymond Knee
University of Houston

Terri L. Orbuch
Oakland University

Although scholars from a variety of disciplines have written and conversed about the importance of personal relationships for decades, the emergence of personal relationships as a field of study is relatively recent. *Advances in Personal Relationships* represents the culmination of years of multidisciplinary and interdisciplinary work on personal relationships. Sponsored by the International Association for Relationship Research, the series offers readers cutting-edge research and theory in the field. Contributing authors are internationally known scholars from a variety of disciplines, including social psychology, clinical psychology, communication, history, sociology, gerontology, and family studies. Volumes include integrative reviews, conceptual pieces, summaries of research programs, and major theoretical works. *Advances in Personal Relationships* presents first-rate scholarship that is both provocative and theoretically grounded. The theoretical and empirical work described by authors will stimulate readers and advance the field by offering new ideas and retooling old ones. The series will be of interest to upper-division undergraduate students, graduate students, researchers, and practitioners.

Other Books in the Series

Attribution, Communication Behavior, and Close Relationships
Valerie Manusov and John H. Harvey, editors

Stability and Change in Relationships
Anita L. Vangelisti, Harry T. Reis, and Mary Anne Fitzpatrick, editors

Understanding Marriage: Developments in the Study of Couple Interaction
Patricia Noller and Judith A. Feeney, editors

Growing Together: Personal Relationships Across the Lifespan
Frieder R. Lang and Karen L. Fingerman, editors

Communicating Social Support
Daena J. Goldsmith

Communicating Affection: Interpersonal Behavior and Social Context
Kory Floyd

Changing Relations: Achieving Intimacy in a Time of Social Transition
Robin Goodwin

Feeling Hurt in Close Relationships
Anita L. Vangelisti, editor

Romantic Relationships in Emerging Adulthood
Frank D. Fincham and Ming Cui, editors

Responding to Intimate Violence Against Women: The Role of Informal Networks
Renate Klein

Social Influences on Romantic Relationships: Beyond the Dyad
Christopher R. Agnew, editor

Positive Approaches to Optimal Relationship Development
C. Raymond Knee and Harry T. Reis, editors

Personality and Close Relationship Processes
Stanley O. Gaines, Jr.

The Experience and Expression of Uncertainty in Close Relationships
Jennifer A. Theiss

Contemporary Studies on Relationships, Health, and Wellness
Jennifer A. Theiss and Kathryn Greene, editors

Power in Close Relationships
Christopher R. Agnew and Jennifer J. Harman, editors

Health and Illness in Close Relationships

ASHLEY P. DUGGAN

Boston College, Massachusetts

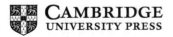

CAMBRIDGE
UNIVERSITY PRESS

CAMBRIDGE
UNIVERSITY PRESS

University Printing House, Cambridge CB2 8BS, United Kingdom

One Liberty Plaza, 20th Floor, New York, NY 10006, USA

477 Williamstown Road, Port Melbourne, VIC 3207, Australia

314-321, 3rd Floor, Plot 3, Splendor Forum, Jasola District Centre, New Delhi - 110025, India

79 Anson Road, #06-04/06, Singapore 079906

Cambridge University Press is part of the University of Cambridge.

It furthers the University's mission by disseminating knowledge in the pursuit of education, learning and research at the highest international levels of excellence.

www.cambridge.org
Information on this title: www.cambridge.org/9781108412643
DOI: 10.1017/9781108325578

© Ashley P. Duggan 2019

First published 2019
First paperback edition 2020

A catalogue record for this publication is available from the British Library

Library of Congress Cataloging in Publication data
Names: Duggan, Ashley P., author.
Title: Health and illness in close relationships / Ashley P. Duggan, Boston College, Massachusetts.
Description: New York : Cambridge University Press, 2018. | Series: Advances in personal relationships | Includes index.
Identifiers: LCCN 2018040392 | ISBN 9781108419932
Subjects: LCSH: Care of the sick – Psychological aspects. | Sick – Psychology. | Interpersonal relations.
Classification: LCC R726.5 . D845 2018 | DDC 610–dc23
LC record available at https://lccn.loc.gov/2018040392

ISBN 978-1-108-41993-2 Hardback
ISBN 978-1-108-41264-3 Paperback

For the Martha's Vineyard Communication Association, the MVCA for short.

My favorite quasi-professional "association," a group of eight women who hold space for each other in the complexities of illness, surgery, new grandbabies, the loss of loved ones, accomplishments, and milestones, all over lots of wine, good food, and laughter. We are connected as communication faculty across different universities through our annual "conference" at Martha's Vineyard, through many years as a collective, and through our shared history of friendship and support. The MVCA is made up of Bonnie Jefferson, Sara Weintraub, Rita Rosenthal, Anne Mattina, Sherry Shepler, Roberta Kosberg, Nancy Willets, and me.

Contents

Acknowledgments   *page* xi

Introduction   1

PART I   THE UNIQUE CONTEXT OF HEALTH AND
ILLNESS IN CLOSE RELATIONSHIPS   17

1 Defining Health and Illness   19

2 Close Relationship Processes   59

3 Attributes of the Health and Illness Context for
   Relationship Processes   109

PART II   HEALTH AND ILLNESS, THE BODY, AND
RELATIONAL PROCESSES   153

4 Relationships as Buffering or Exacerbating Health and
   Illness Outcomes   155

5 Reconsidering Embodiment and Language for
   Illness   193

6 Relationship Theories Applied to Illness
   Transitions   220

PART III   INTEGRATED THEORY OF HEALTH AND
ILLNESS TRAJECTORIES AND RELATIONAL
PROCESSES   261

7 Theorizing Close Relationships and Health and Illness
   Trajectories: Co-created, Co-generative, and Systematic
   Processes   263

8 Integrated Co-generative, Systematic Processes and
   Considerations for Interdisciplinary Understanding   308

   References   327
   Index   366

Acknowledgments

Health and illness trajectories require that we understand beyond what we already know. The story of illness does not end with the completion of medical treatment. Sometimes the vulnerability shatters hope and leaves people feeling fragmented. Other times, the vulnerability shifts understanding such that people find new meaning. Never does it seem that illness is just a point of going through the motions. I am grateful for the many people over the years who have allowed and invited me into their lives as they navigate the complexities of health and illness in their own close relationships. Many people over the last twenty-plus years have shared their stories. Doctors and patients allowed me to videotape their interactions. Patients let me record their conversations as they made decisions with close friends and family members. Doctors wrote reflective journals about their experiences of finding meaning in their own learning about medicine, about patients' lives, and about their own challenges.

My own research on health and illness in close relationships began in 1996 with my master's thesis on nonverbal communication behaviors connected to disclosure about roles and relationships in doctor–patient interactions. I thank Roxanne Parrott for my early experiences in considering the complexities of health and healthcare and Beth Le Poire and Judee Burgoon for my initial foundation in social scientific theory-building and application.

John Caughlin and Chris Agnew approached me about writing a proposal for this *Advances in Personal Relationships* series and, with the series editors, provided feedback as I developed the proposal.

Janka Romero, my editor at Cambridge University Press, gave thoughtful responses throughout the process and offered helpful, particular answers about the production process but flexibility in the creative aspects of writing.

Lauren Alevizos, my research assistant, worked tirelessly on citations and references for this volume.

Martha Bancroft, friend, artist, and photographer, who took the cover photo.

Terri "The Love Doctor" Orbuch, after hearing my comments at the International Association for Relationship Research (IARR) mentorship conference I hosted, asked whether I had noticed I was good at making sense of lots of different strands of research. Her question prompted subsequent commitments to writing projects that integrate many different aspects for a topic. Perhaps in love and in writing, the seemingly small gestures make a difference!

Teresa Thompson shaped my understanding of whether theory can be context specific. In our shared work in connecting interpersonal communication processes with health and illness trajectories we considered how attributes of health and illness context shape relationship processes.

Sandra Petronio, my friend, co-author, mentor, and travel partner, introduced me to IARR, and challenged me to consider privacy boundaries in health and illness.

Allen Shaughnessy, co-author and collaborator, who makes the process of learning and challenging assumptions all the more rich and colorful. Cheers to our next steps in research in family medicine together.

Stan Deetz, with whom I have the privilege of learning what it means to see differently, and who has greatly influenced my understanding of generativity and engagement in theory-building and everyday life.

Todd Miller, spouse, co-parent and life partner, who helps me keep my grounding over time.

I could not do this work without the support of my university, Boston College, where Jesuit traditions shape my thinking and allow me to recognize competing tensions as productive. I am also grateful for my long-standing academic appointment at Tufts University School of Medicine and for my research colleagues there.

Introduction

I am drawn into the context of health and illness because of the vulnerabilities that require us to reconsider assumptions and expectations. When we face serious illness, changes in ourselves and in our close relationships often unfold differently from how we anticipate. Dealing with serious illness brings an increased sense of vulnerability, but also can bring opportunities to heal and grow. This book is primarily intended for scholars and practitioners interested in relationship research and in understanding that health and illness are inherently connected to relationship processes. As issues of health and illness and close relationships are applicable to a far broader audience, I have tried to keep the book accessible to a wide audience by minimizing technical terms and explaining contemporary issues using language that keeps the issues clear to people who are not already familiar with the research.

I write this volume at this time because I've spent the last twenty years listening to stories and experiences of illness. For more than twenty years I've had the extraordinary privilege of integrating my research in communication processes into health-care conversations and decisions. I've had the ongoing privilege of being included in vulnerable conversations people have with health providers, family members, and close friends navigating illness. These conversations are sometimes difficult or painful, and the conversations sometimes evoke closeness and newfound intimacy. I've come to understand that in many friendships and close relationships that indicate a depth of intimacy, people have been there for each other in the disorienting moments of diagnosis or in the decision-making about next steps in treatment (or forgoing treatment). I've come to see differently how my own understanding of research and relationships continues to evolve, how the current answers also translate into new questions. In the years I've done this research, I've learned that one of my strengths as a scholar is integrating multiple strands of thought.

Close relationships require us to be vulnerable, to risk ourselves in ways we cannot fully anticipate. We can sustain relationships over time that are not close, but closeness involves emotional exposure and risks in embracing a co-participation with multiple uncertainties with another person over time. Our close relationships are also not isolated from other parts of life. Illness brings vulnerabilities beyond what people usually experience in everyday life. The diagnosis of serious illness is often painful and disorienting. We do not go through life anticipating serious illness, just as we do not enter marriage anticipating divorce. The experience of serious illness can prompt fear and isolation and can challenge the very cornerstones of what we thought of our close relationships and of ourselves. Desires can shift to instead address the needs of caretaking. Our relational voices can become lost amidst clinical talk of diagnosis, prognosis, surgery, clinical appointments, and chemotherapy. The experience of illness can shrink our horizons. For other people, or at other times, the experience of serious illness becomes a cocoon of moments where we know frailty and uncertainty a bit differently, where the shared experience of illness shifts understanding such that we view ourselves and others with a bit more compassion. Illness does not always challenge relationships, but does change understanding.

We cannot understand health and illness in close relationships without also considering the broader context of health-care structures and distribution of resources to promote health and address illness. Health care in the United States, and perhaps the world, has reached an important juncture. In the last century we have seen vast increases in knowledge and investment in science and technology that allows for more accurate diagnosis and treatment of disease. We also see disparities in wealth and health in the form of access to quality health care such that advances in science, technology, and medicine are unequally distributed. With great variability in the distribution of resources, we also understand how health disparities across communities and countries interconnect with social factors. At the same time the complexities of health-care topics inherently require interdisciplinary explanatory frameworks that are attentive to processes that produce disparities and marginalize some people and relationships. Thus, this volume considers disparities in substantive ways that require us to consider how relationships are tied to resources, to values, and to larger economic motives.

An academic volume brings meaning in intellectual development but also in addressing practical concerns. This book interprets and contributes to a way of thinking broadly about health and illness and about close relationships. My intention is to cut across current theoretical concerns and propositions and to connect with practical issues. Theoretical foundations provide a way of understanding explanatory frameworks. The developments in this book extend what we already know by offering a way of viewing what current interdisciplinary social science offers together. From a practical perspective, identifying productive tensions as communicatively coproduced allows us to question our own roles in the research we produce and in how we together impact each other and the world around us. My intention is to bring a more insightful responsiveness in our research and in our everyday engagement in close relationship processes and in health and illness contexts.

As I complete the revision for this book, I am working with colleagues on unmet needs that are holding back the delivery of relationship-centered, high-value health care in family medicine. My own practical engagement involves improving communication between patients and physicians by designing interactions that foster relationships, improve shared decision-making, and improve patients' and physicians' experiences in health care. We are integrating communication processes with clinicians' evidence-informed decisions, which connects relationship-centered interactions with clinician information sources and sense-making.

I am grateful for the opportunity to develop this book and for my work with research colleagues as we co-envision next steps in implementation of the practical aspects that theoretical vision allows.

CONTRIBUTION TO THE LITERATURE

This book advances the literature in the social and behavioral science connecting health and illness and close relationships by capturing the theoretical and empirical cornerstones in considering how health and illness redefine relationships and by mapping out an integrated, systematic theoretical framework of health and illness trajectories and relational processes as co-generative.

The first purpose is to provide a cohesive understanding of the current empirical and theoretical literature on health and illness in close relationships. To that end, I synthesize empirical evidence and associated theoretical constructs from the literature on health and illness as connected to close relationships. By outlining and comparing foundational assumptions of research on relational processes and research on health and illness, this book provides a cohesive, cross-disciplinary understanding of relevant theoretical and empirical issues and why health and illness provide a unique context for understanding close relationships.

The cohesive synthesis allows for better understanding the empirical evidence indicating features of relationships that can either buffer against or, on the contrary, can further exacerbate the negative consequences of a chronic disease or a health crisis. I describe pathways and processes that exist in current empirical and theoretical work, pathways and processes through which health and illness trajectories are associated with relationship processes. I also illustrate how language shapes health and illness understanding and responses in close relationships. I outline defining characteristics of relationship theories and illustrate how relationship theories provide helpful foundation but miss the holistic complexities of integrating health and illness and relational process trajectories.

The second purpose of this volume is to propose and map out an integrated theoretical framework of health and illness and relational processes as co-generative. To that end, I map out an integrated, systematic theoretical framework that begins with interconnections of individual factors, dyadic factors, turning points in diagnosis, management and treatment of illness, turning points in relationships, and the societal, economic, and cultural factors within which the relationships are embedded. The integrated theoretical framework proposes communicative and embodied processes through which health and illness trajectories and relational processes can be understood as coproduced, co-generative, and inherently systematic. I outline how the integrated theoretical processes pose considerations for the vulnerability of illness as a point of seeing differently the complexities in the bodily experience and in close relationships and for recognizing productive tensions that emerge from the theoretical framework.

SYSTEMATIC INTEGRATION AND CO-GENERATIVITY

When we see the complexities of health and illness trajectories as interconnected with close relationship processes, we unpack theoretical richness for understanding how the integration of research in health and illness and close relationships can potentially uncover, even generate, something new. Instead of refining the process of doing the same thing, we uncover potential to shift and do something different. We have seen a number of excellent edited volumes focusing on some aspect of health and illness and relationships that illustrate how family members and close friends wrestle with the diagnosis of someone they love. In edited volumes we also see how family members and close friends not only provide support, hope, and comfort but also require their own processes and information. The multiple lenses described in each chapter in this volume provide a cohesive synthesis of the interconnected social and behavioral science and map out the systematic theoretical connections to provide an integrated and generative explanatory framework for relational complexities of health and illness trajectories.

This volume pushes forward and articulates a comprehensive theoretical foundation of what it means to study health and illness in close relationships across disciplines and to also integrate a "knowing" that exists in the body. The engaged theorizing offers a way to notice and disentangle complexities. The focus on emergence brings an integrated, systematic, and co-generative understanding to health and illness trajectories in close relationships. Competing lenses offer a way to consider paradigms we might initially see as incompatible as actually offering multiple lenses, each lens with insight that informs contradictions and points of difference.

COHESIVENESS AND CHOICES IN WHAT TO INCLUDE

Within academic communities, we see multiple international, inter-disciplinary conferences and edited volumes focused on health and illness and relationships. For example, the International Association for Relationship Research (IARR) sponsored three conferences within the last ten years on health and relationships (2005, Indianapolis, Indiana: Conference on Exploring Relationships in Health or Health of Relationships; 2011, Tucson, Arizona: Conference on Health, Emotion, and Relationships; and 2015, Rutgers University: Conference on Relationships, Health, and Wellness). A recent IARR mini-conference (2017 Syracuse, New York) similarly focused on interdependence, which speaks to the complex interplay of individuals with their close others, a cornerstone construct for connecting relationship processes and health and illness. Conferences in disciplines including psychology, communication, sociology, and family studies over the last ten years have similarly focused on health and relationships. This solo-authored volume presents a comprehensive theoretical and empirical academic understanding and brings cohesiveness to this research area. The richness and proposed theoretical integration in this volume disentangles conceptual and empirical work within multiple disciplines and across disciplinary boundaries.

The topic of health and illness and close relationships comes with expansive literatures and ongoing interest across a broad range of disciplines. Because of the scope of the literatures, this volume has required decisions about what to include at every turn. Theoretical and empirical literatures included in this volume should be interpreted as illustrative rather than exclusionary of other researchers or literatures. At every stage of writing and across every topic, it has been necessary to make choices about including enough to illustrate the area without getting so caught up in the particulars that we miss the big picture. That said, I've intentionally included enough examples to highlight breadth in each area and to give citations that could guide further reading within any section. I have also reached beyond traditional literatures in the social sciences to integrate lenses that offer a different understanding beyond what is typically included in IARR. I have included literatures on trauma and on reflection as additional lenses of understanding the body in health and illness and in creating or designing interactions for attentiveness to emergence in close relationships.

OVERVIEW

Part I: The Unique Context of Health and Illness in Close Relationships. Before we can understand how health and illness connects to close relationships, we have to first define fundamental terms. That might seem easy, but as soon as we explore further we realize the complexities and competing tensions in definitions. The first three chapters of the book look at the place of health and illness in everyday relational life and together illustrate the unique context of health and illness in close relationships.

Chapter 1 illustrates how defining health and illness involves complexities that exceed initial biomedical orientation. I begin with a summary of the definition of health as provided by the World Health Organization (WHO), which sets the stage for health and illness as first biomedical but also as psychosocial and as including social well-being. The WHO definition sets the groundwork for the complexities of defining health and illness and positioning definitions within

a framework that implies much depth beyond the biomedical orientation of recognizing and treating symptoms. As a starting point, the
definition of health and illness involves the absence of disease or
impairment, but that starting point is only a tiny hint at the necessary
breadth in understanding. Health and illness include both biomedical
explanation and a broader notion of illness as a host of social experiences and social constructions of the concept of malady. Mental
health and social well-being considerations additionally involve coping with the demands of everyday life in such a way that invites
a feeling of (dis)equilibrium with the social and physical environments. Health promotion considerations then introduce additional
layers of the dynamic and ongoing process by which coping capacity
is enhanced or strengthened. Individual-level understanding is not
consistent across people, and human illness or suffering requires taking into account personal meaning. Health and illness considerations
require positioning and recognizing inequalities and disparities. Thus,
we cannot really understand health and illness without also considering entitlements and resources as shaped by social, political, economic, and environmental factors, resources that are unequally
distributed and can be systematically skewed. Social determinants
and social gradients of health are interconnected such that social,
economic, and political circumstances cluster together with psychological challenges. Definitions of health include social determinants,
but cultural contexts pose ongoing implications for well-being beyond
what are currently measured or conceptualized as social determinants. When we consider the breadth of defining health and illness
we move past a biomedical orientation to also considering the social
construction of illness as embedded within cultural meaning and
societal response. Further, health and illness concepts are tied to the
models of health care in which health and illness is diagnosed and
treated.

Chapter 2 presents defining characteristics of close relationship
processes, especially as close relationship processes shift foundations
for considering health and illness trajectories. I provide an overview of

how core principles of relationship science let us understand how relationship processes influence, and are influenced by, health and illness. Close relationships connect to the most vulnerable parts of our lives, to the joys and heartaches. Close relationships can bring out the best in us, but close relationships can also manifest in complicated dilemmas and contradictions where we enact the very behaviors that keep us from getting what we really want. The foundations of Chapter 2 are developed from an interdisciplinary understanding of the scientific study of relationship processes including empirical and theoretical frameworks to explain relationship initiation, development, maintenance, and dissolution of close relationships. Relationship science explicates concepts such as love, commitment, respect, jealousy, willingness to sacrifice, loneliness, disclosure, and positivity in close relationships. Relationships involve cognitive, behavioral, and affective (or emotional) aspects as manifest in a series of interactions particular to the people involved. Close relationships involve mutual understanding of closeness and behavior as developed over time. The foundations of Chapter 2 illustrate how concepts such as relationship commitment, stability, relationship integration, goal pursuit, emotional bonds, and sacrifice translate into the communicative enactment of ongoing relationships. These foundations illustrate how the cornerstones of theoretical and empirical work in close relationships then connect to health and illness trajectories.

Chapter 3 builds on the defining characteristics described in the first two chapters and outlines attributes of the health and illness context that shape and shift close relationship processes. This chapter examines how illness diagnosis and trajectories can shift roles, relationship choices, and relational assumptions. Changes in relationship processes alongside the fragmented uncertainty of health and illness pose implications for coping, for social support, and for the conceptualizations of our closest relationships including shifted understanding of love. I describe how a health and illness crisis requires a recalibration of close relationship processes and ongoing considerations of vulnerability and dependence. Changing expectations include attentiveness to what is manifest in the body at the individual level but also what shifts in the relational and communal dimensions of health and illness. The set of theoretical attributes described in this chapter lets us position how strengths and difficulties inherent in close relationships are magnified by serious illness and situated within a broader community context. Furthermore, I connect communicative processes such as disclosure with ongoing interactions to shed light on how everyday conversations function alongside the explicit relational renegotiations that become necessary in dealing with new relational roles in making sense of illness.

Part II: Health and Illness, the Body, and Relational Processes. In Chapters 4 through 6, I describe links between relationships and health outcomes, outline an expanded conceptualization of illness as embodied more holistically than biomedical markers, and illustrate the current strengths and limitations of applying relationship theories to health and illness trajectories. The three chapters within this section comprise relationships as buffering or exacerbating health and illness outcomes, reconsidering embodiment and language for illness, and relationship theories applied to illness transitions.

In Chapter 4, I synthesize empirical literature linking relationship characteristics with health and illness outcomes to show how relationships can buffer against or, on the contrary, can exacerbate the negative consequences of a chronic disease or a chronic health crisis. I position the complexities of health and illness as interconnected with the broader context of relationships, which co-occur within extensive considerations of social networks and societal-level attributions, particularly as shaped by social and economic conditions. Strong empirical research across many disciplines provides evidence that high-quality relationships and strong social networks are correlated with good physical and mental health. Research in psychology, family studies, communication, sociology, and epidemiology (in addition to other disciplines) provides evidence that the quality and quantity of relationships connects with physical and mental health and with survival. But these outcomes are not equally distributed across communities or across populations. Prior research indicates that features of relationships can be helpful or can further challenge the unfolding complexities of a chronic disease or a health crisis. Relationship characteristics are associated with exacerbating or buffering against physical health including such biomedical markers as blood pressure, ulcers, LDL cholesterol levels, and cortisol levels. Relationship characteristics are associated with exacerbating or buffering against mental health including depression and anxiety. Current theoretical and empirical foundations provide evidence for relationships and social networks as embedded within macro-social environments in which large-scale social forces influence social network structures and also connect to causal processes in which social structures shape and are shaped by psychobiological processes and relationship processes. This chapter addresses the empirical research linking relationships with physical and mental health outcomes that then allows for subsequent chapters to build on what is not currently addressed in the theoretical or empirical literature.

In Chapter 5, I reconsider the notion of embodiment and language for illness to show how the experience of the physical and emotional notions in the body connect to health and illness in close relationships. In unpacking the concept of embodiment, I show how language shapes conceptualization and understanding of health and illness. I illustrate how research on illness in medicine and relationship science sometimes reveals dualism and body alienation in the concepts of self and body and in language of illness and disease. Dualism is observed in biomedical illness diagnosis and treatment that focuses on symptoms such that the body is conceived and described in language implying a material object to which the self happens to be attached. I illustrate how the relational and embodied experiences of people living with illness or disability indicate a more fundamental intertwining of body and self than biomedical language indicates. This chapter on embodiment indicates how close relationship processes involve both the body and the mind such that our instinctive knowing can serve as an intimate and vulnerable point of understanding. What we feel in our physical selves connects to how we make sense of relationships, but the physical aspects of illness symptoms and medical experiences are not yet treated as a holistic part of the pathways between close relationships and health and illness. The foundation for this chapter rests on the tenet that the physical body holds and enables the experience of illness just as the physical body enables touch. The language used to talk about health and illness and to talk about relationships holds consequences and opportunities for broader understanding than currently addressed in the research literature. In considering illness as a qualitatively complex experience that shapes how we interact with other people, I propose how the body serves as meaning-making differently from what is manifest in symptoms. The body in illness shifts understanding of space and time but also shifts understanding of how we connect with other people. In a biomedical orientation to disease, the body can be reduced to a set of measurable symptoms. This chapter offers a glimpse into moving beyond a reduced or dualistic sense of body and self in close relationships and into a way of recognizing wisdom as manifest in the body.

In Chapter 6, I illustrate the current strengths and limitations of applying relationship theories to health and illness transitions. I outline theoretical assumptions for exemplary relationship theories to show strengths and limitations of understanding health and illness trajectories through relationship theories. For example, I show how exemplary relationship theories account for illness as a relational transition, point of turbulence, or relational stressor. I illustrate examples of relationship theories that explain how interactions are constrained or enhanced by the contexts in which they take place. I show the potential for richer explanations by considering interconnectivity between illness trajectories and relational processes over time. The theories outlined in this chapter for the purpose of applying relationship theories to health and illness contexts are all dyadic theories in that they assume a social and interconnected explanatory framework involving multiple people. This chapter then addresses how relationship processes occurring between people hold particular strengths in explaining the science of what is truly social about situations that influence behavior and outcomes. In the application of key relationship theories in the context of health and illness, I illustrate how relationship theories shed light on shifted interdependence processes during illness diagnosis, management, and ongoing sensemaking.

Part III: Integrated Theory of Health and Illness Trajectories and Relational Processes. In Chapters 7 and 8, I propose and map out pathways and processes for an integrated theory of health and illness trajectories and relational processes. I describe how the integrated pathways and processes pose considerations for resilience and flourishing or, on the contrary, for relational and health and illness decline. I discuss interdisciplinary and life-span implications of the integrated theory. Two chapters within this section include mapping out an integrated theory of relational and health and illness trajectories, and integrated pathways and considerations for outcomes.

In Chapter 7, I map out an integrated theory of relationship processes and health and illness trajectories. The cornerstone of the integrated theoretical approach is understanding close relationships and health and illness trajectories as co-created, co-generative, and systematic processes. Co-created theory engages what we currently understand with what we do not yet know and what continues to emerge through co-generative engagement. In close relationships and in health and illness, the subject matter is complex, and the theoretical lens engages the parts of the subjects we know with ongoing unfolding of what is manifest and what is understood over time. In order to outline co-created and co-generative theory, first I describe interconnections of individual factors, dyadic factors, turning points in diagnosis, management and treatment of illness, turning points in relationships, and the societal, economic, and cultural factors within which relationships are embedded. This systematic understanding of close relationships and health and illness trajectories positions social scientific theories and humanistic understanding not as dichotomous but as mutually compatible and as offering different lenses. In outlining systematic understanding, my intention is to recognize and illustrate co-created theoretical process as generative rather than to elaborate two connected hypothetico-deductive models. The communication, behavior, understanding, and choices emerge from the interaction between the health and illness systems and the close relationships systems such that emergence and generativity are the foundation of the theoretical framework. In describing emergence or generativity of interconnected systems, the end goal is not to take into account all of the contributing variables, but to recognize competing tensions and stakeholders and how interactions are communicatively coproduced at particular moments and over time. Instead of attempting to include all variables, we recognize competing tensions and stakeholders that contribute to communicatively producing interactions.

In Chapter 8, I apply the theory to relational trajectories and delineate how the integrated theoretical processes pose considerations for health outcomes including relational and health and illness changes over time. I provide illustrations of health and illness trajectories where close relationships help people successfully find meaning and purpose despite enormous medical challenges and illness-related vulnerabilities. To that end, I show how integrated pathways can promote resilience and relational thriving in the face of adversity. I show how integrated pathways similarly explain other relationships where illness serves as a catalyst for relational decline, for shattered assumptions, or for decreased ability to navigate the relationship instability, disorientation, and disillusionment of the ongoing illness trajectory. I also discuss interdisciplinary and life-span implications of the integrated theory. Interdisciplinary implications include considerations across disciplines and interplay and collaboration in theory and methods. I discuss implications for cross-level linkages between relational theories and macro-level theories of social and economic context within which close relationships are embedded. I suggest considerations for how the theoretical integration provides implications for renegotiating relationships across the life span.

PART I **The Unique Context of Health and Illness in Close Relationships**

I   Defining Health and Illness

SHERRY'S STORY OF FRIENDSHIP AND DIAGNOSIS

At the annual "conference" of the Martha's Vineyard Communication Association, a favorite quasi-professional "association" of eight women, Sherry wondered aloud whether her challenges finding the right word could be something to worry about.

A few days later, Sherry had a meeting with her department chair, who, seemingly out of nowhere, expressed concerns about Sherry's language usage. As evidence, she had printed a series of email messages that Sherry had written over the last few months and suggested that Sherry see a doctor as soon as possible. To the doctor, Sherry confirmed that she too had noticed language difficulty, particularly finding herself mid-sentence, not having words to capture her thoughts. Convincing the doctor to recommend an MRI was no easy task; symptoms were minimal.

Sherry was grateful for the Saturday afternoon MRI appointment. She thought she and her husband Mike would drop in, get the MRI, grab a bite downtown, and head back home to catch the Red Sox. The first sign things would not go as planned was when the MRI tech told Sherry that the doctor wanted to see her ... TODAY ... on Saturday afternoon, and escorted Sherry and Mike down a long hallway, where they were isolated from other patients and staff. That was the moment Sherry knew something was REALLY wrong.

The doctor seemed so young. "I don't want to alarm you, but we saw something on the MRI, requiring additional tests." An ambulance had been summoned to take Sherry to the Beth Israel Deaconess Emergency Room, and the 45-minute wait felt interminable. Mike tried to keep the mood light as they continued to harken back to the young doctor's advice, "There's no need to go all gloom and doom." Holding onto those words, they waited ... and waited.

The long emergency room visit began with Sherry, a nurse, and an intern; Mike joined. Neurosurgery and neurology residents joined. Sherry received a chest x-ray. She was sure she should have eaten; she was not supposed to be here; she felt fine. She worried about her dog; it was well past dinner time, dark, and they had not left the light on for him. The neurology residents returned to explain the diagnosis, but never quite articulated those words with clarity. It was up to the chief of the Emergency Room. Sherry knew the BIG PICTURE, KNEW IMMEDIATELY ... tumor growing in the brain (a pretty large tumor) and it was most likely malignant. Mike remembers the nurse who took Sherry's blood pressure consoling Sherry when Mike moved away to get a full view of the x-ray.

Then Sherry and Mike were left alone, tears streaming. Sherry could not get a grip on reality; it had no real substance. She felt the same; she just had a language problem. The doctors could "fix" that. The mundane helps one cope. Sherry needed to go to the bathroom. Mike had the worst allergy and went through a box of over-dry hospital tissues. It was after 10pm. They were hungry. Sherry was admitted to the hospital and moved into her room. Mike got water and crackers from the vending machine. This was their first intimate view of the hurry-and-wait hospital game. Another MRI was scheduled for the following morning. The depth and size of the brain tumor meant that surgery was not an option. An attempt to remove the tumor could cause irreparable harm to speech, memory, and personality. The neurology and oncology teams recommended a biopsy of the brain.

– Shepler et al., 2013

Sherry's story provides a brief glimpse into the complexities of defining health and illness and the very fine line between wellness and malady. Sherry's story also provides a glimpse into the ways in which health and illness interconnect with close relationships. Being able to name a diagnosis or illness shifts the ways we think of the problem. Language also shapes the ways we talk about ourselves in experiences with illness and with relationships. Language serves an exploratory and constitutive function in that words provide and enact sense-making. The language and experience of diagnosis can put boundaries on what the "issue" is and can sometimes indicate a turning point in next steps in decisions about treatment and/or about relationships. Health and illness provide a unique context for interpersonal issues and relationship processes. The vulnerable state of illness context-shifts expectations and roles in relationships. Friendships developed over many years can provide support to a variety of life challenges that accompany diagnosis and experience with illness. Illness can challenge the circumstances of other relationships. These complexities are prevalent even before considerations of resources including time and travel for appointments and paying for health care: resources for obtaining and paying for medical treatment that can quickly be foreboding.

Before we can understand how health and illness connect to close relationships, we must first consider what it means to be healthy (or, conversely, what it means to experience illness). The World Health Organization (WHO) definition of health provides an initial foundation for defining health as both biomedical and psychosocial. In this chapter, I describe inherent and holistic assumptions of the WHO definition for complete physical, mental, and social well-being. I compare the assumptions and core constructs of social determinants of health and relationship-centered health care to fundamental assumptions about relationship processes as used in relationship research.

As a starting point, note that the WHO defines "health" but that the language implies much more breadth and indicates experience with symptoms or malady. A biomedical orientation as a basis is more consistent with the language of "disease" as a disorder of structure or function as recognized in specific symptoms. The broader experience of malady or disorder is more consistent with the language of "illness," which includes a host of social experiences and social constructions in the context of the malady. Throughout this book, I refer to health and illness as an indication of how language constitutes the experience of reality, but in this chapter, I use language consistent with the cited authors to build foundation.

Defining health and illness might at first seem as simple as having a diagnosis, but upon investigation, understanding health and illness quickly becomes an ambitious and complex goal with interconnected considerations of science and technology, philosophy, core values, psychology, and competing stakeholders. Defining health and illness requires acknowledging the context of culture and economic conditions. Complete mental and social well-being is far-reaching and calls on additional political and economic domains and innovative and imaginative considerations of broader constructs than diagnosis and management of disease.

The biomedical orientation to health and the ability to accurately recognize, diagnose, and manage symptoms is a necessary foundation for understanding the task orientation of medicine. Health, however, is a broader construct, the complexities of which are implied in the extended form in which the WHO definition is written. Beginning by disentangling multiple complexities in defining health gives us a basis for then understanding cornerstone foundations from which more systematic theoretical integration is presented in subsequent chapters.

WORLD HEALTH ORGANIZATION DEFINITION OF HEALTH

The constitution of the World Health Organization (WHO, signed in July 1946 and enacted in 1948) defines health as a state of *complete physical, mental, and social well-being and not merely the absence of disease or infirmity*. The WHO constitution begins by outlining principles perceived as basic to the happiness, harmonious relations, and security of all people (World Health Organization, 2014).

Principles outlined in the Constitution of the World Health Organization include the following:

The WHO constitution asserts that the enjoyment of the highest attainable standard of health is one of the fundamental rights of every human being without distinction of race, religion, political belief, economic or social condition. WHO states that the health of all people is fundamental to the attainment of peace and security and is dependent upon the fullest co-operation of individuals and States. The achievement of any State in the promotion and protection of health is of value to all. Unequal development in different countries, especially communicable disease, is a common danger. Healthy development of the child is of basic importance; the ability to live harmoniously in a changing total environment is essential to such development. The extension to all peoples of the benefits of medical, psychological, and related knowledge is essential to the fullest attainment of health. Informed opinion and active co-operation on the part of the public are of the utmost importance in the improvement of the health of the people. Governments have a responsibility for the health of their people, which can be fulfilled only by the provision of adequate health and social measures.

(World Health Organization, 2014)

The writers of the WHO constitution first defined health as a state dependent on the presence or absence of disease. Health is defined as a state of being but the definition misses the aspects of process or trajectory. The WHO definition includes mental and social well-being, but not the ongoing complex interplay of biological and non-biological factors, the aging population, years of living with chronic illness as the norm, and the inter-individual variability in health priorities.

STRENGTHS AND CHALLENGES OF THE WHO DEFINITION OF HEALTH

Broad and ambitious. The WHO definition is both broad and ambitious, particularly in biomedical scope and in naming not merely the absence of disease or infirmity, but complete physical, mental, and social well-being. Assumptions for defining illness first assume a biomedical basis for disease, a biomedical basis that is consistent with the massive catalogues of medical textbooks and psychological disorder classifications. Although the WHO definition moves toward a broader biopsychosocial model in also including mental and social well-being, the definition suggests a biological foundation dependent first on the presence or absence of disease as measured in biomedical symptoms. This definition as first disease-centered and then holistic in its conception presents a broad understanding of health, which then implies a broad and idealized understanding of well-being.

Physical health as first biomedical. A complete state of physical health is difficult (perhaps impossible) to achieve. The vast notion of health as complete well-being presents an idealized condition. Viewing health with the absoluteness of the word "complete" poses an ongoing emphasis on potential screening for conditions not yet diagnosed. This broad and ambitious view of health is consistent with a medicalized view of society where increasingly sophisticated technology can detect smaller indications of abnormalities over time (Huber, 2011). Pharmaceutical companies produce and advertise multiplicities of drugs for conditions we would not have defined or measured as health problems in years past. Health-care systems expand in scope to treat health problems with lower thresholds for intervention for people with resources for those treatments. The completeness assumed in the WHO definition supports the tendencies of the medical technology, pharmaceutical industries, and providers, to continue to expand the scope of the health-care system (Huber, 2011).

Individuals declared healthy today may be diagnosed with a disease tomorrow, and medical professionals are positioned to declare an individual healthy or to diagnose disease or malady. Defining health as first dependent on the absence of disease presumes a biomedical understanding such that disease is discovered or realized by biomedical markers. The objective of the doctor (or other health provider), then, is to discover and measure symptoms of disease in order to manage disease as presented by patients. Doctors and health providers are trained in clinical identification, diagnosis, and management of diseases. Medical textbooks provide endless classifications of disease. If we define health as the negative state, through the absence of disease or infirmity, then we are healthy until a blood test, an advanced imaging indictor, a genetic analysis, or some other measure of illness lets us know of a measure indicating disease or malady.

The broader concept of health and illness quickly becomes evasive and is not clearly defined by the WHO definition. Instead of clearly outlining the nature of the subject of health, the WHO definition introduces the broader notion of mental and social well-being.

In positioning well-being rather than illness, health is implied as an ideal state. This ideal state seems to leave constant room for improvement. For people who already live with access to resources, one aspect of "privilege" is setting forever unachievable markers of mental wellness and social well-being. At the same time, many other people live without access to health care.

Mental health and well-being as always leaving room for improvement. Complete mental and social well-being involves adequately coping with all demands of life and living in equilibrium with the social and physical environment (in addition to absence of disease or impairment). If complete physical health is difficult to achieve by the implied WHO definition, then perhaps the additional dimensions of complete mental and social well-being leave most of us unhealthy most of the time. That said, understanding mental and social well-being first involves differentiating well-being from disease or malady. The WHO defines mental health as a state of being in which people realize their own abilities, can cope with the normal stresses of life, can work productively and fruitfully, and are able to make a contribution to their community (World Health Organization, 2014).

Defining mental health by positive dimensions can be considered consistent in terms of health as well-being and adapting to diversity and demands in the environment. Concepts measured to indicate well-being include such dimensions as self-esteem, internal locus of control or mastery, optimism, and sense of coherence (World Health Organization, 2015b). Defining mental health through (lack of) negative dimensions of psychological distress or mental disorders poses different implications. Mental disorders, on the contrary, are defined through classifications such as the International Classification of Diseases (ICD10) or the *Diagnostic and Statistical Manual of Mental Disorders* (DSM). Mental disorders are broadly categorized as organic deficiencies and dementias (apart from their cause), psychotic disorders, depressive and anxiety disorders, substance use disorders, personality and conduct disorders, and eating disorders (World Health Organization, 2015b). The continuous dimensionality of psychological distress poses difficulties in the subjective elements of defining mental and social well-being. An individual can score highly on psychological distress following a negative or stressful life event or over a longer period of time and not meet the categorical diagnoses measured through diagnostic instruments. Complete mental health is connected to, and influenced by, a wide range of biological and psychological factors, social interaction, societal structures or resources, and cultural values that necessitate understanding mental health and well-being within the context of broader social structures.

Misses co-existing components. Critics of the WHO definition of health suggest that its emphasis on complete well-being is no longer fit for helpful purpose given the rise of chronic disease, and critics note the counterproductive nature of declaring people with chronic disease and disabilities as definitively ill (Huber, 2011). Seeking complete absence of disease or infirmity poses difficulties for our aging populations and for living with chronic illness or disability. People who have abnormalities that are measured as symptoms of disease are measured as "ill" but might feel well, and people who feel ill and do not function well but whose biomedical markers do not indicate abnormality are measured as "well" (Sartorius, 2006). Many people find ways to live productively for many years following a diagnosis.

Because people are living significantly longer, because technology enables more sophisticated diagnoses, and because pharmaceutical advances allow for treating more and more medical conditions, people can live for decades with a chronic disease or disability. The WHO definition suggests definitive illness diagnosis for people with chronic disease or disability. To that end, the definition suggests a need for medical treatment instead of recognizing the capacity for people to accept chronic disease or disability as a natural part of the human condition. In defining health as complete physical, mental, and social well-being, potential co-existing dimensions in which health can co-occur with the presence of a disease, disability, or impairment are not included (Sartorius, 2006). The definition was written at a historical time when acute illness led to early death and when public health measures such as improved hygiene, sanitation, and powerful health-care interventions were far less developed in their sophistication (Huber, 2011).

Health promotion considerations for dynamic components. The WHO definition of health also misses explicit health promotion components. In first defining health as the absence of disease, promotion of health then is an effort to remove disease and diminish the number of people who suffer from disease (Sartorius, 2006). Numerous attempts to adapt the WHO definition also include a promotion or functioning aspect, in which the promotion of health then becomes a dynamic and ongoing process by which the capacity of individuals to cope is enhanced or strengthened (Sartorius, 2006). Thus, recommendations to improve the treatment of disease would be considered alongside removing risk factors of disease (e.g., hygienic measures such as washing hands, limiting exposure to toxic chemicals, environmental conditions without pollution) and addressing lifestyle factors such as sedentariness, smoking, and eating habits.

A well-known attempt to adapt the WHO definition comes from the Ottawa Charter for Health Promotion, which conceptualizes health as a positive resource for everyday life, emphasizing social and personal resources in addition to physical capacity. The definition of health promotion provided in the Ottawa Charter is, seemingly, the most widely accepted. In the Ottawa Charter, health promotion is defined as "the process of enabling people to increase control over, and to improve, their health" (World Health Organization, 1986). Adding health promotion components moves from defining health or illness as a static state to instead considering a dynamic state. The dynamic state suggests the potential for individuals to act with resilience in their capacity to cope and maintain and restore their integrity, equilibrium, and sense of well-being. The static nature of the WHO definition misses the capacity for adaptability and self-management inherent in health promotion efforts. Health promotion assumptions suggest enabling people rather than diagnosing illness. Living with a chronic illness or disability under the Ottawa Charter definition requires an ability to adapt to the environment and self-manage.

Health as individual experience. In the narrowest interpretation of the WHO definition of health, how an individual feels about his or her state of health and illness is not relevant to the paradigm (Sartorius, 2006). To define health as a negative state (the absence of disease) fosters thinking about health in terms of disease, and disease is generated by the ability to recognize a biological dysfunction or pathology across people. A broader philosophical view such as Immanuel Kant's suggestion that every person has a particular way of being in good health would offer a broader definition of health. To some extent, the WHO definition emphasizes individual subjective experience as well-being, such that a condition of little impact to one person may have substantial impact on the life of another person. The physical condition might be the same, but the impact on well-being varies across individuals. The broadest interpretation of health integrates the experience of a relative balance of dynamic interactions between biological, emotional, social, and sense-making (cognitive) dimensions affecting the individual person in all of the context of that person (Sturmberg, 2009). Integrating the overall health experience means that people seek to stabilize immediate life-threatening pathological processes and then seek to understand illness experience in order to regain a new equilibrium of health experience (Sturmberg, 2009).

Understanding human illness or suffering requires taking into account personal meaning as a fundamental dimension. Patient experiences reinforce the personal meaning or sense-making in understanding health. An approach of reducing complexities to a set of measurable variables and regarding those variables as representing the whole is epistemologically and sometimes statistically flawed or biased. The process of quantitative measurement can focus on variables that can more clearly be measured. Understanding health as individual experience means also recognizing the experiences and values of patients, societies, and cultures. Disease then might be observed as disruption and as an interruption in the ability of the person to cope (Sturmberg, 2009).

The complexities in the meaning of health are subject to change at the individual level, at the community level, and at the society level. The notion of health as a state of balance and adaptation between the person and the social and physical environment means that health is an individual dimension of human existence regardless of the presence of disease (at least apart from measurement of disease as biological). From this understanding of health, disease does not replace health but instead shapes the ability to balance. Observed through this lens, people work to alleviate disease but also to achieve a state of balance within themselves and with their environment. Diagnosing disease then implies that technology to measure biological symptoms is considered within the context of a person's judgment about his or her level of health. To that end, the body is less a transport of biological markers potentially indicative of disease, and instead people determine the balance of the complex adaptive personal and experiential nature of their health.

Public health considerations of inequalities. Public health is grounded in the premise that adaptation and self-management are important, but within the context of considering that health is also a fundamental human right protected by entitlements, and a resource for life shaped by social, political, economic, and environmental factors. These core values are outlined in reading further the WHO definition for health but less frequently included in shorter definitional excerpts. Public health emphasizes population-based health and works on the premise that changes to social, political, economic, and environmental factors translate into greater health gains than individual action. Because of inequalities, many problems driving illness in low- and middle-income countries are outside the control of the dispossessed, the poor, and the disenfranchised (Shilton et al., 2011). In addition, in resource-rich countries, inequalities are manifest in disparities such as food desert communities lacking fresh fruits, vegetables, and other health-ful whole foods due to the absence of quality grocery stores within convenient distance. People in these communities are often also impoverished in other ways, such as having limited access to medical centers. Public health advocates consider adaptation and self-management desirable for wealthy developed countries, but more importantly, public health advocates suggest that health must recog-nize and address implications of fundamental and growing inequality (Shilton et al., 2011). Understanding health and illness through the lens of public health necessitates systems approaches to policy, legis-lation, and environments, as well as a definition of health highlighting underlying determinants that are less amenable to self-management; health and illness are then embedded in policy and inequality (World Health Organization, 2003). Health then is created when individuals, families, and communities are afforded the income, education, and power to control their lives, and their needs are supported by systems, environments, and policies that are enabling and conducive to better health (Institute of Medicine, 2003; World Health Organization, 2003). Inequalities in health among populations are better understood through social determinants of health and illness.

THEORETICAL FRAMEWORK ON THE SOCIAL PRODUCTION OF HEALTH AND DISEASE

In considering the social production of health and disease, the WHO poses that conceptual frameworks in a public health context should ideally serve the purposes of both guiding empirical work to enhance our understanding of determinants and mechanisms of health and guiding policy-making to illuminate entry points for health interven-tions and policies (Diderichsen, 2010). Effects of social determinants on population health and health inequalities are characterized by long causal chains of mediating factors, many of which cluster together among individuals already living in underprivileged conditions (Diderichsen, 2010). Theories on the social production of health and illness include psychosocial approaches, frameworks that address social production of disease and the political economy of health, and eco-social frameworks (Diderichsen, 2010). Across these three theoretical traditions, pathways and mechanisms link social determinants to health and illness outcomes. The frameworks include explanations for social selection or social mobility, social causation, and life course perspectives. Each of these theoretical traditions and associated pathways and mechanisms emphasizes the concept of social position. Social position places emphasis on power such that the central role of power is not necessarily about domination but also to do with more positive and creative aspects, such that communities can express their collective social power (Diderichsen, 2010). The central role of power in the understanding of social pathways and mechanisms means that tackling the social determinants of health inequalities involves political process that engages both the agency of disadvantaged communities and the responsibility of the state (Diderichsen, 2010).

In Diderichsen's public health model of health inequality, social contexts include the structure of society and social relations in society. Social contexts create social stratification and assign individuals to different social positions (Diderichsen, 2010). Social stratification engenders differential exposure to health and illness and to health-damaging conditions and differential vulnerability in terms of health conditions and material resource availability (Diderichsen, 2010). Social stratification then determines differential consequences of illness for more-advantaged and less-advantaged groups including economic and social consequences of health outcomes (Diderichsen, 2010).

The role of social position in generating health inequalities then necessitates understanding the central role of power. Social, economic, and political mechanisms give rise to a set of socioeconomic positions whereby populations are stratified according to income, education, occupation, gender, race, ethnicity, and other factors (Diderichsen, 2010). These socioeconomic positions, in turn, shape specific determinants of health status reflective of people's place within social hierarchies based on their respective social status (Diderichsen, 2010). Individuals experience differences in exposure and vulnerability to illness conditions. Illness can feed back on a given individual's social position (Diderichsen, 2010). For example, by compromising employment opportunities and reducing income, illness can feed back to shape the functioning of social, economic, and political institutions (Diderichsen, 2010). Context includes social and political mechanisms that generate, configure, and maintain social hierarchies, including the labor market, educational systems, political institutions, and other cultural and societal values (Diderichsen, 2010). Structural mechanisms generate stratification and social class divisions in society that define individual socioeconomic position within hierarchies of power, prestige, and access to resources (Diderichsen, 2010). Structural mechanisms are rooted in the key institutions and processes of the socioeconomic and political context (Diderichsen, 2010).

Together, context, structural mechanisms, and the resultant position of individuals are structural determinants and essentially function as what public health refers to as "social determinants." As summarized in the WHO report on a conceptual framework for action on the social determinants of health, definitions then address material circumstances, psychosocial circumstances, behavioral factors, and biological factors (Diderichsen, 2010). Material circumstances include factors such as housing and neighborhood quality, consumption potential (the financial means to buy healthy food and warm clothing) and the physical work environment. Psychosocial circumstances include psychosocial stressors such as stressful living circumstances and relationships, and social support and appropriate coping (or lack thereof). Behavioral and biological factors include nutrition, physical activity, tobacco consumption and alcohol consumption, which are distributed differently among different social groups. Biological factors also include genetic factors.

SOCIAL DETERMINANTS OF HEALTH AND ILLNESS

This section provides a brief overview of social determinants and then distinguishes social determinants of health and illness from relational processes and relationship-centered health care in social relationships. The goal of this overview of social determinants of health and illness is to acknowledge the broader economic and policy systems within which close relationships are embedded. The subsequent two chapters then further elucidate how close relationships serve as a unique context for health and illness trajectories.

Defining and understanding health and illness requires also acknowledging the complex social systems and environmental influences of health and illness. The WHO identifies social determinants of health as the conditions in which people are born, grow, work, live, and age, and the wider set of forces and systems shaping the conditions of daily life (World Health Organization, 2003). These forces and systems include economic policies and systems, development agendas, social norms, social policies, and political systems.

Understanding social determinants of health and illness involves addressing the complex aspects of people's living and working circumstances and people's lifestyles (World Health Organization, 2003). Social determinants of health and illness concern the health implications of economic and social policies, as well as the benefits that investing in health policies can bring (World Health Organization, 2003). Social determinants include such areas as stress, early life experiences, social exclusion (or inclusion), work or unemployment, social support, addiction, food, and transportation (World Health Organization, 2003).

Even in the most affluent countries, people who have access to fewer resources have substantially shorter life expectancies and more illnesses than people who have more money and better access to education and resources (Institute of Medicine, 2003). Recognizing social determinants of health and illness provides foundation for understanding differences in health and illness as an ethical dilemma and as a social injustice (Institute of Medicine, 2003). Social determinants are connected to understanding the sensitivity of health and illness to the social environment.

Social determinants are included in health promotion and public health considerations for understanding health and illness. Considering social determinants poses concerns for the health implications of economic and social policies and the benefits that investing in health policies can bring. Although categories of social determinants vary depending on aspects of health promotion or public health efforts and on the desired outcomes for understanding population-based implications of health, the field of social determinants of health concerns key aspects of people's living and working circumstances and their lifestyles. Considering social determinants of health and illness allows for prioritizing and developing health promotion interventions to address disparities in economic and social policies and systems (World Health Organization, 2003). For example, the WHO Centre for Urban Health develops tools and resource materials in the areas of health policy, integrated planning for health and sustainable development, urban planning, governance, and social support (World Health Organization, 2003).

At the individual level, social determinants of health and illness include demographic characteristics such as race, class, and ethnicity. Evidence from around the world shows that health outcomes are patterned by aspects of social class including access to material resources, education, and occupation (World Health Organization, 2003). Disadvantaged groups are more likely to suffer from higher rates of mortality and morbidity. Furthermore, patterns of disparities typically reveal gradients in which each additional increase in income, education, or occupation grade confers additional health protection (World Health Organization, 2003).

Poor material circumstances are harmful to health. The social gradient includes advantages such as education, occupation, housing, social inclusion, unemployment, social inclusion (or exclusion), social support, addiction, food access (or scarcity), and transportation (World Health Organization, 2003). Moreover, the social meaning of being poor, unemployed, socially excluded, or otherwise stigmatized also matters (World Health Organization, 2003). From a positive frame, social determinants allow for feeling valued and appreciated, having friends, living in sociable societies, feeling useful, and implementing control over work that feels meaningful. Without those qualities, people are more prone to negative issues such as depression, drug use, anxiety, hostility, and feelings of hopelessness, all of which are also connected to physical health. Social and psychological circumstances such as social isolation and lack of control over work and home life, especially over time, are correlated in large-scale studies with increased chances of poor mental health and premature death (World Health Organization, 2003).

Social determinants also predict well-being as connected to resilience, health assets, capabilities, and positive adaptation that enable people to cope with adversity and reach their full potential and humanity or, on the contrary, limit opportunities for well-being (Friedli, 2009). The chronic stress of struggling with material disadvantage is intensified with larger social hierarchy; the distribution of economic and social resources predict health beyond individual pathology. Self-damaging behaviors and violence may function as survival strategies in the face of multiple sources of anger and despair related to occupational insecurity, poverty, debt, poor housing, exclusion, and other indicators of low status (Friedli, 2009). In addition, psychobiological studies provide evidence of chronic low-level stress influencing neuro-endocrine pathways to influence poorer cardiovascular and immune systems such as cortisol levels, cholesterol levels, blood pressure, and inflammation (Friedli, 2009).

Health and illness differences between different social groups widen or narrow as social and economic conditions change. Although understanding genes holds promise for understanding and treating specific diseases, genetic susceptibilities to disease are conceptualized at the individual level; at the societal and population levels the common causes of illness are also environmental (World Health Organization, 2003). Genetic factors can interact with environmental factors to exacerbate disparities. Policies in government, in public and private institutions, in workplaces, and in the community pose responsibility for creating healthy societies at the societal levels. Recognizing social determinants of health and illness emphasizes the need to understand how health behavior is shaped by the environment, and thus how social and environmental changes could lead to healthier behavior (World Health Organization, 2003). Furthermore, economic and social advantage or disadvantage is interconnected to both resources and social meanings.

Defining health and illness in terms of diagnosis (and provision) of medical care allows for addressing symptoms and survival once illness or disease is diagnosed. Once we move beyond individual-level understanding, defining health and illness means also considering social and economic conditions that shape illness vulnerabilities. Access to medical care is presumed in defining health and in the scope of the WHO definition of health provisions. Social determinants of health and illness provide context to recognize the wider set of forces and systems shaping the conditions of daily life, the conditions in which people are born, grow, work, live, and age.

Health policy is inherently connected to social determinants of health because social determinants move beyond the provision and funding of medical care to addressing survival and serious disease alongside the health of the population as a whole (World Health Organization, 2003). Social and economic conditions can be the cause of what makes people ill in the first place as well as the context for access to medical care. Tackling material and social injustices can improve health and well-being and may also reduce a range of other social problems that develop and grow alongside illness (World Health Organization, 2003).

SOCIAL GRADIENT OF HEALTH AND ILLNESS

Social determinants do not simply suggest that poor material circumstances are harmful to health, but instead that we also need to consider the social meaning of *being* poor, unemployed, socially excluded, or otherwise stigmatized (World Health Organization, 2008). The report from the WHO Commission on Social Determinants of Health defined health inequalities as systematic differences in health considered to be avoidable by reasonable action and therefore unfair (World Health Organization, 2008). Access to material goods is not enough; people need to feel valued and appreciated from early childhood. People need friends; people need to feel useful; people need a significant degree of control over meaningful work (World Health Organization, 2008). Without social meaning conceptually connected to good health, people become prone to depression, drug use, anxiety, hostility, and feelings of hopelessness which then further rebound on physical health (World Health Organization, 2008).

Poor social and economic circumstances affect health and illness throughout life. Life expectancy is shorter and most diseases more common further down the social ladder in each society (World Health Organization, 2008). People further down the social ladder run at least twice the risk of serious illness and premature death as people near the top of the social ladder (World Health Organization, 2008). These effects are not confined to the poor; the social gradient in health runs across society such that lower-ranking staff among middle-class office workers suffer more disease and earlier death than higher-ranking staff (World Health Organization, 2008). Differences are attributed to both material and psychosocial causes, and effects extend to most diseases and causes of death. Disadvantage may be absolute or relative (World Health Organization, 2008). For example, disadvantage can be manifest in having few family assets, having a poorer education during adolescence, having insecure employment, becoming stuck in a hazardous or dead-end job, living in poor housing, trying to raise family among difficult circumstances, or living on inadequate retirement money (World Health Organization, 2008). Disadvantages tend to cluster among the same populations, and deleterious effects accumulate over the life course (World Health Organization, 2008). The longer people live in stressful economic and social circumstances, the harsher their psychological challenges and the less likely they are to be healthy in older age (World Health Organization, 2008). To that end, a life span perspective must consider social gradients built across a lifetime as well as critical transitions in life circumstances.

Critical transitions can be powerful moments of social injustice. Critical transitions include emotional and material changes in early childhood, moving from primary to secondary education, starting work, leaving home and starting a family, changing jobs, facing possible job redundancy, downsizing or loss, and retirement (World Health Organization, 2008). Each of these life transitions marks a moment where people who have been disadvantaged in the past are at greater risk in a subsequent transition (World Health Organization, 2008). Addressing earlier disadvantage requires offsetting subsequent transitions and requires societal consideration of (un)employment, (lack of stable) housing, and considerations of social, economic, and cultural life connected to insecurity, exclusion, and deprivation (World Health Organization, 2008).

Stressful circumstances where people feel worried, anxious, and unable to cope can damage health and can predict premature death (World Health Organization, 2008). Lack of perceived control over work or over home life can affect physical and mental health by activating hormones and nervous system response that divert energy and bodily resources away from physiological processes important to long-term health maintenance (World Health Organization, 2008). The cardiovascular and immune systems in people who feel tense too often, or who experience tension over a long period of time, become more vulnerable to a wide range of illness conditions including infection, diabetes, high blood pressure, heart attack, stroke, depression, and aggression (World Health Organization, 2008).

THE CULTURAL CONTEXT OF HEALTH AND ILLNESS

The 2014 report from the Lancet Commission on Culture and Health argued that the systematic neglect of culture in health and health care is the single biggest barrier to advancement of the highest attainable standard of health worldwide (Napier et al., 2014). The first WHO meeting of experts on the cultural context of health and well-being was convened in 2015 to consider a working definition of culture, to rethink data and evidence needs for well-being, to suggest ways to report more effectively on well-being, and to identify gaps in relation to culture and well-being (World Health Organization, 2015a). Their report begins with an illustration that the percentage of people successfully treated for diabetes is only a fraction of the total diabetes population, mainly because of sociocultural factors (World Health Organization, 2015a). Even where multibillion-dollar budgets are spent on diabetes and diabetes-related complications, hardly any of this money is invested in understanding the sociocultural factors preventing people from getting successful treatments (World Health Organization, 2015a). In addition to the economic argument to focus on cultural contexts of health, recognizing the impact of culture on health connects policy to people's agency, their beliefs and values, and the meanings they construct from their experiences of health and illness (World Health Organization, 2015a).

The WHO group agreed to embrace the United Nations Educational, Scientific and Cultural Organization's (UNESCO) conceptualization of culture as a way of life rather than defining culture simply as religious, social or ethnic characteristics delimited by geopolitical boundaries, thus acknowledging the presence (and importance) of dynamic microcultures (World Health Organization, 2015a). The committee noted that even the process of focusing on well-being can lead to developing particular cultural artifacts. The UNESCO definition defines culture as a set of distinctive spiritual, material, intellectual, and emotional features of society or a social group, and in that, culture encompasses, in addition to art

and literature, lifestyles, ways of living together, value systems, traditions, and beliefs (World Health Organization, 2015a). Thus, the WHO
committee considered culture as a shared social construction, as
a dynamic process, as striving for something new, as well as preserving
tradition; culture functions as forward-looking, even visionary (World
Health Organization, 2015a).

Assumptions and implications of the study of culture and well-
being pose implications for empirical and theoretical study of health
and illness across disciplines (World Health Organization, 2015a).
The cultural context of health and illness then assumes that values,
including values of health and illness, do not exist in a social vacuum.
Instead, values change over time and are perpetuated in practice
(World Health Organization, 2015a). Boundaries of cultural groups
are fluid. Studying values, then, requires studying agency and practice.
Furthermore, all forms of knowledge are culturally connected, including scientific knowledge and medical practice.

The committee of experts on the cultural context of health and
well-being posed questions about how the concept of culture is
defined and relates to health and well-being. They also explored
whether cultural bias factors connect to social indicators, and how
cultural factors might introduce measurement error in any form of
self-reported survey data (World Health Organization, 2015a).
The report offers implications for what subjective well-being data
can tell us about the impact of culture on health and well-being
(World Health Organization, 2015a). Factors that may affect cross-
cultural comparability of subjective well-being data include language
and translation issues in which semantic and conceptual equivalence
challenges should be considered; the choice of terms and semantic
structures do not necessarily ensure equivalent translation, and the
concept does not necessarily exist, even when the words are similar
(World Health Organization, 2015a). Cognitive challenges and
response bias vary across cultures.

Cross-cultural comparability poses questions for translation
and measurement error (World Health Organization, 2015a).

Moreover, deeper cultural differences may operate below emotional reporting styles. For example, the group identified positivity bias in North American responses to well-being, as compared to modesty bias from Confucian cultures; these different cultural conceptions of well-being also indicate types of mental states that are most highly valued (e.g., excitement vs. calmness) (World Health Organization, 2015a). Defining the concept of well-being in terms of human flourishing poses considerations for cultural bias in that the modern, secular, European definition of well-being may be similar to human flourishing but not necessarily aligned with a spiritual dimension that offers a different lens (World Health Organization, 2015a).

The committee of experts on the cultural context of health and well-being advocates multidisciplinary approaches that allow for compelling and localized well-being narratives to complement existing, international data sources, especially where developing and implementing resource-intensive, country-specific well-being surveys is not an option (World Health Organization, 2015a). The committee also advocates more culturally specific sources of evidence gathered from traditions and symbols, especially those that give voice to people whose views are systematically left out of national and global well-being surveys and assessments (World Health Organization, 2015a). Finally, the committee advocates integrated, multidisciplinary approaches that are open to insights from the human and wider social sciences that encourage exposing the systems of values in which information is obtained and promoting reflexivity that facilitates better understanding (World Health Organization, 2015a). For example, this approach might address case studies of counterintuitive subjective–objective well-being data contradictions such as Denmark's higher premature mortality rate including suicides compared to its high levels of life satisfaction and happiness scores (World Health Organization, 2015a). Statistical reports build evidence for policy but also must be supplemented with other forms of evidence. Top-down frameworks and definitions for well-being may be reductionist and may not leave room for the rich diversity of cultural contexts within which health and well-being are situated (World Health Organization, 2015a). The expert group suggests that policy initiatives should be participatory and interactive, allowing room for choice and creativity, and integrating communication pathways that empower communities to share their stories of well-being in ways that make a difference in conceptualization and in impact (World Health Organization, 2015a).

The WHO expert group recommends exploring culture-centered, participatory approaches that engage local communities in sensitive ways, that understand and measure what it means to be well and healthy in communities, and that foster avenues of communication and for sharing resources of health and well-being (World Health Organization, 2015a). The report poses particular implications for defining health. Specifically, defining and understanding health and illness involves two-way communication and listening. Additional information is likely needed and can likely produce additional insights when counterintuitive information emerges.

THE SOCIAL CONSTRUCTION OF HEALTH AND ILLNESS

Social constructionism provides an important counterpoint to biological medicine's largely deterministic approaches to disease and illness. A social constructionist perspective on illness allows for recognizing the ways some illnesses are particularly embedded within a cultural meaning that can then shape how society responds to people and influences the experience of their illness (Conrad & Barker, 2010). The social construction of illness cannot be fully disentangled from biomedical markers but recognizes that symptoms of a social problem are not a "given" but conferred within a social context of how claims about behaviors and experiences are made and inferred (Conrad & Barker, 2010). Social construction of health and illness places the exploration of illness within the experience of daily social interaction, which can also be enacted and appropriated by people as they make sense of their illness and cope with, manage, and interact with physical and social restrictions (Conrad & Barker, 2010). Social construction of illness provides a broad understanding of how signs or symptoms get to be labeled or diagnosed as illness or disease based on social ideas about what are treated as valid medical categories and medical knowledge (Conrad & Barker, 2010).

Viewing health and illness through the roots of a social constructionist perspective contributes to understanding the social dimensions of illness and falls within the work of medical sociology and medical anthropology as well as interdisciplinary work. Social constructionism as a conceptual framework emphasizes the cultural and historical aspects of phenomena, with emphasis on meanings as developed through social interaction. In contrast to a biomedical model, a social constructionist approach is rooted in the widely recognized conceptual distinction between the biological condition of disease and the social meaning of illness (Conrad & Barker, 2010). Social constructionists emphasize how meaning and experience of illness are shaped by cultural and social systems. Social constructions of illness help shed light on the cultural landscape and meanings embedded in illness, of what is stigmatized, of what gets noticed, and of what policies are created concerning the illness (Conrad & Barker, 2010). For example, one lesson from a social constructionist perspective is that there is nothing inherent about a condition that creates stigma, but instead the social response to the condition or to some manifestation can translate into the illness being stigmatized (Conrad & Barker, 2010).

The social construction of illness sheds light on the broader experience of illness and considers how people construct and manage their illness and with what consequences the illness experience connects more broadly to individual experience (Conrad & Barker, 2010). Recognizing the social construction of illness allows for systematically collecting and analyzing the experiences of people living with illness in order to focus on the meaning of illness and on strategies for adapting to illness (Conrad & Barker, 2010). To that end, the social aspects of surviving or thriving during experiences of illness are captured in research grounded in the thick, rich examples of social constructionism.

The viability of the idea of disease or illness (rather than the validity per se) is connected to the social construction of health and illness (Conrad & Barker, 2010). A social constructionist perspective brings aspects of illness that the tools of medicine are unable to reveal and examines with serious rigor the personal and social meanings of illness and how illness is managed in the social context (Conrad & Barker, 2010).

Including a section on the social construction of health and illness in this chapter does not deny or ignore the biophysical world but acknowledges that experiences of health and illness include elements that can be biologically measured, while recognizing that social forces constructing the definition and treatment of illness can be studied empirically. From a social constructionist perspective, the idea instead is to investigate how something comes to be defined as a disease or illness. The language of health and illness can be perceived as medical discourse that shapes the bodily experience, shapes identity connected to illness, and shapes perceived legitimacy of medical interventions. Language and social construction of health and illness are closely connected.

FURTHER DEFINING HEALTH AND ILLNESS COMPLEXITIES THROUGH NARRATIVE RESEARCH

Patient narratives can affirm the humanity of the person with an illness and can provide information that can be missed in other measures. Patient narratives can authenticate the existence of pain and limitation and can offer context beyond the limitations of high-tech medical measurements. Patient narratives also offer a lens for understanding culture as connected to health and illness, shedding light on definitions of health and illness and posing implications for the use of narrative forms of evidence. As noted by the WHO expert group on cultural contexts, the conventional hierarchy of evidence-based policy privileges randomized control trials, case control trials, and other statistical forms of quantitative data that limit access to subjective meanings of experiences, the contextual nature of knowledge production, and dominant discourses for policy and research (World Health Organization, 2015a).

Upon recommendation of the expert group on cultural contexts for health, a subsequent group was commissioned to look at new types of scientific evidence, particularly qualitative and narrative research from a larger variety of academic disciplines and from a wider array of cultural contexts. The resulting synthesis report from the Health Evidence Network addressed the use of narrative research in the health sector (Greenhalgh, 2016). Narrative storytelling is an essential tool for reporting and illuminating the cultural contexts of health, for illuminating the practices and behaviors that groups of people share and that are defined by customs, language, and geography (Greenhalgh, 2016). Storytelling and story interpretation as understood in humanistic lenses can complement social science, and established techniques of social science can be applied to ensure rigor in sampling, validity, and data analysis.

Narrative conveys individual experience of health and illness and of well-being, complementing, and sometimes challenging, epidemiological and public health evidence (Greenhalgh, 2016). A narrative (story) is a subjective, experiential version of events told to a listener or reader; narrative research includes the gathering of new stories, the collation and reanalysis of existing stories, the use of ethnography to study enacted stories, the construction of organizational or community case studies, and the study of policy as discourse (Greenhalgh, 2016). Narratives can complement other forms of evidence but must be collected and analyzed with careful attention to quality. Attention to quality includes measures to ensure trustworthiness, plausibility, and criticality (Greenhalgh, 2016). Listening to patients' stories has long been a key element of clinical medicine, but the use of narrative research as connected to cultural contexts of health is more recent (Greenhalgh, 2016).

Strengths of narrative research in health and illness contexts include sense-making characterized by nonlinearity, fluidity, memorability, and capacity to convey the perspective of disadvantaged people (Greenhalgh, 2016). Narrative research sometimes brings the inherent limitation that stories are not necessarily "true" in a direct sense and are open to multiple, sometimes competing, interpretations (Greenhalgh, 2016). Narrative research in health and illness highlights the distinction between the *biomedical* world of biology, physiology, biochemistry, and pathology studied by scientists and biomedical clinicians, and the world of behavior, culture, society, and experience (Greenhalgh, 2016). For example, people usually eat food because it has meaning or relational connection for them rather than eating food purely for nutritional value; people who seek to change a community's eating behavior must consider the social and cultural aspects of why, when and with whom people eat the foods they do (Greenhalgh, 2016). Narrative provides contexts for food choices.

Narratives also illustrate concerns in the measurement of well-being, which has been dominated until recently by quantitative metrics and survey questions (Greenhalgh, 2016). Narratives can also illuminate the dramatic and often tragic life experiences of people whose lived experiences can be missed or obscured at the individual level and in relation to diasporas of cultural groups; for example, mental health in refugees and asylum seekers can be invisible in dominant quantitative metrics (Greenhalgh, 2016).

Stories are subjective in that they convey an individual experience or a collective experience. A story is not intended to convey an explicitly objective version of truth, but to convey a lived experience (Greenhalgh, 2016). Stories are subjective in that they convey a particular version of events using language, metaphors, images, and styles that hold meaning for the storyteller(s) (Greenhalgh, 2016). Stories are inter-subjective in that they connect and respond to the subjectivities of the readers or listeners and are embedded in institutional and social practices (Greenhalgh, 2016). Even the same story told again is not quite the same. Different people tell different stories about their experiences with the same event.

Stories hold meaning because of their potential to illustrate some part of life and because of their poignant or emotional impact on the reader or listener (Greenhalgh, 2016). The impact is achieved through literary features, through genre or metaphor, through how a story rings true for a listener, or through illustrating just rewards or punishment. Scholars of narrative focus on the act of storytelling, the circumstances of the storytelling, and the shaping of the story (Greenhalgh, 2016). Scholars of narrative explore why this person has told *this* particular story to *this* particular person or audience; similarly, scholars consider why someone has *not* told a story in this particular setting or to this audience (Greenhalgh, 2016).

The practice of medicine depends on the clinical case history. Patients' stories about their symptoms or experiences resonate to a greater or lesser extent with patterns about diseases and allow for accurate diagnosis (and subsequent treatment). The patients' clinical case history also indicates their lived experience with the symptoms or illness, and the case history illustrates how their lived experience connects to other parts of their lives. Individual accounts of illness are also captured through qualitative interviews. Case studies of narratives of health-care organizations provide institutional context for health care.

Narratives also provide cultural and historical information within which particular illness narratives are embedded and thus illustrate the meta-narratives of disadvantaged or displaced people who might not be included in traditional, quantitative measures of health (Greenhalgh, 2016). Narratives provide policy discourses though language and communicative process connected to action, to justify inaction, or to encourage or constrain further conversation (Greenhalgh, 2016). Narratives show the social drama of participatory research and the manifestation of online communities and social movements (Greenhalgh, 2016). Narrative research includes gathering stories written for another purpose (e.g., online blogs or complaint letters), stories elicited using an established method for narrative interviewing, observing the enactment of real-life and real-time stories as ethnography, story interpreting using an explicitly narrative approach, or analyzing the storyline of a text using discourse analysis (Greenhalgh, 2016). Scientific and linguistic methods can be applied in the collection and interpretation of text to anchor multiple voices by collecting multiple stories about the same event, to link the story to other sources of empirical data, or to include a thorough and critical review of relevant literature (Greenhalgh, 2016).

Narrative research should not be equated with anecdote any more than quantitative data should be equated with truth (Greenhalgh, 2016). Epidemiological studies and trials help people make predictions about the frequency of events in populations and the likelihood of particular outcomes. Narrative research helps people make sense of experiences. Both can be done well or badly, and both methods can produce findings that are more or less trustworthy.

A narrative approach in health care and related fields includes several strengths, as summarized in Health Evidence Network Synthesis Report 49 (Greenhalgh, 2016). Stories are sense-making devices that enable people to look back and make meaning of their health and illness experiences by retrospectively structuring events and actions. Stories are inherently nonlinear in that stories can be powerful tools for making sense of the emergent interplay of actions, relationships, and context. Stories can be evocative and memorable, offering rich images and easier recall than graphs or numbers. Stories can convey nuance including mood, tone, and urgency. Stories allow for modifying experience by conveying another perspective. Stories capture knowledge that moves beyond formal and explicit information. Stories are nested within wider narratives and thus provide a broader context for understanding organizations, communities, and cultures. Stories have an ethical dimension; for example, stories incur desire to relieve pain, to heal the sick, or to protect the vulnerable. Stories are open-ended in that they create possibilities for further imagination, a different person, or a different question.

Stories shed light on the dynamic and complex role of messages in physical, psychological, social, and spiritual dimensions of health and health care (Yamasaki, Geist-Martin, & Sharf, 2017). When people tell a story that explains what has occurred or what we hope will happen, the story illustrates a point of view or exemplifies something about the person, and narrative has special salience for communication in health- and illness-related contexts (Yamasaki et al., 2017). Stories of illness illustrate a rupture or turning point in a person's life, and illness narratives contribute to understanding and articulating the meanings of illness for the storyteller and listeners (Geist-Martin, Ray, & Sharf, 2003). Stories of illness function as sense-making in the chaos of serious diagnosis or health risk; stories of illness provide implicit accounts for cause, remedy, and outcomes of illness; and stories of illness infer warrants or reasons for decisions and enable a sense of control in the face of illness threat and disorder (Geist-Martin et al., 2003). Stories of illness can help enact transformation in individual identity in providing language for how people view others. Narratives can create identification and social support in a sense of community among people experiencing similar problems (Sharf & Vanderford, 2003). Storytelling around health and illness helps to humanize the practice of medicine (Sharf et al., 2011). Stories function as sense-making and identity as illness-related changes to the physical body, to psychosocial elements, and to relationships become an ongoing and integral feature of a person's personal narrative. For example, from his studies of stories written by people with life-threatening illnesses, sociologist Arthur Frank (1995, 2002) describes stories of restitution where people strive to return to their pre-illness identity, stories of chaos in disorder, lack of control in diagnosis, and recurrence of illness, and stories of quest in searching for deeper existential significance of undergoing illness or suffering. In addition to his stories of life-threatening illness, narratives can help in sense-making for people living with chronic but not life-threatening illness and stories of recovery and continued good health (Geist-Martin et al., 2003).

Although a narrative approach has much potential to inform and to co-construct experiences of health and illness, some narratives cannot be told, and some people cannot tell the story that needs to be told. A person may be so profoundly traumatized that the story is repressed or too distressing (Greenhalgh, 2016). Ethics of research involve careful interplay between eliciting stories and allowing the stories to come from the person or group to whom the story belongs. Narrative interviewing and analysis are specialist skills. Narrative research by untrained or poorly trained researchers is no more reliable than epidemiological research done by people ignorant of basic statistics (Greenhalgh, 2016). Eliciting or sharing stories of vulnerability can cause harm, and the specialty skill of learning the interplay between respect for the person and the story and when the story should be told involves walking a fine line. The ethical responsibility lies with the research team to know when to prompt questions and when to terminate the interview.

RELATIONSHIP-CENTERED PROCESSES IN HEALTH-CARE DELIVERY

Health and illness concepts are inherently tied to models of health care in which health symptoms (or illness symptoms as the contrary) are diagnosed and treated. The conceptualization of health care in medicine and biomedical care has shifted over the last two decades to a model of "relationship-centered" health care. In this volume about close relationships and in a chapter addressing the social context of health and illness, it is important to distinguish the social context of health and illness from relationship-centered health-care constructs. In health-care delivery, relationship-centered processes are more about shared power between health providers (usually physicians) and patients than about the concepts or processes of close relationship. The goal of this section is to provide an overview of relationship-centered health care. This section is included in defining health rather than in the next chapter on close relationship processes because the task dimensions of diagnosis and management of health and illness are always inherently connected to the health-care inter-action. Thus, any shift to "relationship" orientation falls quite short of conceptualization of close relationship processes as described in reciprocal relationships in the next chapter. Relationship-centered health care cannot be removed from the task-driven objectives of diagnosis and making treatment decisions.

The extent to which there is a distinction between patient-centered and relationship-centered health care is considered by some researchers as an important shift in the development of the construct, where "relationship-centered" care is the more recent development and acknowledges the mutual interaction between patients and clin-icians as central to the delivery of health care (Beach et al., 2006). Other researchers continue to use the term "patient-centered" care with similar conceptual meaning as relationship-centered care. Thus, patient-centered care also focuses on patient behavior as vital to med-ical care, research, education, and delivery. Organizations involved in the transformation of health-care delivery may be more likely to use the term "patient-centered."

The shift to patient-centered or to relationship-centered lan-guage in health care can be understood as moving from a traditional biomedical model of health care that addresses pathology and physiol-ogy of disease to a psychosocial model that addresses both biomedical and psychosocial health in accordance with patient preferences (Institute of Medicine, 2001). In light of the definitions included in this chapter, the traditional biomedical model is absence of disease or infirmity, and a broader biopsychosocial model also integrates mental and social well-being. Defining and treating health and illness func-tions as a dynamic process means that the health-care interaction is conceptualized as ongoing relational integration of patient prefer-ences and concerns with managing and treating illness symptoms. In clinical medicine, the world of behavior, culture, society, and experience is also manifest and described as the life world or as lived experience and usually describes the world of the patient. The language, organization, and delivery of relationship-centered health care is intended to integrate biomedical orientation with patient experiences of health care and patient concepts of the preferences and goals for health care.

Relationship-centered health care is historically conceptualized alongside the biopsychosocial model of health care. Illness diagnosis represents a shift from a biomedical explanation for illness to a biopsychosocial model that considers the patient's subjective experience of illness as inherent to treatment and health-care delivery and to shared decision-making. The biopsychosocial model offers a holistic alternative to the traditional biomedical model that historically dominated medical education and illness explanations. The biopsychosocial model can be traced to the late George Engel, who suggested that responding to patients' suffering required giving patients a sense of being truly understood in their psychological and social dimensions in addition to a biological explanation for symptoms (Engel, 1977). Engel's influential conceptualization poses the need for considering physicians' expanded roles as active participants in the unfolding of interactions rather than detached observers of biomedical information.

Balint (1969) originally coined the term "patient-centered medicine" to describe examining the whole person in order to form an overall diagnosis based on the unique attributes of the patient as a human. Later, the patient-centered care group (which was subsequently renamed the relationship-centered care group) articulated patient-centered care as including both physicians' and patients' agendas, finding and exploring common ground, and integrating both the disease and the broader illness experience (Beach et al., 2006). Stewart and her colleagues are part of the Academy on Communication in Healthcare (formerly the American Academy on Communication in Healthcare) and the European Association for Communication in Healthcare, which are two branches of interdisciplinary nonprofit sister organizations including researchers, trainers, and clinicians in the field of communication in health care. These organizations have provided an institutional framework for the foundation for research, teaching, and developing curricula for defining and teaching relationship-centered health care, and for advocating positive outcomes associated with relationship-centered health care.

Although the biopsychosocial model of illness serves as a foundation for a relationship-centered model of health-care delivery, recognizing the ways physicians and patients co-construct the dynamics through communication extends beyond the theoretical scope of the biopsychosocial model. The foundations of relationship-centered care represent a fundamental shift from the traditional bio-medical model of medicine that addresses pathology and physiology of disease, and from the paternalistic model of Western medicine that advocates the provider's role as gathering information, and the patient's role as responding to questions. Much like other supportive interpersonal interactions, relationship-centered health care focuses on the primacy of patient autonomy, preferences, and well-being. The biopsychosocial model explains illness much more broadly than as a set of symptoms, and assumes a "whole person" approach, such that patients come to the interaction as experts in their own life world and illness experience, and poses that patient emotions, roles, and experiences are integral to negotiating treatment decisions.

Relationship-centered health care integrates a biopsychosocial framework and poses joint creation, responsibility, and attribution for the meaning of communication in medical encounters. Thus, the model of relationship-centered care conceptually expands patient-centered care to include a philosophy of shared power between health-care providers (usually physicians) and patients, and acknowledges the *mutual interplay* between providers and patients, and patients' families (Beach et al., 2006). Relationship-centered health care vali-dates the importance of relational processes, shared decision-making, self-awareness, reciprocal processes, difference and diversity, and authentic and responsive participation (Suchman, 2006). More broadly, relationship-centered health care recognizes that the nature and quality of provider–patient relationships are central to diagnosis and health-care delivery. Relationship-centered health care values the individual characteristics and concerns of patients, acknowledges affect and emotion as important components of relationships, considers processes of reciprocal influence, and places moral value on the formation and maintenance of genuine provider–patient relationships (Beach et al., 2006).

Research and practice continue to examine the interconnection between establishing a correct biomedical diagnosis and interpreting illness and health by fully exploring patients' concerns, understanding patients' expectations, and recognizing the human element of the health professional (Borrell-Carrió, Suchman, & Epstein, 2004). Inherent in the relationship-centered model is the assumption that the interaction is co-created by provider and patient, such that the physician comes to a shared understanding of the patient's narrative through negotiated dialogue with the patient; thus, one of the central concerns is removing judgment and developing empathy that allows for solidarity with the patient and respect for his or her humanity (Borrell-Carrió et al., 2004). Care, trust, and openness serve as the foundations for relationship-centered care. Relationship-centered health care promotes the physician's ability to play a role in relational dynamics and finding common ground (Frankel, Eddins-Folensbee, & Inui, 2011).

Research and clinical work explicate the interconnection between a correct biomedical diagnosis and fully exploring the human element of providers' and patients' concerns, understanding, and expectations (Borrell-Carrió et al., 2004). Communication within a relationship-centered care model would account for both health-care providers' and patients' explicit and subtle expressions of concerns, values, and preferences.

Although the concepts of relationship-centered care are philosophically embraced in medical education and practice, models of how relationship-centered care manifest in clinical settings remain a work in progress. Medical education about relationship-centered care theoretically addresses mindful practice (active awareness), integration of reflection into medical training, and communication skills training as core foundations for teaching relationship-centered care (Frankel et al., 2011). The ideals of relationship-centered care were considered radical not so long ago, but now have become a core component of quality recognized by the Institute of Medicine. The ideals are assumed to translate into patient health behaviors by addressing the patient not as a collection of symptoms to be treated but as a person to be cared for, such that obstacles to health behavior change should be addressed within a trusting relationship with a primary caregiver. Nationally standardized, publicly reported evaluations of patient experiences allow for measuring experiences with health-care providers. The practical aspects of what it means to be relationship centered are less clear, and organizations struggle with actualizing and implementing the concepts.

When we recognize medical interactions as serving a relational function in addition to attending to the tasks of addressing symptoms, we are also better equipped to explicate the *meaning* of communication messages. In other words, the meaning of the interaction requires considering health and illness as a larger-scale context and process that acknowledges multiple functions of the encounter. The goal of shaping health behavior poses implications for parallel, even competing, communication functions.

RELATIONSHIP-CENTERED HEALTH CARE VERSUS CLOSE RELATIONSHIP PROCESSES

Interpersonal communication is associated with health outcomes relevant to daily life, including quality of life, illness symptoms, and even death (Duggan & Thompson, 2011). Social determinants shape interpersonal communication and health, including the social environment such as education, income, employment, and occupation, as well as social determinants of place including neighborhood and urban vs. rural environment (Ackerson & Viswanath, 2009). Relevant relationship factors move beyond social determinants to consider the influence of close relationships on health and the influence of illness on close relationships. Relationship-centered health care is quite different from the conceptualizations of close relationship processes. In the health-care literature, relationships are often treated as a topic to be included in conversation. Scripts for relationship-centered health care have become mainstream for providers and patients, but these scripts miss the *process* of communication. For an example analysis, see the comparison of script vs. process in Chapter 7 in this volume. Communication research illustrates how interpersonal communication behaviors shape relational processes when someone is dealing with illness and influence health behavior change.

Relationship theories are grounded in a fundamental assumption that relationships between people are at the heart of identity and behavior, where expectations for behavior are a product of the relationship. Expectations for relationships are usually defined implicitly and develop over time, and theories of communication in relationships explain how communication serves as the manifestation of the relational co-construction of people involved. Considering interpersonal communication in the context of health education and behavior means recognizing an inherent interconnection between the roles and relationships of health providers, friends, and family members in their attempt to influence health and illness (Duggan & Thompson, 2014). Considering close relationship processes as interconnected to health and illness recognizes a broader, systematic interconnection between the emerging experiences of diagnosis and treatment of illness and changes in close relationship processes.

Theories of interpersonal communication focus on explaining how relational processes are manifest in behavior and messages. In essence, relational processes involve the expression and interpretation of messages in personal relationships. In the health context, a foundation in interpersonal communication theories allows for understanding how relationships are interconnected with the goals and tasks associated with health behavior change. For example, in physician–patient interactions, the foundation of trust and rapport can promote (or on the contrary, can inhibit) disclosure about illness behaviors (Duggan & Parrott, 2001). Communication in physician–patient interactions influences decision-making and adherence to medical regimens. Trust and rapport may be a better predictor than biomedical markers of symptoms in predicting the degree of honest disclosure and openness within the physician–patient interaction, as well as subsequent behaviors and outcomes. Similarly, in families, health behavior change often requires that family members interact around a health issue and may shift how they relate to each other (Duggan & Thompson, 2014). Relationships with health providers, family members, and friends can provide support and enhance the efficacy of behavior change. Conversely, relationships can exacerbate the emotional toll of illness and can inhibit behavior change.

In health-care interactions, improving health outcomes requires recognizing and attending to both the task functions of health behavior and the relational functions of attending to human elements, such as emotion, rapport, and fear. In essence, interpersonal communication becomes the manifestation of the interconnection between biomedical or technical information and the complex roles and relationships within which health behavior is negotiated. Although theories of interpersonal communication are not necessarily context specific, the attributes of the context shape the application of theory (Duggan & Thompson, 2014). Interpersonal communication is relevant to behavior change in professional relationships, in families, in romantic relationships, and in friendships, and the attributes of those contexts need to be considered in order to understand health behavior change within any of those contexts. The physician–patient context provides a rich illustration of the interplay between the professional tasks of treating biomedical symptoms (or lack thereof), and the relational goals of attending to the whole person and the breadth of the illness experience (Duggan & Thompson, 2014). However, the physician–patient relationship misses the fundamental assumptions of researchers focused on close relationships. A primary distinction is that the physician–patient relationship is role-driven and does not constitute a reciprocal relationship. Although relationship-centered health care assumes a valid provider–patient partnership as the foundation for symptom reduction and behavior change, as well as prevention behaviors such as advice on smoking and physical activity, the physician–patient interaction is first defined by the roles of *being* physician and patient. Furthermore, the tasks of health care also involve a biomedical orientation (even when the "relationship" is fulfilling), and changes in health behavior involve more than a good relationship with a health provider.

HEALTH AND ILLNESS CONTEXT FOR RELATIONSHIP RESEARCH

Relationship research does not define health, but health and illness are important contexts for relationship researchers. Social relationships are related to physical and mental health outcomes and well-being. Relationship research indicates features of relationships that can predict health or illness and turning points in illness diagnosis that shape relationship processes. Features of relationships can buffer against the negative consequences of a chronic disease or a health crisis. Conversely, features of relationships can exacerbate the challenges of illness. Relationship science does not define health, but relationship processes connect to health and illness contexts in ways that shift the focus for relationship researchers and uncover new processes. The next chapter outlines defining characteristics of close relationships in order to delineate how these characteristics are foundations for understanding relationship processes interconnected with health and illness.

2   Close Relationship Processes

I constantly tried to let go of resentments over his poor control and his constant denigration and despair. I could feel his depression; we couldn't live together, but we couldn't live apart either. It was worse when people would tell me he's mentally ill and I should leave. They wouldn't tell a woman whose husband had cancer to leave him. We didn't have good answers, but we were a couple. When I tried to let him go, I knew it just wasn't right. I couldn't be there for him, but I couldn't be without him. I could hear in his voice when he was in trouble.

    I internalized how to handle the reality for him, how to avoid arguments, and how to acknowledge his feelings without getting caught up. I said loving things about how much I cared about and loved him. Sometimes it was too much to take; I would get really angry and fight with him. He would remind me this makes him more depressed, and so I would apologize for exploding, and help get the chemical condition under control. I think of myself as a loyal person, and we have so many good memories.

– Duggan & Le Poire, 2006.

CONCEPTUALIZING CLOSE RELATIONSHIPS AND HEALTH AND ILLNESS EXPERIENCES

As this brief illustration of a couple including one depressed individual indicates, close relationships shift the understanding of illness, and the understanding of illness connects to our sense of ourselves in our close relationships. When we are committed to a close relationship, we work through issues that we did not envision. Like the couple in this illustration, we do not have easy answers, and difficult choices are not apart from caring. We might experience illness after first developing our many good memories, with a foundation for the relationship during times of health. We might experience illness in a close relationship after a longer history of our own illness or a family illness. As this story begins to illustrate, relationship processes are not apart from the unfolding illness.

In this chapter, I describe defining characteristics of close relationships, and then I delineate how close relationship processes shift foundations when also considering health and illness. Examples of defining characteristics of close relationships include mutual influence (see also the theory chapter on interdependence), relational stability and commitment, emotional bonds (positive and negative emotions), and mutual influence and interconnected interaction patterns. Close relationships include, but are not limited to, intimate relationships, close friendships, and partnered romantic relationships. Summarizing defining characteristics of close relationships puts parameters on non-reciprocal relationships (i.e., professional caretaking, doctor–patient interactions, and broader community networks) that are not the focus of this volume. Understanding relationship processes allows for recognizing how health and illness trajectories are interconnected with close relationships.

The scientific study of personal and social relationships involves theoretical and applied explanations for core principles and constructs of relationship development, maintenance, and dissolution and provides extensive exploration of the nature of close relationship processes. This chapter is not intended as exhaustive but instead provides an overview of how core principles of relationship science connect to understanding how relationships influence, and are influenced by, health and illness behaviors and trajectories. This chapter focuses in particular on health and illness as manifest in *ongoing interactions* in close relationships in order to illustrate how relationship concepts can translate into communicative complexities and dilemmas that emerge around health and illness. The next chapter then focuses on theoretical attributes that shape relationship processes following diagnosis of a serious health condition.

CONCEPTUALIZING RELATIONSHIP SCIENCE

Childhood friends. School friends. Neighborhood friends. College friends. Work friends. Best friends. Boyfriends. Girlfriends. When people describe what makes life meaningful, what contributes to their happiness, and what they most value, they identify close relationships. Close relationships are vital to well-being, including happiness, mental health, physical health, and longevity. On the other hand, close relationships can challenge everything we thought we knew about our well-being, emotions, and mental health! Close personal relationships have a holistic quality that meets more than a need to belong and that is conceptually bigger than shared goals. Close relationships conceptually are more cohesive than a set of interactive moments and more complex than any set of variables. Many of the variables of interest in conceptualizing close relationships, and in the scientific study of close relationships, are causally bidirectional and highly correlated with each other (e.g., trust, love, commitment) (Attridge, Berscheid, & Simpson, 1995). Close relationships can bring out the best in us, but close relationships can also manifest complicated dilemmas and contradictions and paradoxical patterns where we unwittingly enact and encourage the very behaviors we wish to control and curtail.

Close relationships connect to the most vulnerable parts of our lives, to our greatest joys and our deepest disappointments. Colloquial definitions and descriptions of close relationships capture the joys and heartaches associated with intimacy and vulnerability. Songwriters, poets, novelists, theologians, and philosophers have long acknowledged the centrality of relationships to human existence. People sometimes describe their romantic partner or close friends as "part of me," as "attached at the hip," as "soul sisters," as "the family we choose." Conversely, anyone who has felt the poignancy of deep loneliness can describe the desire for meaningful human connection.

The essence of a close relationship comes from the interactions that take place between the particular people and can only be understood by considering the qualities of the people involved as well as the unique dyadic context generated by the combination of behaviors of the particular people. A relationship functions on the specific qualities of each person and on the unique interaction patterns that emerge when people interact (Finkel, Simpson, & Eastwick, 2017). The defining hallmark of the interactions is influence specific to the relationship; each partner's behavior influences the other person's subsequent behavior (Reis, Collins, & Berscheid, 2000). Statistical models address uniqueness at the dyadic level by measuring the unique individual effects of each person in addition to the interaction of both people (partners) in order to indicate relationship variance in social interactions as predicted by individual and partner interactions (Garcia, Kenny, & Ledermann, 2015; Kenny & Kashy, 2011). Empirical support provides evidence for relationship uniqueness and suggests that considering the unique dyadic context better predicts outcomes than individual measures. For example, relationship variance explains most of the total variance in perceptions of mate value (the degree to which a person is able to provide a long-term relationship) and long-term attraction, indicating that romantic evaluations really are in the eye of the beholder (Eastwick & Hunt, 2014). A relationship is more holistic than the sum of its constituent interactions, and relationships are inherently temporal in that current interactions are influenced by past interactions (Hinde, 1979). Close relationships involve strong mutual influence on each other's behavior for an extended period of time and the individuals' mental representations of the relationship are idiosyncratic to the relationship among several dimensions (Kelley et al., 1983a).

Interdisciplinary understanding. The scientific study of relationship processes often includes an interdisciplinary understanding from research in psychology, communication, sociology, family studies, anthropology, philosophy, and other related disciplines. Relationship science is characterized as a multidisciplinary field of interpersonal relationships and human behavior and is grounded in empirically informed frameworks. At the professional level, scholars and practitioners focused on the scientific study of personal and social relationships come from around the globe and across disciplines. The International Association for Relationship Research (IARR) is a scientific and professional organization focused on stimulating and supporting the scientific study of personal and social relationships. It sponsors interdisciplinary conferences, journal publications including *Personal Relationships* and the *Journal of Social and Personal Relationships*, and this *Advances in Personal Relationships* book series. The IARR endeavors to translate scientific research into mainstream media and publicly accessible research summaries. For more information see the IARR website (www.iarr.org).

Relationship science includes interdisciplinary empirical methods and theoretical frameworks to explain relationship initiation, development, maintenance, and dissolution. Relationship scientists explicate concepts such as love, commitment, respect, jealousy, willingness to sacrifice, loneliness, disclosure, and positivity in close relationships. Although the term "relationship" is part of common language, relationship scientists addresses the complexities in relationship *processes* beyond common use of the term. A close relationship extends over some period of time and involves a mutual understanding of closeness and mutual behavior. A key part of this definition is an interconnection in people's thoughts, feelings, and behaviors such that two people's lives in a close relationship are intertwined in a myriad of ways (Harvey & Pauwels, 1999). Relationship scientists have written extensively about definitions of terms such as "close" and "relationship" (Berscheid & Regan, 2005; Kelley et al., 1983b).

Relationships involve cognitive, behavioral, and affective (or emotional) aspects connected to a series of interactions two (or more) people share. A pervasive concept that characterizes attempts to define close relationships is that two people are dependent on one another to obtain good outcomes and facilitate the pursuit of their most important needs and goals (Finkel et al., 2017). Formal or role relationships are distinct from personal relationships in that the end goal or the task at hand defines many of the relationship processes. For example, the health-care provider–patient relationship or caretaker–care recipient relationship is considered a formal or role relationship because the connections are sustained around meeting the particular health needs of the patient or individual and would not necessarily sustain the relationship apart from that particular need. Another feature of the formal or role relationship is lack of reciprocity in relationship processes, for example, such that the patient discloses disproportionately more personal and larger amounts of information than the health-care provider or caretaker.

CLOSE RELATIONSHIP PROCESSES INSTEAD OF RELATIONSHIP FORMS

In the early days of interdisciplinary research on close relationships, contributing disciplines tended to focus on a particular type of relationship (Berscheid, 1996). Sociologists tended to focus on marital and family relationships; social psychologists largely investigated romantic premarital relationships and friendships; marital and family therapists, as well as clinical and counseling psychologist, tended to focus on distressed marital relationships; and developmental psychologists typically examined parent–child and child–peer relationships (Berscheid, 1996).

Researchers interested in relationship phenomena outline validity problems of identifying relationships in terms of relational type or form (Berscheid, 1996). Close relationships cannot necessarily be identified with type or form of relationship. For example, identifying close relationships with reference to relationship type (i.e., spouse, friend, romantic partner, parent) misses relational process components and imposes assumptions that may be invalid. We cannot assume that family relationships are close, or conversely, that most close relationships are family relationships. Relationships between biological parents and their children can be superficial and distant. Positive sentiment, emotion, and feeling are not necessarily associated with kinship relationships. Relationships between people who are unrelated by blood or by contract might be the closest, most meaningful, and most significant relationships. Similarly, we cannot assume that married people are necessarily close. The context in which relationships occur does provide a framework for how the patterns of relationships are revealed over time and across situations. Relationships are temporal, and the time and situation shed light on different aspects of relationship processes.

CONCEPTUALIZING RELATIONAL CLOSENESS

The dimension of closeness is a cornerstone for most relationship phenomena of interest. More reliably than any specific relationship type, close relationships are especially likely to reflect high interconnectedness or interdependence and the degree or frequency with which people influence each other's behaviors, the diversity of the kinds of behaviors that are affected, and the strength of influence, with these properties being characteristic of the interaction patterns over some duration (Kelley et al., 1983b). Interdependence is viewed as involving months or years rather than days and translating into a recursive feedback loop of interaction forces and bonding (Harvey, 1995).

A simpler approach to defining a close relationship is that the relationship has extended over some period of time and involves a mutual understanding of closeness and mutual behavior that is seen by the people involved as indicative of closeness (Harvey, 1995). A close relationship is a process with varying degrees of intensity and various turns that have consequence in the minds and actions of the people involved (Harvey, 1995). People might feel different degrees of closeness or exhibit different behaviors indicative of closeness.

Some indication of reciprocity in feelings or behavior is necessary to develop and maintain a close relationship; closeness with another person cannot be done alone. Similarly, closeness cannot be accomplished by strong feelings and expressions of closeness that paint a picture of ambivalence (i.e., "I love you but I don't know whether I want you in my life"). Some degree of ambivalence and vacillation exists in close relationships, but a high degree of ambivalence by one or both people does not translate well into closeness over time (Harvey, 1995).

Relationships do change over time, and mutuality in feelings and behaviors may ebb and flow over a long relationship at different points in time, where one or both people may act as if no close relationship exists, but then come back together and reconnect (Harvey, 1995). A serious diagnosis can pose challenges for commitment in close relationships (i.e., "I am not sure whether I can go through this serious and sometimes difficult path with you"), and changing health behaviors can challenge perceptions and behaviors in close relationships (i.e., "I want to support you in the weight loss but get frustrated when you skip exercise or eat those desserts").

RELATIONSHIPS AND CONTINUED ADULT HUMAN DEVELOPMENT

Relationship scientists would describe human behavior and development that neglects the influence of close relationships as inaccurate and incomplete. Explanations for relationships are grounded in the assumption that humans' omnipresent relationship context strongly influences each individual's behavior and development through adulthood and over their life span (Reis et al., 2000). Empirical evidence offers support for the theoretical contention that relationships influence human behavior and life span development (Reis et al., 2000).

Positioning adult development and behavior within a relationship context means recognizing relationship cognition, intrinsic emotional links to relationships, and relationship changes across the life span. Relationship cognition reflects how social life is organized around interactions with others with whom one has ongoing association and the social-cognitive processes that connect to dealing with major life tasks (Reis et al., 2000). Chronically accessible negative interpersonal beliefs and expectations are associated with challenges such as increased depression, insecure attachment, loneliness, low self-esteem, higher divorce rates, and poorer self-regulatory processes. Relationship cognition includes expectations we hold for others and adds a dynamic, interactive component to the mental representations of others. For example, the same behaviors may be interpreted more negatively to the extent that spouses have negative expectations of each other (Bradbury & Fincham, 1991). Relationship cognition is about relationships with particular people in particular contexts and not just about chronic tendencies in perceiving others, even close others (Reis et al., 2000). Similarly, cognition about the self often depends on relationship context including social cues and feedback such that different aspects of the self may be expressed with different partners or during different interactions with the same partner. Relational cognitions are not isolated and independent structures but networks activated by ongoing, interdependent relationships that continue to depend on how people process information when thinking about partners and while interacting with them.

Relationships may alter the very processes by which social perception and cognition operate. Relationship cognition is interconnected with motives, emotions, communication, and conflicts of interest, while simultaneously being affected by each other's behavior and representing a history of interaction with each other and with other people. Relationships change as people also mature and develop over their life span. Relationships change with shifting human capacities, needs, and activities; as we consider health and illness trajectories we also must consider involuntary restrictions and changes to the relationship context.

RELATIONAL COMMITMENT AND STABILITY

Relational commitment represents the degree to which people experience a long-term orientation toward a relationship, including intention to proceed through good and lean times, feelings of psychological attachment, and sometimes an implicit recognition of "needing" the relationship (Kelley & Thibaut, 1978). Commitment is argued to emerge with specific circumstances of interconnectedness that characterize a given relationship. In particular, commitment is argued to develop alongside increased satisfaction, especially when the relationship gratifies important needs such as the need for intimacy or security. In romantic relationships with some (often unwritten or without explicit negotiation) expectation of exclusivity, commitment is also argued to develop with the decline in quality of alternatives (Rusbult & Buunk, 1993). Commitment is an emergent property also connected to interdependence, reflecting more than the sum of the component parts from which the commitment arises. Numerous studies demonstrate that satisfaction level, quality of alternatives, and investment size predict commitment (Rusbult & Buunk, 1993). Moreover, commitment is the strongest predictor of persistence in a relationship; commitment better predicts persistence than relationship satisfaction, plausibility of alternatives, or investment in the relationship (Rusbult, 1983; Rusbult & Buunk, 1993).

Sometimes people in close relationships are able to coordinate their behavior in such a manner as to achieve good outcomes; when people share the same interests and goals, achieving desirable outcomes can be relatively easy to coordinate. When interests are at odds in close relationships, when something is good for one person but not good for the other person, people then face choices about what they are willing to sacrifice. In research examining the plausibility of a model of willingness to sacrifice, commitment accounts for an important part of the variance in willingness to sacrifice (Van Lange et al., 1997). Lagged associations indicate the significance of time such that earlier commitment accounted for significant change over time in willingness to sacrifice; commitment was also positively associated with satisfaction level and investment size and negatively associated with quality of alternatives (Van Lange et al., 1997).

People in close relationships indicate that close relationships entail some willingness to set aside personal interests that conflict with the well-being of the relationship overall. Sacrifice includes giving something up for another person, being devoted with loss, or forgoing something valued for the sake of having something more pressing. In the context of close relationships, willingness to sacrifice is defined as the propensity to forgo immediate self-interest to promote the well-being of a partner or a relationship (Van Lange et al., 1997). Sacrifice may involve forfeiting of behavior otherwise described as desirable (passive sacrifice), enacting behaviors that otherwise are undesirable (active sacrifice), or both. The experience of sacrifice may take a variety of forms and may range from minor sacrifices to more substantial, extended sacrifices. Sacrifice refers to behavior that departs from direct self-interest. Sacrifice may or may not be consciously experienced as costly and may or may not be described as substantial. Acts of sacrifice are intended to further positive goals, or to promote the well-being of the other person in a close relationship (Van Lange et al., 1997). Acts of sacrifice involved departures from individual, self-interested preferences, such that individuals take broader considerations into account to maintain a long-term relationship.

Commitment and willingness to sacrifice are likely to co-occur for multiple reasons. Commitment and willingness to sacrifice both consider sustaining long-term relationships over self-interest. Commitment and willingness to sacrifice both involve long-term orientation in looking beyond the present and anticipating future situations. Reciprocal cooperation can involve acts of sacrifice as conscious or unconscious means to maximize long-term interests by smoothing the bumps in an undesirable outcome such that the longer-term cooperation is more reciprocal over time (Van Lange et al., 1997). Also, because commitment involves psychological attachment to another person, people may feel linked, such that benefits for the other person may not be experienced as departure from individual self-interest but broader relational interest (Aron et al., 1991). Good outcomes for the other person may be perceived as inseparable from good outcomes for oneself. Similarly, strong commitment can feel collectivist and communal in orientation, as seen in tendencies for some romantic partners to address the other's needs or desires in an unconditional manner (Van Lange et al., 1997). Commitment is observed in language tendencies to describe the relationship in a relatively collectivistic, pluralistic manner with language such as "we," "us," or "our" rather than "I," "me," or "mine" (Agnew, Van Lange, Rusbult, & Langston, 1998). In highly committed relationships people may exert effort or endure cost without counting what they receive in return and without calculating whether their acts will be reciprocated (Van Lange et al., 1997). The act of sacrifice in the context of a generally committed relationship may increase the probability that the other person will reciprocate in the future. Sacrificing immediate self-interest might create better options for the future in promoting trust and cooperation and other pro-relationship transformation including patterns of interaction for which little or no sacrifice is required (Van Lange et al., 1997).

RELATIONSHIP INTEGRATION AND SHARED GOAL PURSUITS

Relationship theories address the principle of relationship uniqueness directly in measuring the unique individual and collective features, and indirectly in addressing how people in particular relationships negotiate turning points or dilemmas. For example, interdependence theory emphasizes specific qualities and characteristic of relationship partners and desired outcomes from the particular interaction (Kelley et al., 2003). As an extension of interdependence to consider shared goals, transactive goal dynamics theory argues that successful goal attainment depends on features of the self (e.g., a person's desire to lose weight) in conjunction with features of the partner (e.g., the spouse's training as a dietician) (Fitzsimons, Finkel, & vanDellen, 2015).

In close relationships, the cognitive, affective, motivational, and behavioral boundaries between people become blurred (Finkel et al., 2017). As people become closer, they also spend more time together, share a variety of interactions together, and perceive mutual influence on each other's decisions, activities, and plans. The self-concept can be deeply embedded in and altered by close relationships.

Representations of the self are linked to complex relational associations such as sister/brother, spouse, lover, best friend, parent/mother/father, or daughter/son, associations so fundamental that distinctions between the self and the other person cannot be meaningfully disentangled. People indicate relationship integration through plural pronouns such as "we," "us," and "our," indicating committed romantic partners view themselves as a self–other collective (Agnew et al., 1998).

As a close romantic relationship develops, and as desire to maintain the relationship increases, individual self-concept becomes increasingly intertwined with the partner and the relationship (Aron, Aron, & Smollan, 1992). Self-expansion theory describes how people seek to expand their self-concept as they also acquire new skills, characteristics, and resources. As people feel closer and behave in ways that interconnect the self and other, self-concept includes the partner (Aron et al., 1992). Emotional reactions in close relationships are connected to the integration of routines, plans, and goals (Berscheid & Ammazzalorso, 2001).

Self-regulation and goal pursuit can become embedded in close relationships. Transactive goal dynamics theory presents a relational perspective on self-regulation and suggests that people in close partnered relationships form a single self-regulating unit that involves a complex web of goals, pursuits, and outcomes (Finkel et al., 2017; Fitzsimons et al., 2015). Instead of functioning as individual, independent, self-regulating agents, the people form a relationship identified by the theory as the regulating unit in which resources are pooled (Fitzsimons et al., 2015). The shared constellation of goals, pursuits, and outcomes then resides collectively within people in a close relationship. Although individuals can behave independently of their close relationships, the extent and complexity of overlap and interaction among the partners' goal dynamics can be great enough to form a relational system of goal pursuit.

The authors of transactive goal dynamics theory describe the goal of losing weight (a health-promoting behavior) to illustrate the theory. People possess goals for themselves, for their partners, and for the relationship. The goal becomes part of the relational system not only when an individual sets the goal, but when the partner (or other person in a close relationship) also possesses the goal. Alice might set a goal to lose weight herself, or for her partner John to lose weight; she might then pursue this goal by buying healthier snacks, and John might pursue the goal by skipping desserts. Alice might also set a goal for herself, such as submitting a work project on time, which John helps her pursue by additional solo parenting so she can focus on the work. The goals might compete and conflict, and the goals people hold for their partners shape the goals they hold for themselves (Fitzsimons et al., 2015). All goals, regardless of who possesses them and whose outcomes are targeted by them, can potentially be pursued by all people in the system.

Research on social support provides evidence that people pursue goals held by their partners and that this pursuit shapes outcomes (Overall & Fletcher, 2010; Uchino, Cacioppo, & Kiecolt-Glaser, 1996). For example, social support and behavioral monitoring can be helpful in encouraging health behavior. Transactive goal dynamics theory moves beyond social support and beyond the idea of monitoring a partner-oriented pursuit. Goals for the self or the partner and shared goals are subparts of the dyadic (or relational) unit of interest. Goals targeted toward both partners' outcomes and toward the system as a whole are common in everyday life, and the outcomes cannot necessarily be individually measured (Fitzsimons et al., 2015). For example, relational partners might possess a goal of buying a house or starting a family. Partners can possess parallel goals when the goals match in content but not target, or they can possess shared goals held by two partners for the same target. For example, John and Alice might both want John to lose weight. Shared health-behavior goals are common in health care and health psychology.

Partners' goals cannot be understood in isolation; instead, partners' goals, pursuits, and outcomes affect each other and create a dynamic system of mutual influence that draws on shared resources

(Fitzsimons et al., 2015). Partners can share resources (time, energy, skills) and can rely on each other. Goals may be linked across partners in a number of ways such that multiple distinguishable influences may operate in concert. When goal coordination is strong, partners can achieve a level of goal success that would have been impossible if they were single or had a less compatible partner (Finkel & Campbell, 2001; Fitzsimons et al., 2015). Research indicates that people who think about the ways their romantic partner is helpful in their pursuit of a goal work less hard at pursuing that goal, which frees resources for other goal pursuits (Fitzsimons et al., 2015). Research supporting transactive goal dynamics theory suggests that people in close relationships performing joint tasks who desire a communal relationship behave in ways that maximize shared dyadic contribution (Fitzsimons et al., 2015).

Relationships with a longer shared history and more frequent interaction (such as established romantic relationships) might already function to promote interdependent goals. Two people are in a relationship with one another if they have an impact on each other, if they are interdependent in the sense that a change in one person causes a change in the other and vice versa (Kelley et al., 1983b). Kelley et al. (1983b) defined a close relationship as one of strong, frequent, and diverse interdependence (between two people) that lasts over a considerable period of time. Interdependence is the extent to which two people's lives are intertwined, in terms of their behavior toward one another and thoughts and feelings about one another over time (which is conceived as months or years rather than days). Contextual or environmental factors can also enable partners to become interdependent in their goal pursuits. Relevance of a person's resources might promote opportunity for shared goals.

SHARED HEALTH PURSUITS AS SHARED GOALS OF RELATIONSHIP INTEGRATION

Transactive goal dynamics theory is a relational theory that describes the structure of interdependent goal pursuits, predicts the emergence of shared goals, and predicts circumstances where shared goals promote (versus impair) goal outcomes and relationship persistence (Fitzsimons et al., 2015). The theory poses implications for health behavior and health outcomes and can shed light on shared goals in coping with illness trajectories. Consider that health outcomes, like other goal outcomes, reflect a complex and dynamic system of goals and goal pursuits in interdependent relationships (Lakey & Orehek, 2011). The question to consider in applying transactive goal dynamics theory is the extent to which people share the same goals and can coordinate where the goals might be in conflict with other goals. For example, recovering from serious surgery involves the need for social support, but we know less about how support is connected to partner-oriented pursuits and individual self-oriented pursuits of health goals. Partners may be more supportive of an individual who seems to be engaging in successful behaviors moving toward pursuit of a health goal. Partners may also be more supportive when a person is pursuing a goal they share for themselves (Fitzsimons et al., 2015).

Although the examples of transactive goal dynamics theory in this chapter are limited to romantic partners, friends and broader social networks of people can share goals. In the context of health and illness diagnosis and trajectories, considering friends and broader social networks is helpful, even necessary. Spillover effects from one relationship to another may shape shared goals differently from considering the dyadic level. Effects of the romantic relationship might ripple more broadly throughout other close relationships over the course of illness. Close friends might engage in shared goal pursuits that free the spouse to engage in other pursuits or to tend to other aspects of home life while other close friends engage in shared goals throughout the course of treatment. Coordinating goals requires considering a broader theoretical and applied context than interpersonal pursuits. Theoretical attributes about coordinating health goals are helpful in explaining health behavior, since people who are in a position to make choices about undertaking new activities for the purpose of getting healthier or preventing disease can share or coordinate goals to maximize benefit.

EMOTIONAL BONDS (BOTH POSITIVE AND NEGATIVE EMOTIONAL CONNECTIONS)

In close relationships, people experience strong emotions, both positive and negative. Close relationships can be a frequent or intense context for the experience of negative emotion, as observed in distressed and dysfunctional close relationships. Strong emotions can also be regularly observed in non-distressed, happy, and functional relationships. An individual's strongest negative emotions are most frequently precipitated by close relationships (Berscheid, 1996). The association between interdependence and negative emotion is also illustrated by the well-established empirical support that increasing closeness is usually accompanied by increasing frequency and severity of anger and the experience of other negative emotions (Berscheid & Ammazzalorso, 2001). Although some people manage to resolve their conflicts through negotiation and compromise over time, others continue close relationships with ongoing conflict and intensity. Communication that validates emotion is necessary in developing and maintaining social relationships both in early years of development and throughout adulthood. Emotional development includes both positive and negative affect, and experiences appear to interact with age of the relationship such that emotional connection and relationship outcomes vary over the course of relationships (Berscheid & Ammazzalorso, 2001). Consistent with a widespread assumption that close relationships are characterized by positive sentiment, the positivity of emotions and feelings experienced in the relationship sometimes has been used by relationship scholars to classify relationships as close or distant. Sometimes this assumption is inaccurate. Colloquial language also tends to classify the closeness of relationships with reference to the positivity of the emotions and feelings experienced in association with another person.

Within close personal relationships, people experience a broad range of emotions, from the mildest feelings of contentment, annoyance, and anxiety to the most profound experiences of love, rage, and despair (Fitness, 2015). Close relationships including romantic partners, parents, children, friends, siblings, and enemies possess the greatest power to facilitate or frustrate people's needs and desires, and close relationships also function as a primary attribution for the source of people's emotions. Relationship research conceptualizes emotions as having an evolutionary history in that people depend on others for their physical survival and psychological well-being. The preferences, desires, frustrations, and sorrows, as well as the experiences of joy and love, fear and anger, and shame and grief, constitute the currency of human relationships (Fitness, 2015). Feelings and emotions prompt people to act in the service of their needs, desires, and goals (Fitness, 2015).

The social-functionalist view of emotions addresses how emotions serve critical interpersonal functions in people's lives. Emotions such as joy and anger have contributed to the evolutionary history of human survival over thousands of years (Fitness, 2009). For example, anger is hardwired and serves the survival function of alerting individuals to the fact that their desires or goals have been blocked, and motivates and energizes people to attack and remove the perceived source of obstruction (Fitness, 2009; Fitness, 2015). Other emotions similarly motivate adaptive behaviors. Fear motivates escape and avoidance behaviors that keep people safe; happiness motivates adaptive behaviors that build resources and strengthen social bonds; parental love motivates nurturing behaviors that increase likelihood of offspring survival (Fitness, 2015). Emotions that may have been adaptive during evolutionary history may be less adaptive in functions currently served in people's daily lives. The evolved capacity to feel anger and respond by removing the obstruction can be adaptive, but people also must learn how to regulate the expression of anger so that they behave according to the rules of the culture and the context (Planalp & Fitness, 1999). The social-functional perspective suggests that emotions are neither positive nor negative, not good nor bad, but instead that emotions motivate and help people solve survival and personal welfare-related problems, most of which involve their relationships with other people (Fitness, 2015). Sometimes emotion scholars describe emotions as positive or negative, but the social-functional perspective instead considers how emotions can be potentially adaptive.

In addition to motivating adaptive behaviors by understanding our own needs, desires, and goals, the social-functional perspective describes how the expression of emotions plays the critical function of informing people how they are doing (Fitness, 2015). Expressing a range of emotion allows for adapting relationship behaviors. From a functionalist approach, people experience emotions in close relationships when interruptions to expectations or experiences occur; the relatively undifferentiated state of psychological arousal is interrupted by emotional experience. Events capture attention because emotions disrupt the smooth running of the person's life. Ellen Berscheid and colleagues describe a seminal model of emotion solicitation in relationships where relationship partners develop interdependent routines, plans, and goals and depend on each other to keep both of their lives running smoothly, and when each partner behaves as the other expects, the relationship is emotionally tranquil and without interruptions. When a partner does something unexpected or fails to do what is expected, interruptive events may be extremely powerful and may generate strong emotional arousal (Berscheid, 1983; Berscheid & Ammazzalorso, 2001). The model proposes that increasing interdependence prompts greater potential for experiencing emotions in close relationships. Better synchronized routines and plans pose less interruption and less emotion on a daily basis (Berscheid, 1983; Berscheid & Ammazzalorso, 2001). However, without interruptions indicated through emotions, positive and quality-enhancing emotions, as well as painful or disruptive emotions, people miss the potential to better adapt to others' desires and needs. This model of emotion generation in relationships provides foundation for understanding the conditions under which people respond with relatively undifferentiated feelings or upset or happiness in response to another person's daily behaviors (Berscheid, 1983). People appraise interruptive events in terms of motivational relevance ("to what extent does this matter to me?"), and motivational congruence ("to what extent is this helpful or harmful to me?"). Knowing how another person in a close relationship will appraise an event or behavior alongside other dimensions allows one to evaluate the relevance and congruence for the other person, for the self, and within the relationship.

Studies of cognitive appraisal elucidate the ways in which individuals' interpretations of events elicit different kinds of emotional responses, including in the context of close relationships (Fitness, 2015). For example, appraisals that characterize anger include perceptions of injustice and partner blame (Fitness, 2009). Appraisals eliciting hurt were associated with perceptions of relationship devaluation and perceived lack of caring from the partner (Fitness & Fletcher, 1993). Hurtful events were viewed as more unexpected, effortful, and difficult to understand than anger-eliciting events (Fitness & Fletcher, 1993). Emotions prompt distinct motivations to confront, to cry and withdraw, or to seek comfort. Emotions do not function in isolation, but instead people can experience simultaneous multiple emotions (Fitness, 2015). Emotions are elicited cognitively in relationships when partners perceive an interruptive event that they view as congruent or incongruent with their needs, desires, plans, or goals. To the extent that people cognitively evaluate dimensions such as perceived cause, fairness, controllability, and intentionality, different kinds of emotions are elicited along with their associated motivational features (Fitness, 2015). The appraisal process is sequential and dynamic, with emotions having potential to shape ongoing cognitive appraisals (Fitness, 2015). Elicited emotions may then shape perceptions and interpretations of future interruptive events.

Overall, the social-functionalist view of emotion suggests that the experience of emotions serves important intrapersonal functions, and the expression of emotions serves important interpersonal and relational functions. Emotions signal internal and relational responses about how people are doing, and that can be helpful in better meeting needs, desires, and goals. Meeting the needs of others in close relationships further strengthens the bonds between people (Fitness, 2015).

Love. Colloquially, people often equate love with close relationships. Among varieties of love assessed within close relationships, friendship and compassionate love particularly connect to the self-sacrifice that can be manifest during an illness trajectory. Companionate love, conceptualized as strong liking or friendship love, appears in virtually all taxonomies of love and is prominent in lay vocabularies and language about love. Friendship is a comfortable, affectionate, trusting love for a likable partner or person, based on a deep sense of friendship and involving companionship and the enjoyment of common activities, mutual interests, and shared laughter (Fehr, Sprecher, & Underwood, 2009; Neff & Karney, 2009). This type of friendship love may be described as friendship laced with fondness and admiration and is described across a variety of studies. For example, Orbuch and colleagues asked newlyweds to talk about their relationship history after the time of their marriage and then assessed their marital satisfaction two years later. In their studies, Orbuch and colleagues expressed surprise in discovering that having a highly romantic reconstruction of courtship does not predict marital well-being. Instead, a general positive tone without romanticism seemed to be important and is consistent with companionate love (Orbuch et al., 2002; Peterson, Orbuch, & Brown, 2014).

Compassionate love is also described in language such as agape, caregiving love, selfless love, sacrificial love, pure love, true love, unconditional love, altruistic love, and communal responsiveness. This kind of love is described in religious literature and across types of love literatures. Compassionate love in ongoing relationships can be described as an attitude toward another that contains feelings, cognitions, and behaviors that are focused on caring, concern, tenderness, and an orientation towards supporting, helping, and understanding the other, particularly when the other person is perceived to be suffering or in need (Sprecher & Fehr, 2005). In compassionate love, acts of responsiveness are given without demanding or expecting future benefits in return.

Respect. Mutual respect is another foundational component of power-balanced relationships. Respect as an affective component of close relationships includes content components of equality or mutuality and carrying or support of this mutuality as a central relationship feature (Hendrick & Hendrick, 2006). Much more literature describes disrespect, particularly as it pertains to injustice, professions of power and status, and violations of a group's moral norms (i.e., Miller, 2001). Respect (and the lack of it) has been viewed as important to individual identity, individual success in the work world, and general regard for one's humanity (Hendrick & Hendrick, 2006). Respect comes into play among perceptions of equality or balanced power in a close relationship. Respect can be seen structurally as an attitude, consisting of affect, cognition, and behavioral tendencies. Dimensions of respect might be observed in curiosity, attention, empowerment, and reciprocal and validating dialogue. Respect is correlated with positive constructs such as commitment (Hendrick & Hendrick, 2006).

Emotional suppression and sacrifice. Although sacrifice can be good for relationships, not all sacrifices are equal. Some sacrifices inspire feelings of joy, but other sacrifices leave lingering feelings of frustration or resentment that detract from relationship quality (Impett et al., 2012). Regulating emotions by suppressing or inhibiting their overt expression can have negative consequences including lower personal well-being, decreased closeness with others, and lower responsiveness to partners' needs. Emotional suppression when people sacrifice for a romantic partner can indicate less authentic feelings and, in turn, poorer personal well-being and romantic relationship quality (Impett et al., 2012). However, emotional suppression might feel authentic and may sometimes be beneficial. In highly interdependent relationships, people might suppress negative emotions during a sacrifice and instead emphasize the importance of maintaining harmony in the relationship. Engaging emotional suppression for pro-social reasons, such as to avoid harming one's relationships, may be a key motivation for people in developing interdependence (Butler, Lee, & Gross, 2007). Because expressing negative emotions can communicate that one feels troubled or inconvenienced, suppressing emotions during sacrifice can prompt interdependence in people feeling that they have authentically chosen to prioritize their relationship over their own personal concerns (Le & Impett, 2013). In other words, suppressing negative emotions in the specific context of sacrifice can enable people in highly interdependent relationships to experience a sense of congruence between their outward behavior of sacrificing for the good of the relationship and their internal desires to prioritize interpersonal harmony over their own concerns (Le & Impett, 2013). For example, in a daily diary experience study of people in romantic relationships, people with higher levels of interdependence experienced boosts in personal well-being and relationship quality if they suppressed their negative emotions during sacrifice, whereas people who construed the self in the least interdependent terms experienced lower well-being and relationship quality if they suppressed their negative emotions during sacrifice (Le & Impett, 2013). Feelings of authenticity for the sacrifice mediated those associations.

INDIVIDUAL DIFFERENCES IN RELATIONSHIP PROCESSES AND RELATIONAL AMBIVALENCE

Personality and close relationship processes. Although understanding close relationships involves acknowledging the extent to which people mutually influence each other's thoughts, feelings, and behaviors, people do not behave simply in response to each other's behavior. People bring their individual personalities and individual differences into each relationship as well (Gaines, 2016). The enormously complex attributes of the individual selves include a multitude of personality characteristics, including traits, values, attitudes, motives, and emotions that contribute to the selves' richness (Gaines, 2016). Understanding the intersection of individual characteristics and relationships involves an explanatory framework that addresses each person's dispositions, motives, goals, and needs, as well as the interconnection of situations that interfere with dispositions and activate specific relational schemas.

In his thorough integration of the theoretical and empirical strands of literature on personality and close relationship processes, Gaines (2016) provides evidence that interpersonal aspects of personality consistently are related to one or more interdependence phenomena. The interpersonal trait of nurturance (i.e., positive femininity), the interpersonal attitude of positive evaluation concerning significant others (i.e., secure attachment), the interpersonal motive of intimacy, and the interpersonal emotions of life experiences (i.e., affection) all covary with accommodation, satisfaction, and/or commitment in close relationships (Gaines, 2016). Gaines also extends his analysis beyond the purely individual to illustrate how individual differences also translate into differences in how people connect with others. To that end he describes how traits of agreeableness and conscientiousness (and extraversion to a lesser extent), the "me-value" of individualism and various "we-values" such as collectivism, familism, and romanticism, the attitudes of eros and ludos (and the attitudes of mania, pragma, and agape to a lesser extent), and emotional jealousy appear to be related to interdependence (Gaines, 2016). Gaines suggests that personality characteristics beyond the interpersonal processes in close relationship processes likely reflect *combinations* of interpersonal constructs. For example, emotional jealousy is likely part of a broader emotional climate of marriage in which emotional jealousy represents a combination of antagonism and affection and also includes additional emotions (Gaines, 2016).

Gaines' comprehensive review of the literature on personality constructs and close relationships highlights how understanding the interpersonal domain is necessary in understanding differences in interdependence variables such as accommodation, commitment, and satisfaction across individuals. However, personality variables do not explain the entirety of either close relationship processes or interdependence variables. Overall, as seen in Gaines' (2016) volume, personality constructs are important components for understanding close relationship processes. The traits of agreeableness and conscientiousness, the value of romanticism, the attitudes of eros, ludos, mania, and agape, the motive of intimacy, and the emotions of love, jealousy, and anger provide a solid foundation to explain individual differences in close relationship processes (Gaines, 2016). Additional personality explanations where people are simultaneously both producers and products of social systems (e.g., communal values, power motivations and manifestations, and experiences of anxiety) deserve additional examination (Gaines, 2016). The major theme throughout Gaines' (2016) integrated volume is the relevance of the interpersonal domain of personality to close relationship processes such as interdependence; this domain of personality is operationalized as trait, attitude, value, motive, or emotion dimensions. Gaines' review further provides evidence that various aspects of personality may be more intricately woven to provide a better understanding of both investment and interdependence. An interdependence framework allows for relationship scientists to gain substantial insight into the ways in which personality affects the ways in which partners relate to each other.

ATTACHMENT THEORY AND RELATIONAL AMBIVALENCE

Attachment theory (Bowlby, 1982) has been a cornerstone theory in explaining how the formation and quality of emotional bonds and the interplay between individual- and relationship-level processes is manifest across phases of the life span (Hazan & Shaver, 1987). One of the basic assumptions of Bowlby's attachment theory is that interactions with significant others (attachment figures) are represented in internal working models of the self and others. These models include expectations, strategies, and procedures that shape a person's goals, thoughts, feelings, and behaviors in interpersonal situations across the life span (Hazan & Shaver, 1987; Mikulincer et al., 2010). People are motivated to seek proximity and comfort from attachment figures in times of need.

The attachment process was originally proposed and tested to explain when frightened children seek proximity to their caregiver, and when caregivers respond by providing comfort and reassurance, helping infants regulate distress and regain a feeling of security. Adults who are distressed may similarly seek out someone else in an attempt to restore emotional well-being, and adult partners may respond by providing care through reassurance, comfort, and/or tangible support (Collins & Feeney, 2000). Attachment-related relationship dynamics require an ability to regulate behavior (seeking proximity, for example), and deciding when to disengage from a goal. The attachment system works together with other biobehavioral systems. For example, the adult caregiving system leads individuals to attune to their relationship partner's distress signals and triggers behavior that will protect, support, and promote the well-being of the relationship partner. In adult relationships both partners may rely on each other to fulfill attachment needs and both partners may act as caregivers; attachment and caregiving processes in adults are highly interrelated (Collins & Feeney, 2000).

Security-enhancing interactions with available and responsive attachment figures promote a positive view of others. Repeated interactions with available and responsive attachment figures create both a persisting sense of attachment security and positive working models of the self as being loved, and of others as being reliable, helpful, and loving (Mikulincer et al., 2010). Frustrating, emotionally painful interactions with unavailable or rejecting attachment figures weaken a person's sense of security and contribute to negative views of others (Hazan & Shaver, 1987). When relationship partners are repeatedly rejective, unresponsive, or unavailable in times of need, however, the rejections undermine attachment security, and serious doubts can arise about others' availability and support and potentially about one's own value and lovability.

Individual differences are reflected in working models that consist of expectations about the worthiness of the self in relation to significant others and the availability and responsiveness of attachment figures (Bowlby, 1982). Working models show some continuity from childhood to adulthood, but they may change as a function of experience and across different relationships (Mikulincer, 1998). Individual differences in attachment can roughly be measured along two dimensions: anxiety and avoidance (Mikulincer & Shaver, 2007). A person's position on the anxiety dimension indicates the degree to which he or she worries that a partner will not be available or responsive in times of need. A person's position on the avoidance dimension indicates the extent to which he or she distrusts relationship partners' goodwill and strives to maintain behavioral independence and emotional distance from partners (Mikulincer & Shaver, 2007). The two dimensions can be measured with reliable and valid scales and are associated in theoretically predictable ways with relationship quality and affect regulation (Mikulincer & Shaver, 2007).

A person's location in the two-dimensional concepts of attachment anxiety and avoidance reflects both the person's sense of attachment security and the ways in which he or she deals with threats or distress (Mikulincer & Shaver, 2007). People who score low on both dimensions tend to employ constructive affect-regulation strategies; people who score high on either the attachment anxiety or the avoidant attachment dimension tend to rely on deactivating strategies, trying not to seek proximity, denying attachment needs, and avoiding closeness and interdependence in relationships (Mikulincer & Shaver, 2007). These strategies develop in relationships with attachment figures who express disapproval or punish closeness or expressions of need or vulnerability. People scoring high on attachment anxiety tend to rely on hyper-activating strategies, energetic attempts to achieve proximity, support, and love, combined with lack of confidence that these resources will be provided and anger when they are not.

Relationships where an attachment figure is sometimes responsive but not reliably responsive function as partial reinforcement from a learning-theory perspective, because sometimes people are successful at having their needs met. Anxious attachment is associated with complex views of other people; people scoring high on attachment anxiety have a history of frustrating interactions but believe that if they intensify their proximity-seeking efforts, they may compel relationship partners to provide adequate support (Mikulincer & Shaver, 2007). Even when they are angry, attachment-anxious people take some of the blame for the partner's unreliable attention and care (Mikulincer & Shaver, 2007).

Attachment anxiety may translate into relational ambivalence as marked by conflicting relational goals and action tendencies and by ambivalent attitudes toward relationship partners (Mikulincer et al., 2010). Attachment-anxious people are strongly influenced by their desires for security and closeness, which can translate into their over-focusing on the potential rewards of intimacy and their attitudes toward relationships and relationship partners (Mikulincer et al., 2010; Hazan & Shaver, 1987). Attachment-anxious people are also driven by fears of rejection and abandonment and by memories of frustrating attachment relationships, which lead them to overemphasize risks of intimate interactions and the potentially negative traits and intentions of the relational partner. Although attachment-anxious individuals are interested in developing and relying on relationships with people they view as attractive and desirable, when such people show signs of interest or support, the signs of interest may arouse fears of being rejected or disliked (Mikulincer et al., 2010). Implicit motivational conflicts seem to plague attachment-anxious individuals. Moreover, relational ambivalence may underlie the well-known tendencies to ruminate obsessively about how to react in social situations in relationships; attachment-anxious individuals may lack relational intimacy despite their desire for closeness; and they may be reluctant to seek a partner's support despite strong needs for reassurance and comfort (Mikulincer et al., 2010). In the context of health and illness, individual attachment processes predict how people regulate their emotions and behavior. The communicative processes serve as a pathway linking individual self-regulation and health behaviors.

COMMUNICATION PROCESSES AND CLOSE RELATIONSHIPS

Communication is the process through which people enact and define relationships, and communication can indicate whether a relationship will continue or end. Within the study of personal relationships, communication is the means by which people construct and maintain relationships, along with a set of skills or skill deficits that contribute to relationship adjustment (Burleson, Metts, & Kirch, 2000). Integrative frameworks to organize a coherent understanding of communication in close relationships consider communication as strategic and consequential (Burleson et al., 2000). Communication is *strategic* in that it involves message production intended to achieve a goal or desired end. Goals may be organized hierarchically, or goals can be situation specific. Considering communication as strategic assumes purposeful and intentional messages. Of course, messages might not always be consciously or intentionally created, but the strategic perspective of communication assumes that people use messages generally to pursue goals and that people vary in their ability to effectively achieve goals through communication. Understanding communication as functional stresses communication as a central means through which people pursue and maintain desired goals in relationships. People expect different relationships to do different things for them, and communication functions to provide distinct sets of material, as well as social, emotional, and psychological goods (Burleson et al., 2000). Communication behavior includes the verbal and nonverbal actions or messages people use in a particular context, in this case the context of close relationships.

Communication is *consequential* in that messages externalize and structure the relationship in which it occurs. Communication enacts the relationship, expresses images of the self, of other people, and of the relationship; communication creates patterns, routines, and rituals; communication establishes and perpetuates shared codes and meaning systems; communication establishes and reinforces communal norms and rules (Burleson et al., 2000). Communication creates, maintains, and modifies the dynamic, evolving processes of close relationships. Communication messages create and maintain meaning systems as well as norms and rules that organize, sequence, and control behavior and role structures that organize situated identities. Relational structures are not typically the intended result of strategic actions but are outcomes or consequences of day-to-day communication within relationships (Burleson et al., 2000). The symbolic properties of language and nonverbal behavior enable people in relationships to construct a shared meaning system such that people simultaneously construct and participate in systems as well as align their perceptions and channel their behaviors as fits their meaning system.

The basic properties of communication in close relationships, as outlined in Vangelisti's (2015) chapter on communication in personal relationships, comprise communication interdependence, reflexivity, complexity, ambiguity, and interdeterminacy. These properties elucidate the ways in which communication shapes the enactment and interpretation of messages that create and sustain close relationships (Vangelisti, 2015). Interdependence as a property of communication refers to the mutual influence process in shaping and responding to verbal and nonverbal messages (Vangelisti, 2015). In close relationships, messages across interactions create coherence and function to enact individual and relational goals and relationship choices and trajectories. The patterns and ongoing processes of close relationships, as well as the patterns indicating understanding in close relationships, are manifest in communication. The developmental interconnection begins at birth, as can be observed in the mutual regulation of infant–parent communication such that infants imitate adults' facial expressions, vocalizations, and response latencies. Interdependence in messages translates into explanatory frameworks focusing on patterns of interaction over time rather than on individual messages (Vangelisti, 2015). Patterns of interaction in relationships are structured and coherent such that people can carry on conversations because they understand the rules and routines that typically structure interactions between them. People in close relationships respond to the communication sequences and interaction patterns that exist within their relationships but also shift patterns over time such that communication is also dynamic and flexible.

Interaction patterns of communication in relationships change with relational events, with external pressures, and with time, but the patterns and structures are patterned and sequenced enough to study interactions that characterize particular relational experiences (Vangelisti, 2015). Patterns of interaction also are shaped by time and place, by the relational history of people, and by the patterns that preceded the current interaction. People in close relationships interpret messages by other communication behaviors that preceded the message and by the temporal environment and other contexts of the message (Vangelisti, 2015). The relatively stable styles or patterns of behavior also represent adaptations to relational features. For example, parents and children create patterns of behavior that adapt to features of their relationship and to the context of their relationship (Bugental, 2000). Communication in close relationships reflects behavioral sequences that mediate relationship quality (for better and for worse) (Vangelisti, 2015). For example, couples' interaction patterns can predict relational outcomes beyond overall base rates, as observed in demand–withdraw patterns as a behavioral sequence that occurs when one partner demands or tries to engage when the other partner tries to avoid conversational interaction (Caughlin & Huston, 2002).

Communication reflexivity means that communication simultaneously creates structure and is constrained by structure (Vangelisti, 2015). Communication reflexivity in close relationships means that communication enacts relationships and is also shaped by the relationship. People in close relationships might respond to normative practices that become scripted within the relationship but also by intentional choices in enacting particular goals. The communication history establishes the boundaries of communication in close relationships but also people have some flexibility and fluidity in creating dynamics (Vangelisti, 2015). In close relationships, people discuss and interpret topics and language in unique ways that reflect their relational history. Conversation in relationships also influences subsequent talk, in that dialogue shapes the quality of people's connections over time and shapes their ongoing relationship narratives and stories (Vangelisti, 2015). Individuals' descriptions of their relationships then can further influence how they subsequently behave in the relationships. For example, people who describe their relationship as affectionate and resilient are likely to then interpret the relationship partner's behavior in light of that description and are also likely to then behave in ways that support their description of the relationship (Vangelisti, 2015).

Communication complexity refers to the idea that communication conveys multiple meanings simultaneously on multiple levels of analysis (Vangelisti, 2015). The literal content level of the meaning of the words exists alongside the relationship level (also called command level, illocutionary level, or episodic level). These multiple meanings exist between people and denote the action as content as well as the context or relationship meaning of the broader context. The relationship level can include symmetry or dominance in meaning; for example, an apology can simultaneously function as a "one down" communication move. The process of communication is manifest in how communication complexity takes shape. For example, literature on couples' conflict focuses on the acts of communication rather than the content of the messages and on how people negotiate conflict rather than what they fight about (Sillars & Canary, 2013). Other qualities of communication can further complicate the relationship level of meaning and the content level of meaning. A message may serve multiple functions at the same time. For example, a messages can simultaneously create intimacy as well as exert control and indicate social support. Describing the multiple functions offers an indication of complexity, but the multiple functions at the same time can translate into noticing complexity as more apparent (Vangelisti, 2015). Communication can also function to enact and achieve multiple goals simultaneously. For example, people can seek to indicate competence and self-sufficiency potential as well as to obtain social support that may initially be interpreted as in direct contradistinction with the indication of competence and self-sufficiency.

Communication ambiguity involves the idea that messages can only partially encode the meanings they are intended to express, and instead people have to make inferences to understand intent, even in close relationships (Vangelisti, 2015). Interpreting the relational aspects of a message requires people to make inferences about goals, attitudes, and relational history in order to deduce meaning, which can be ambiguous (Vangelisti, 2015). People in more intimate relationships typically have more contextual information and shared history that serves as context to interpret messages. Shared knowledge and understanding help people understand the implicit meanings in their verbal and nonverbal messages (Vangelisti, 2015). On the other hand, shared relational history can complicate and distort the meaning of messages because people can assume a close relationship partner can better understand them, even when the understanding is an inaccurate assumption (Vangelisti, 2015). Incongruity in partners' interpretations of each other's behavior can be explicated (at least in part) by the weak association between the amount of information partners disclose to each other and their perceived mutual understanding (Vangelisti, 2015).

Communication outcomes indeterminacy refers to the effects of messages on individuals or relationships being variable rather than fixed (Vangelisti, 2015). Communication indeterminacy means that communication messages pose contextual, historical, personal, and cultural meaning, and must be interpreted within applicable contexts instead of an individual predicting a certain outcome (Vangelisti,

2015). For example, people can use different messages to persuade each other, to disagree with each other, or to hurt each other's feelings (Vangelisti, 2015). Similarly, the same message in a different relationship can result in different outcomes. A message or sequence of messages interpreted as humorous or affectionate in one relationship might instead be interpreted as insulting in another relationship (Vangelisti, 2015). The same message might also be interpreted differently at different points in the same relationship.

COMMUNICATION AS PERPETUATING RELATIONSHIP INSECURITIES

The consequences of communication are important for understanding how dyadic messages contribute to behaviors that promote or interfere with everyday functioning. The consequences of communication pose implications for understanding vulnerability in close relationships. In some relationships, people chronically doubt that their partner values, accepts, or cares for them. Doubts about the relationship can exist regardless of partners' actual thoughts and affections. Pessimistic interpretation of a partner's thoughts and feelings can undermine the quality of the relationship for both the self and the partner (Lemay & Clark, 2008). The expression-based authenticity doubts model suggests that, paradoxically, revealing to someone in a close relationship that one feels insecure can generate additional insecurities in being perceived as an insecure person (Lemay & Clark, 2008). When people feel insecure about a partner or close friend's regard or acceptance, they typically believe that they have behaved in ways that have communicated insecurity and emotional vulnerability to the partner or close friend. These beliefs about expressing insecurities and vulnerabilities trigger other cognitions that ultimately perpetuate relationship insecurities (Lemay & Clark, 2008). Knowing that a person has communicated relational vulnerabilities about acceptance and rejection in the past prompts reflected appraisals of vulnerability. These reflected appraisals include beliefs that the other person perceives the individual as relationally vulnerable, easily hurt, emotionally volatile, and overly dependent on approval and positive feedback (Lemay & Clark, 2008). Because of the perceptions of reflected appraisals, hearing encouraging words from the person will be less likely to make people who feel insecure about a partner's acceptance feel good about themselves because they dismiss the positive words as being insincere. People then have authenticity doubts in believing that a partner expresses more positive regard and conceals more negative regard than he or she actually feels (Lemay & Clark, 2008). Paradoxically, expressing feelings of insecurity in a particular relationship can trigger overreactions to fears of rejection, and expressing insecurities can make the relational concerns worse in perceiving the partner is just "walking on eggshells" trying to spare the person's ego and not saying what he or she really feels (Lemay & Clark, 2008). Doubts about the authenticity of the partner's expressions of regard maintain the expressed insecurities.

The theory proposes that people who feel insecure about a partner's acceptance doubt that they are truly accepted by the partner and behave in ways that express this insecurity and vulnerability to the partner when they feel especially emotionally vulnerable to the prospect of rejection (Lemay & Clark, 2008). This idea is consistent with dependency regulation, where people defensively reject the partner by distancing from the partner and from the relationship when they anticipate rejection (Murray, Holmes, & Collins, 2006). When people perceive high threat, they communicate and behave in ways that seem to function as self-protective such as derogating their partner and denying the importance of the relationship and enacting cold and hurtful behaviors toward the partner through criticism or insults (Murray et al., 2006). Instead of translating into desired closeness and reassurance, the rejecting messages predict feelings of anger and hostility.

Once people think they have expressed heightened vulnerability or sensitivity, they may tend to believe that the partner views them as particularly sensitive or vulnerable (Lemay & Clark, 2008). A person's behavioral reactions to insecurity about their partner's acceptance are manifest in such forms as hinting for a compliment, privately derogating the partner following a perceived transgression, avoiding the partner, directly seeking reassurance about the partner's affections, or openly insulting the partner. The behavioral reactions are likely salient responses to insecurity in one's own mind. However, the partner may not notice the particular behavior or may not interpret it as relational vulnerability but instead may view the behavior as evidence of a situational state (e.g., he or she "had a bad day"). Still, the focus on one's own reactions to insecurity may be viewed as especially vulnerable through egocentric perception (Lemay & Clark, 2008). The reflected appraisals of vulnerability then prompt doubts about the authenticity of the partner's expressions of positive regard. A person who is suspicious that their partner expresses insincere positive thoughts and feelings then may suppress negative thoughts and feelings, and may behave generally with caution. As people become more cautious about perceiving that their partner exaggerates positive thoughts and feelings and carefully monitors negative expressions, they may further elicit reassurance but continue to interpret the partner's positive expressions as inauthentic (Lemay & Clark, 2008). Doubting the partner's authenticity can undermine confidence and can create a disjuncture between the partner's positive expressions and one's inferences of the partner's true thoughts and feelings. Believing that a partner is concealing some negative sentiment or is expressing unfelt positive sentiment can encourage a person to perceive more negative regard and less positive regard than is indicated by the actual messages (Lemay & Clark, 2008).

In response to a partner's compliment, the person might think the partner is just being nice, or just being polite. The authors of the theory distinguish between the interpersonal/relational processes in a close relationship as posited by the model and effects of trait insecurity or chronic tendencies to feel insecure regarding acceptance by others in general (Lemay & Clark, 2008). A series of studies provided evidence that people believe expressions of regard toward relationally insecure others are relatively inauthentic. Thus, walking on eggshells seems to be a common perception of explanatory frameworks for how people who express insecure messages make sense of the messages received from others in close relationships (Lemay & Clark, 2008). Independent of self-esteem and attachment anxiety, reflected appraisals of vulnerability may induce one's own prior expressions of insecurity, which appear to predict the expectation of walking on eggshells and induce suspicion about the degree to which positive messages are actually positive. In addition, doubts about the authenticity of a partner's or of a friend's authenticity predicted more pessimistic perceptions of the other's regard and caring (Lemay & Clark, 2008).

People do not consciously wish to undermine their own security, but they may unwittingly perpetuate their own insecurity because they are unaware of how their behavioral responses may focus on their present need for security or self-protection. Their responses might temporarily protect them from negative feedback but might serve to reinforce the very behavior from which they seek to protect themselves. The expression-based authenticity doubts model addresses expressions of insecurities about the relationship per se. The model posits that relationship processes can be initiated by and perpetuate relationship-specific insecurity (Lemay & Clark, 2008). The model may especially pertain to the relationship dynamics of people who tend to behave with greater insecurity in relationships because they doubt authenticity and express vulnerabilities more frequently. Understanding insecurities within a framework of experience and expression of emotion allows for a broader lens for expressing and moving through vulnerabilities in close relationships. Theoretical and empirical explanations for disclosing emotions in close relationships provide evidence for enhanced experiences of intimacy through sharing emotions (Reis & Shaver, 1988).

DYADIC COMMUNICATION PROCESSES AND HEALTH BEHAVIORS

In social science literature addressing self-regulation and health behaviors, communication processes contribute to adult health behavior in areas such as weight control, curtailing substance abuse, and managing depression. Understanding dyadic communication processes offers a glimpse into the complexities in health and illness behaviors as interconnected with identities and competing goals in close relationships. Social support from others can predict a healthier diet and more frequent exercise behaviors (Verheijden et al., 2005). Assessing the quality of communication between partners provides insights into how partners impact each other's weight management. In one study, the more partners exhibited warmth and support as well as pushed them to do better, the more individuals felt their partners were effective in helping them to enact healthy diet and exercise behaviors (Dailey, Romo, & Thompson, 2011). In another study, acceptance defined as the degree to which a relational partner shows positive regard, care, warmth, and attentiveness during interactions about weight management, and challenge as defined as the degree to which a relational partner pushes the other person to enact healthy behaviors, both predicted weight management outcomes (Dailey, McCracken, & Romo, 2011). Acceptance provides validation and security and indicates the other person is valued and cared for, and not judged. Acceptance and challenges are proposed to work together; consistent acceptance in the absence of challenge may lead individuals to believe they do not need to change their diet or exercise behaviors. In an analysis of confirming or disconfirming messages during conversations about weight management, high challenge combined with low acceptance predicted the lowest levels of exercise self-efficacy (Dailey, Richards, & Romo, 2010). Weight management messages higher in both acceptance and challenge were perceived as more effective than messages lower in these components (Dailey et al., 2010). In addition, people who were more satisfied with their communication about weight management with relational partners perceived challenging messages as more effective and messages lower in acceptance as less effective (Dailey et al., 2011). People who perceive the conversations as instigating negative conflict or feel they are not successful in accomplishing their goals may avoid discussing weight management issues, which could ultimately impact their health outcomes.

THE DARK SIDE OF CLOSE RELATIONSHIPS: COMMUNICATION AND RELATIONSHIP PARADOXES IN HEALTH AND ILLNESS BEHAVIORS

Research in substance abuse treatment provides a poignant example of communication in the family system as connected to substance abuse treatment, as well as the family circumstances promoting continued alcohol and drug use (Miller-Day & Dodd, 2004). Relational effects point to the need to study the reciprocal impact of family members and continued substance abuse. Living with a substance-abusive romantic partner, or a depressed partner, poses demanding challenges. Research indicates that close relationships can interfere with health outcomes and can paradoxically unwittingly encourage the very behaviors people seek to curtail (Duggan, Dailey, & Le Poire, 2008; Duggan & Le Poire Molineux, 2013). Spouses and people in close relationships share the pain of the problems associated with health and illness contexts such as substance abuse and depression, as well as the gain of recovery. Substance abuse problems are manifest in the ways family members approach, maintain, and communicate about drug and alcohol use within their relationships. Family members may play a role in initiating alcohol or drug use, in the choice of substances, in the intensity of substance use, and in the decision to use or abstain from substances (Rodriguez, Knee, & Neighbors, 2014).

Alcohol abuse is described as both a predictor and a consequence of marital stress, spousal abuse, and other marriage challenges. The spouse is often the focus of research and clinical work both because of the relational complications inherent in substance-abusive marriages and because of the ways communication with family members becomes ingrained with ongoing substance use. The patterns in which couples communicate about substance abuse may exacerbate the problem, or on the contrary, may lead to greater abstinence and improved family functioning. People in close relationships may enable drinking or drug using through learned behavioral responses that increase the probability of further substance use, such as drinking with the spouse or minimizing negative consequences. Family interventions can involve family members encouraging substance-abusive individuals to participate in treatment, joint involvement of family members in the treatment, and responding to the needs of family members.

INCONSISTENT NURTURING AS CONTROL

Inconsistent nurturing as control (INC) theory asserts that significant others (romantic partners, spouses, or family members) in relationships with substance-abusive individuals unintentionally and subtly encourage substance-abusive behavior through their well-intentioned efforts to curtail this behavior (Duggan et al., 2008; Duggan & Le Poire Molineux, 2013). Dyadic communication dynamics can predict sustaining or deterring family members' substance abuse. Originally written to explain relationships between substance-abusive individuals and their non-addicted relational partners, subsequent theoretical and applied research provides evidence that daughters with eating disorders face similar patterns with mothers' inconsistent attempts to control disordered eating, depression, and spousal violence (Duggan et al., 2009).

Inconsistent nurturing as control theory is based on the assumption that functional partners (partners of substance abusers or individuals who otherwise engage behaviors that interfere with everyday functioning) have competing goals of nurturing the partner and controlling the negative behavior (Duggan & Le Poire Molineux, 2013). Inconsistent nurturing as control theory argues that there are several paradoxical injunctions in relationships that include partners who struggle with a behavior that interferes with everyday functioning (e.g., drug abuse, depression, or an eating-disorder) and that these paradoxes ultimately impact expressions of control by the functional family member (i.e., the partner without a particular problem inter-fering with day-to-day functioning) in the relationship. The contradictory nature of the functional family member's nurturing and subsequently controlling behavior is at the heart of the most problematic paradox in the relationship. Specifically, simultaneously, functional family members wish to retain their relationship *while* they attempt to extinguish the undesirable behavior, which translates into competing goals (Duggan & Le Poire, 2006). In addition, the nurturing behavior can be highly rewarding, particularly during times of crisis (Duggan & Le Poire Molineux, 2013). These assumptions lead to the paradoxical conclusion that if functional family members actually control the undesirable behavior, they also lose their ability to utilize their nurturing resource base in response to that undesirable behavior. Thus, functional family members who seek to curtail the negative behavior may ultimately be driven by fear that extinguishing the undesirable behavior will decrease the other person's dependency on them (Duggan & Le Poire, 2006). These competing goals could lead to the inconsistent use of reinforce-ment and punishment of the change attempts. This inconsistency is at the heart of INC theory and could lead to decreased effectiveness of control attempts.

Inconsistent nurturing as control theory argues that the func-tional family members' initial nurturing behavior may reinforce the drug or alcohol use, depression, or eating-disordered behavior. In contradistinction to the goal of reducing the negative behavior, inconsistent influence may actually increase ongoing substance abuse (Duggan & Le Poire Molineux, 2013), depression (Duggan & Le Poire, 2006), or disordered eating (Duggan et al., 2009). Even more problematically, functional family members may intermittently rein-force substance abusive behaviors. This intermittent reinforcement may ultimately strengthen abusive behavior, depression, or disor-dered eating because intermittent reinforcement predicts more long-term, non-extinguishable behavior than continuous reinforcement. Unfortunately, INC theory argues that similar to intermittent reinforcement, the intermittent nature of this punishing behavior should actually increase the substance abuse, depression, or disordered eating as well. Inconsistent nurturing may ultimately strengthen the likelihood of the behavior people seek to curtail in close relationships through the learning theory processes of both intermittent reinforcement and intermittent punishment.

This inconsistency manifests itself within communication behavior over the life span of the relationship (Duggan & Le Poire Molineux, 2013; Duggan & Le Poire, 2006). Before labeling their partners as substance abusive, functional partners more often reinforced the problematic behavior (e.g., offering a drink when they got home from work, using substances with the person, telling the depressed person the negative behavior is a pain). Subsequent to a significant event that promoted labeling of their partners as substance abusive (e.g., a car accident, missing weeks of work, violence, etc.), partners dramatically shifted their behavior to punish their partners (e.g., calling the police, threatening to leave, removing substances from the house). In sum, applications of INC theory provide evidence that functional partners changed their strategy usage over time so that they (a) reinforced substance-dependent behavior more before their determination that the behavior was problematic than after; (b) punished substance-dependent behavior more after they labeled the drinking/drugging behavior as being problematic than before; and (c) upon frustration, reverted to a mix of reinforcing and punishing strategies, resulting in an overall pattern of inconsistent reinforcement and punishment (as summarized in Duggan & Le Poire Molineux [2013]). Thus, as expected by INC theory, reinforcement is followed by punishment, which in turn is followed by reinforcement mixed with punishment.

With regard to effectiveness, partners who were more consistent in punishing substance abuse and reinforcing alternative behavior (e.g., encouraging attendance at Alcoholics Anonymous meetings) had substance-abusive partners who relapsed less. Moreover, more successful partners also reported less depression than those with partners who relapsed more (Duggan et al., 2008). This suggests that partners of substance-abusing individuals can aid in reduced recidivism, and this assistance can also translate into better mental health outcomes for the partners (Duggan & Le Poire Molineux, 2013).

Because INC theory provided evidence linking interpersonal influence in relationships over time, the researchers' next studies examined INC theory during ongoing interpersonal influence episodes between substance-abusive individuals and their romantic partners and explored the role of interpersonal communication in sustaining or deterring substance abuse in married or cohabiting couples including one substance-abusive individual (Duggan et al., 2008). In their examination of videotapes of conversations about substance abuse, the researchers analyzed nonverbal and verbal communication patterns. Results reveal consistent verbal punishment of substance abuse (e.g., threats, nagging) predicted lower relapse, while verbal reinforcement (e.g., telling the partner they are more fun when they use) predicted higher relapse (Duggan et al., 2008). With regard to nonverbal communication, vocalic punishment and vocalic reinforcement predicted relapse and persuasive effectiveness (Duggan et al., 2008). Results suggest the combination of behaviors resemble intermittent reinforcement and punishment and should actually strengthen the substance-abusive behavior the partner tries to curtail.

Depression poses unique challenges for interpersonal communication in romantic relationships, so a subsequent study provides insight into the ways depression serves to challenge researchers' assumptions about confrontation and control strategies. Illness increases vulnerability and changes the ways roles are negotiated, and depression serves as an example of an illness that is attributed to both a biomedical condition and to psychosocial interpretation of events. In applying INC to depression in romantic relationships, overall patterns of reinforcement and punishment originally examined in substance abuse provided evidence for individual and relational differences in reinforcement and punishment patterns of partners of depressed individuals (Duggan & Le Poire, 2006).

Application to the context of depression also provided evidence that partners of depressed individuals change their strategies across time (Duggan & Le Poire, 2006). Specifically, non-depressed partners *actively helped* the depressed individual more after labeling depression problematic than before, and decreased their active helping attempts once they were frustrated their control attempts were not working. For example, partners brought the depressed individuals gifts to cheer them up, listened when the depressed individual wanted to talk about the depression, offered to go to doctors' visits, and helped with depression treatment exercises following the labeling, but eventually reduced their helping behaviors. Similarly, partners *encouraged alternative emotional outlets* most immediately after labeling depressive behaviors problematic. For example, partners encouraged retreats, journaling time, exercise classes, or special dinners for emotional expression. Partners encouraged alternative emotional outlets least when they became frustrated their control attempts were not working, suggesting they were reluctant to invest time, energy, or money into these outlets without seeing results for their efforts (Duggan & Le Poire, 2006).

Conversely, partners used the fewest negative strategies following the labeling but reverted to more negative strategies once they were frustrated with their control attempts. Partners *reinforced depression* the least following the labeling and reinforced depression the most when they felt their attempts at controlling depression were not working. For example, partners used negative, labeling language, negative behaviors (drinking "when he/she was a pain"), and ignored the depressive behaviors (avoided the issue, or monitored conversation topics) most in the post-frustration period. Similarly, partners *withheld rewards* the least following the labeling and the most when they felt their attempts at controlling depression were not working. For example, partners expressed anger about the cost of "extravagant pick-me-ups," went on vacation without the depressed individual, refused to "cater to the needs" (of the depressed individual), refused sex, had affairs, and limited the depressed individual's access to finances after they perceived their attempts at helping were not successful (Duggan & Le Poire, 2006).

Overall patterns of reinforcement and punishment were associated with health outcomes, and the next studies examined individual and relational differences in reinforcement and punishment patterns of partners of depressed individuals (Duggan, 2007). Female partners of depressed individuals used more strategies to actively help their partners get well before labeling the behavior problematic and then reverted to a mixture of reinforcing depression and helping partners get well, but male partners actively helped partners get well after labeling the depressive behavior problematic and eventually decreased helping and instead contributed to depressive behaviors (Duggan, 2007).

If the relationship dynamics are shaped by negative behaviors that interfere with everyday functioning more generally, then strategies to curtail the behavior should be similar across contexts. In order to examine this question, we conducted a qualitative analysis of communicative strategies partners use to control compulsive behaviors. Analysis suggests thematic similarities for partners of both substance-abusive and depressed individuals (Duggan, Le Poire, & Addis, 2006). Specifically, partners of substance-abusive individuals and partners of depressed individuals supported the compulsive behavior by giving up their own time needs to accommodate the partner; ignored or avoided the problem by withdrawal, denial, or avoidance; and attempted to help end undesirable behavior by involving professionals, offering advice, and setting relational boundaries (Duggan et al., 2006). This research lends support to the claim that the paradoxical nature of the functional-afflicted relationship restricts the use of verbal references to the problem and cultivates a reliance on non-verbal strategies of control (Duggan et al., 2006; Duggan & Le Poire Molineux, 2013).

An integrated analysis of INC theory investigated the unique dynamics of relationships with a person who engages in a behavior that interferes with everyday functioning. This analysis suggests people in these relationships invoke particular paradoxes in the ways individuals subvert their own needs to help curtail the negative health behavior of a relational partner or family member in ways that make it difficult to assist in changing behavior (Duggan et al., 2009). Four contexts of interpersonal influence are examined to explore relational dynamics in the reasons why communication behaviors result in less than effective persuasion attempts in reducing substance abuse, increasing eating behavior of anorexics, altering violent tendencies, and curtailing depression (Duggan et al., 2009). Inconsistent nurturing as control theory and application brings to light the unique power dynamics of helping-type relationships and the ways relationship dynamics are shaped by the influence attempts. As predicted by INC theory, partners across these four relationship types who try to change their partner's behavioral patterns are often nurturer-controllers who believe that change will enhance overall mental and physical health and improve their relationships but end up using helping and controlling behaviors simultaneously (Duggan et al., 2009; Duggan & Le Poire Molineux, 2013). These mixed messages problematically serve to intermittently reinforce and intermittently punish the substance abuse, eating disorders, violent behavior, and depression (Duggan & Le Poire Molineux, 2013).

INCONSISTENT COMMUNICATION AND EATING DISORDERS

Family communication patterns around eating disorders also indicate mixed strategies in control dynamics. Issues of family interaction and environment may contribute to the development and progression of eating disorders. Family environments provide a context for interpersonal communication connected to multiple areas of mental health problems and family problems (Segrin, 2000). The ongoing interdependence and long-term commitment of family members poses rich implications for the interconnection of intentional and unintentional messages among parents and siblings aimed at curtailing disordered eating. Relapse of eating disorders is common, and the trajectory of an eating disorder can span across a lifetime. Parental involvement in eating disorder treatment can improve outcomes, but parents also may become resentful of neglecting their own well-being during treatment. Eating-disordered individuals may resist treatment, and caregiving can involve prolonged, challenging processes of care. Furthermore, attributions for eating disorders can blame eating-disordered individuals and their families. Family members navigate difficult treatment processes, such as refeeding after meals and careful monitoring to discourage purging. Parents' development and maintenance of adaptive coping and self-care may be an important foundation for their ability to provide needed ongoing support for the eating-disordered child, but parents may be confined by stigma, or by the eating-disordered child not wanting people to know about the condition.

Therapeutic interventions for eating disorders often involve multiple family members in treatment. However, relationships and control dynamics within families may actually impede treatment, and instead exacerbate disordered eating. Research provides evidence that families with eating-disordered children overall are more conflicted, dysfunctional, and chaotic, with less support and involvement than families without anyone with an eating disorder. Perfectionism and a sense of control are identified as additional features of families with eating disorders (Miller-Day & Dodd, 2004). Family interaction patterns about eating disorders provide a rich context for examining the dark side of family communication. Recent research extends applications of INC theory (Duggan & Le Poire Molineux, 2013) to the domain of eating disorders and examines the interplay between parental and sibling behavior as connected to eating-disordered daughters (Duggan & Kilmartin, 2016).

Daughters with eating disorders were interviewed about strategies each family member used to help curtail the eating disorder, and about changes over time in the strategies used. Based on INC theory, this research poses that parents and siblings of daughters with eating disorders have competing goals of nurturing the daughter and controlling the disordered eating behaviors. Inconsistent nurturing as control theory poses that paradoxical injunctions ultimately impact expressions of control in relationships with an individual who engages in behaviors that interfere with everyday functioning (in this case, the eating disorder). Qualitative empirical evidence in this study provides evidence of interplay between parent and sibling strategies of punishment and reinforcement of eating-disordered behavior that are likely to ultimately encourage disordered eating (Duggan & Kilmartin, 2016).

Interviews of eating-disordered daughters provide evidence of family members' inconsistency in the strategies they use over time to curtail disordered eating. In addition, interviews provided evidence of inconsistency among family members. Such family dynamics provide evidence of simultaneous punishment and reinforcement (Duggan & Kilmartin, 2016). Mothers used nonconfrontational subtleties and questions before the disordered eating was labeled problematic; mothers used intentional support and strategically encouraged healthy eating after labeling the disordered eating problematic; and mothers used emotional confrontation and intervention mixed with support once they became frustrated their attempts to curtail the disordered eating were not working (Duggan & Kilmartin, 2016). Fathers seemed not to notice potential disordered-eating behaviors ahead of labeling; fathers expressed concerns alongside the mother but with distinctions in intensity from the mother after labeling the disordered eating problematic; and fathers used stronger shifts in emotional intensity once they became aware that attempts to curtain disordered eating were not working (Duggan & Kilmartin, 2016). Siblings actively confronted and tried to control indications of disordered eating before labeling the eating disorder problematic; siblings threatened to take more extreme action after labeling the disordered eating problematic; and siblings used emotional reactions and expressions of their own frustration once they became aware that attempts to curtail disordered eating were not working

(Duggan & Kilmartin, 2016). Results support predictions for INC theory and provide evidence for inconsistency in family members' strategic attempts to curtail disordered eating as well as inconsistency among family members within each time period (Duggan & Kilmartin, 2016).

COMPETING DEMANDS IN CLOSE RELATIONSHIPS

Theoretical and empirical research on close relationship processes and health and illness behavior poses implications for influence and for other cornerstone relationship processes. Addressing an ongoing attempt to change health behavior may shift both research assumptions about close relationships and the communicative manifestation of influence. Addressing health behavior change in a close relationship potentially brings perceptions of biomedical information and illness management. Relational dynamics in dealing with ongoing attempts to change health behavior may be challenged further by lack of reciprocity, rigid family boundaries, potential stigma, and different goals in the relationship.

Health and illness behaviors pose unique challenges for close relationships. Illness increases vulnerability and can change the ways roles are negotiated. A diagnosis of obesity, substance abuse, depression, or an eating disorder can serve as an example of an illness that is attributed to both a biomedical condition and to psychosocial interpretation of events. The cycling between positive support strategies and negative control attempts may be a product of people in close relationships experiencing tension between the biomedical explanation for illness behavior, and the relational dynamics of illness episodes. Over time, attributions for illness may influence cognitive and affective responses in close relationships. Furthermore, the interplay among theoretical constructs identified in this chapter sheds light on the potential tension between curtailing the illness itself and redefining relational roles to cope with illness. People in close relationships may acknowledge a person as "sick" following diagnosis, but the nuances of the ways illness interferes with everyday functioning may be interpreted as lack of relational reciprocity over time rather than understood in terms of a biological "sickness." Dealing with a major health issue changes additional theoretical attributes addressed in the next chapter.

3 Attributes of the Health and Illness Context for Relationship Processes

WHEN ILLNESS STRIKES

Couples drift from moment to moment, sometimes embracing, sometimes accusing. They count on the illusion of control while ignoring the ubiquity of chaos, the better to chart lives with a sense of continuity and security. We like to feel like we have it all figured out; when we will buy our first home; when the first baby will arrive, and the second. We plan on satisfying careers, traveling, growing old with dignity, and retiring with secure income streams. Instead, some of us separate or divorce, endure boring jobs, and wind up with cats instead of kids. But that is not the script we write for ourselves. And nowhere in the story is there a placeholder for the intrusion of illness.

Sudden trauma or a terrible diagnosis slams into us like a stray bullet. It penetrates our core in an instant, in the space between two breaths. Illness fades our dreams. It shoves our idealized images of our partner off their pedestals and immerses us in the reality of our own fragility. The patient is not the only casualty. Illness also attacks our belief in the future and in the promise of love.

When illness strikes, it inevitably becomes the hub around which your new life revolves, and your activities are tethered to its mighty pull. Illness determines how far from home you can venture, whether you can continue to work, if you can eat the foods you enjoy, and whether and how you can be intimate with your lover. Partner becomes patient, and as if wearing a carnival mask, the once-familiar face can become a somber profile of disease. Illness is a demanding taskmaster. As exhaustion sets in, resentment can supplant compassion, and passion and humor can vanish. It is possible to emerge from this dark tunnel by separating idealized image from reality and damaged body from person.

– Kivowitz & Weisman, 2013. *In Sickness as in Health: Helping Couples Cope with the Complexities of Illness.*

DIAGNOSIS CHALLENGES ASSUMPTIONS

> *Suddenly at 35 I get this stage IV cancer diagnosis. It was just like a bomb went off. And I'm thinking, did I actually maybe expect that everything was going to work out for me? That I was the architect of my own life? That I could overcome anything with a little pluck and determination? I pictured my life like this bucket, and I'm supposed to put all things into this bucket, and the whole purpose is to figure out how to have as many good things co-existing at the same time. And then when everything falls apart, you totally have to switch imagination. Maybe instead life is just vine to vine, like grabbing onto something hoping for dear life it doesn't break.*
>
> *Maybe I realized a little too late that sometimes it's people's love for you that makes them want you to be as certain as they hope to be. Because the diagnosis was so bad and I went from feeling like a normal person to – all of a sudden – like this spaghetti bowl of cancer; I was trying to learn how to give up really quickly, immediately trying to say all the stuff to my husband you're supposed to say, like I have loved you forever and all I want for you is love. And you're trying to learn to give up these. You have these impossible thoughts, like you will live without me, and please take care of our kid.*
>
> *And you're trying to do all that hard work, and at the same moment, friends and family are trying to rush in and say 'we're going to fight this.' They want to pour their certainty into you, like to remake the foundation. There's this almost terrible exchange where you are trying to remake the world as it was, but it's all come apart.*
>
> – Bowler, 2018. *Everything Happens for a Reason, and Other Lies I've Loved.*

These two brief excerpts provide everyday illustrations into the process by which health and illness shift the life context for everyday explanations and predictions, the processes by which people diagnosed with serious illness find new ways of conceptualizing, thinking, and talking about life events. People approach life as if we can predict what will happen, but a serious diagnosis changes that assumption and instead force us to recognize our own fragility. Similarly, researchers approach theory development and testing as if we can account for life connections. What we know about health and illness in close relationships is that the unfolding vulnerabilities rarely can be predicted. Instead, the trauma or disaster of serious illness shifts in "our core in an instant" what we thought we knew about ourselves and our close relationships. We learn how to give up quickly our current assumptions and adjust to newfound understanding. As Bowler (2018) describes, we cannot pour additional certainty into the picture of our life we thought we could imagine before the illness. These illustrations indicate how illness provides a context to understand the world differently. In the language of social science theorizing, these illustrations indicate how theoretical attributes of health and illness shift the foundational assumptions of our explanatory frameworks.

THEORETICAL ATTRIBUTES OF CLOSE RELATIONSHIPS IN HEALTH AND ILLNESS

Attributes of the health and illness context can shape and shift relationship processes. For example, as the "demanding taskmaster" described in the first passage above, illness diagnoses can shift roles, relationship choices, and relational assumptions. In challenging assumptions as described in the second passage above, fragmented uncertainty at each turning point, and the (sometimes invisible) aspects of illness, pose implications for coping. Romantic partners may shift from passionate to compassionate love. Social support functions shift with nonlinear needs and ongoing renegotiation as new issues arise. Choices about disclosure shift with changing needs, sometimes in response to stigmatized responses to revealing information.

Examining theoretical attributes of the health context allows for continued development of frameworks for explaining the interconnections between relationship processes and health consequences (Duggan & Thompson, 2014). Confronting physical symptoms such as vomiting, mobility issues, and a multitude of other symptoms brings a need to respond to immediate presenting concerns, and when physical symptoms take precedence, negotiating complex relational processes becomes a secondary priority, and navigating the nuances of communication becomes more difficult (Duggan &

Thompson, 2014). In romantic relationships, close friendships, and families, illness can frame relational interactions and shift fundamental assumptions in ways people do not necessarily expect or anticipate, and the shifts can accompany increasing and fragmented uncertainty. Moreover, illness brings to the surface a multitude of constructs that (re)frame perceptions of what is important in relationships and in coping with longer-term possibilities of death or disability. Thus, this chapter describes theoretical attributes (and usually combinations of these theoretical attributes) of the health and illness context that shape relationship processes.

CHANGING EXPECTATIONS. FINDING A NEW NORMAL. AND THEN ANOTHER NEW NORMAL

With medical, financial, and logistical concerns of illness that require immediate attention, close relationships can be an unforeseen casualty of illness or injury. As indicated in the opening passages, we cannot remake the foundation as it was before the illness. A health crisis requires a recalibration of close relationships. Health and illness considerations shape relational processes in multiple ways that first require understanding illness diagnosis and progression as a trajectory. Finding and accepting a new normal shifts roles and expectations in close relationships, but changes at one point then require additional changes over the course of the illness. Interconnected responsibilities keep changing with the demands of next steps in treatment. The new normal might mean sleeping much more, walking with a limp, using a wheelchair, or constantly feeling exhausted. The body might shift from healthy to sick in a short amount of time. Close friends who had been connected socially before illness might learn to administer medications. The new normal might be drastically different from what we hoped.

The new normal might not feel so normal at all. Illness considerations can shift expectations for relationships, and for interconnected roles and responsibilities. In close relationships, illness brings an imposed vulnerability, which is different from the safer vulnerability of intentionally sharing more and more of ourselves in a close relationship. When people cannot do things for themselves, they may depend instead on others. Vulnerability and dependence connect to a sense of identity, confidence, and self-worth. Adapting to diagnosis and changes in the body also means shifting the ways relational roles are negotiated. And just when the body and those in a close relationship have adjusted to a new normal, things can change again, or our understanding or feelings about things can change again. Close relationships can be challenged by resources shifted to address emerging symptoms and limitations. Family members and friends absorb additional responsibilities and also learn technical skills of caretaking such as to inject blood thinners or insulin, to give pain medications, or to perform new tasks. Family and friends assume new roles in daily activities like bathing, cooking, toileting, dressing, and feeding.

Changing expectations for dealing with health and illness require addressing changes in the body at the individual level, but also understanding the relational and communal dimensions of health and well-being. Changes in physical health shift personal, social, and environmental well-being and our broader communities in creating healthy living conditions that enable healing and wellness. Sometimes people experience additional health setbacks. Other times people are doing better than in the past, at least for the current time. The process is not necessarily linear, and even improvements in health can create challenges for relationships; a partner might want to revert to the "old normal" but the person who had been a patient feels like their identity has changed in ways that make the "old normal" now ill fitting (Miller & Caughlin, 2013). Couples and close friends can experience a changed sense of identity long after the completion of treatment.

Health is connected to physical environment and is achieved not only by individuals, but also by relationships, families, groups, neighborhoods, and societies (Klein, 2004). Thus, changing expectations also must be situated within changing community variables including shelter, education, food, resources, and equity as the fundamental prerequisites for health and well-being (Klein, 2004). Challenges in changing expectations at the individual level might be magnified in difficulty when considering additional changes in broader communities. For example, cancers can be connected to environmental exposures within communities; natural disasters shift available community resources; and traumas, bombings, and other threats bring ongoing challenges to communities. Community-wide disasters require the ongoing changing of expectations at multiple levels beyond dyadic considerations.

Changing expectations and finding a new normal can be hard and demanding. Changing needs can bring heavy workload; the physical, environmental, and emotional workload can take further toll on the health of everyone involved. Family members and friends might reduce their work hours or quit their jobs as the illness continues and intensifies, which can pose an additional burden on finances and resources. Strengths and difficulties inherent in close relationships are magnified by serious illness and situated within a broader community context.

UNCERTAINTY

Illness brings multiple, fragmented ambiguities that change across an illness experience. "How will this next step in treatment feel?" "What will the future hold with this new illness?" "What should I share about my experiences?" "How will the new circumstances challenge each of my relationships?" "Will my partner be able to go through this with me?" "Who can I ask for what I need and want, and when might the asking be too much?" "How will this set of choices shape the next few months and years?" "Will I ever get back to normal?"

A fundamental goal of close relationships is achieving understanding and shared meaning, but ambiguity and uncertainty about a partner or about the relationship can often thwart this goal (Theiss, 2018). The experience of uncertainty can accompany a restricted range of acceptable behavioral options for interaction and a struggle to judge the probability of particular outcomes. Behavioral constraint, doubt over interpretations of actions in a close relationship, or questioning meaning in a conversation also undermines the ability to achieve the goal of shared understanding with a partner or in a close relationship (Theiss, 2018). Uncertainty compromises people's ability and willingness to be fully engaged in the pursuit of relational closeness, so understanding the conditions that give rise to the uncertainty, the makers of uncertainty, and the best strategies for mitigating uncertainty can be helpful for people in overcoming trepidation and taking a next step in a close relationship with confidence (Theiss, 2018). Established relationships are not free from uncertainty, and the illness context brings unique aspects of uncertainty.

In close relationships, people experience at least three relational sources of uncertainty. *Self uncertainty* refers to a lack of awareness about the self and an inability to describe, predict, or explain one's own cognition or behavior (Knobloch & Solomon, 1999; Theiss, 2018). "Do I still want this relationship now that I know about the illness [the illness of the self or in the partner]?" "Can I see myself continuing this relationship for the long term with this illness?" Under conditions of self uncertainty, people struggle to identity their own goals for the relationship and struggle to identify the attitudes and behaviors that will be necessary for their relational goals. Thus, self uncertainty reflects an orientation toward the self and questions of one's own thoughts, actions, and involvement in a close relationship (Theiss, 2018). *Partner uncertainty* involves lack of confidence in perceptions of another person's involvement in a relationship (Knobloch & Solomon, 1999; Theiss, 2018). Partner uncertainty reflects a general lack of knowledge or understanding of the other person. "Does this person see a future for the relationship with the illness [again, illness of the self or the partner]?" "Is this person able to be satisfied in the relationship with me with the illness?" Partner uncertainty reflects sources of ambiguity focused on the other person in the relationship. *Relationship uncertainty* represents a third relational source of uncertainty and exists at a broader level of abstraction. Relationship

uncertainty involves lack of confidence in perceptions of the relationship as an entity unto itself and integrates questions of the self and the
partner in the context of the particular relationship (Knobloch &
Solomon, 1999; Theiss, 2018). Relationship uncertainty includes
questions about norms for behavior in the relationship, mutuality of
feelings in the relationship, the future of the relationship, and how
people should behave toward each other in the relationship (Theiss,
2018). Self, partner, and relationship sources of relationship uncertainty have been examined in multiple aspects of close relationships,
but especially in courtship and dating (perhaps because of the ambiguity about long-term compatibility with a partner in courtship and
dating) (Theiss, 2018).

The diagnosis of illness brings fragmented uncertainty in
response to the distinct relationship experiences of illness. People
face unique uncertainty in making sense of their relationship(s) at
each point connected to illness diagnosis and trajectory. For example,
in the context of one or both people in a close relationship coping with
depression, analysis of online discourse among individuals coping
with their own or a partner's depression revealed specific sources of
uncertainty related to this context (Knobloch & Delaney, 2012).
Researchers identified depression uncertainty in concerns that
a partner might physically harm himself or herself, questions about
the origin of the depression, and fears that a lack of understanding of
the condition could create problems for the relationship (Knobloch &
Delaney, 2012). In that study, themes of uncertainty included feeling
helpless to improve the relationship and fearing that the mental illness challenged the relational identity (Knobloch & Delaney, 2012).
Although many of the specific sources of uncertainty in the context of
depression (or other illness) can be classified under the broader constructs of self, partner, and relationship uncertainty, the catalyst for
new questions stems from circumstances specific to the conditions
associated particularly with depression (Theiss, 2018). Close relationships are especially prone to experiences of uncertainty, and the specific illness context connected to the specific relationship(s) brings

many specific aspects of ongoing choices and turning points that cannot be fully known. Coping with uncertainty in the context of close relationships goes beyond strategies for personal information management and instead requires complex plans that take into account one's own goals, the desires of the other person, and the stability or trajectory of the relationship itself.

SOCIAL SUPPORT

With illness trajectories, physical and emotional needs change. Priorities for close relationships can change to allow provision of additional support. People in close relationships might provide emotional support through expressions of empathy, love, trust, and caring. Friends and family might provide instrumental support through tangible aid and service such as driving the person to medical appointments. People in close relationships provide informational support by gathering information on treatment processes or information on options available for addressing needs. Friends and family provide appraisal support through information intended to enhance self-evaluation. In addition to social support functions, illness diagnosis sometimes requires evaluating social networks, which are understood as links among people who might provide support. Illness can be stressful, and explanations for social support depict social support functions both mediating the effects of stress on illness and directly affecting illness.

Social networks. Theories of health behavior distinguish between the functions of social support and the broader social networks. Social networks are measured by density (the extent to which network members know and interact with each other), homogeneity (the extent to which network members are demographically similar), geographic dispersion (the extent to which network members live in close proximity), and directionality (the extent to which power and influence are shared) (Valente, 2015). In addition, social network analysis considers characteristics of specific relationships between social networks including network reciprocity (the ability to both give and receive resources), network intensity/strength (the extent to which social relationships offer emotional closeness), complexity (the extent to which social relations serve many functions), and formality (the extent to which social relationships exist in the context of organizational or institutional roles) (Valente, 2015). The connections of people in social networks have patterns and structures that can have profound and enduring influences on health behaviors; considering the conditions under which people are connected can improve our understanding of how populations can be healthier and more productive (Valente, 2015).

Social support functions. Overall, epidemiological research provides evidence that distinct measures of social support are related to positive health outcomes. Social support can be a buffer for stress. The buffer argument of stress suggests that stress does affect some individuals severely, but that people with social support or other coping resources can be relatively resistant to the deleterious effects of stressful events (Schwarzer & Leppin, 1991). A major variant in the stress-buffering model is the matching hypothesis that predicts that stress buffering is most effective when the type of support matches the needs or challenges of the stressful event; this is one of the few theoretical models that highlight how different functional components of support might be related to outcomes based on the nature of the stressor (e.g., controllability of the stressor) (Holt-Lunstad & Uchino, 2015). Social science theories and empirical evidence suggest that social support is a heterogeneous concept and that there are multiple pathways by which social support may influence mental and physical health (Holt-Lunstad & Uchino, 2015). As opposed to social structures in social networks, social support functions are measured by the actual or perceived availability of support, aid, or resources from relationships (Holt-Lunstad & Uchino, 2015). The broad approach of structural and functional social support describes how aspects of social relationships may influence health and the interconnection among these constructs; however, such an approach makes it difficult to identify what particular aspects of support are related to health outcomes (Holt-Lunstad & Uchino, 2015). Social support is linked to health-relevant outcomes including health behaviors (e.g., smoking cessation), adherence to medical regimens (e.g., medication), development of and the course of specific chronic conditions (e.g., cardiovascular disease), and all-cause mortality (Holt-Lunstad & Uchino, 2015; Uchino, 2006).

Understanding close relationship processes provides additional insight into what we know from epidemiological and experimental research on social support functions. For example, we know that individuals with few or no social contacts have an increased risk of dying prematurely from coronary disease, but relationship research indicates that social relationships may be less health protective in women than in men. One study of women's cardiac health patients who received a one-year cognitive stress-reduction and support-strengthening program indicated that the effects of social support and cardiac health evidenced in population-based studies, clinical observation studies, and controlled interventional studies are stronger for men than for women (Orth-Gomér, 2009). Negative social ties may sometimes be harmful for women's cardiac health (Orth-Gomér, 2009). Relationships among gay and bisexual friends provide evidence of friendship and caregiving in network groups in assuming responsibility for providing care because "that's what friends do" (Muraco & Fredriksen-Goldsen, 2011).

IDENTITY AND ILLNESS PROGRESSION

Living with a serious illness diagnosis involves integration of the experience into one's self-concept, including adapting identity. A person who feels ill or has been recently diagnosed adopts a sick-role identity and engages in behaviors to remedy the presenting concerns. Over time, people integrate the sick role into other aspects of identity, including relational identity. Feeling ill, facing diagnosis and illness progression, and dealing with post-treatment experiences change how we see ourselves in close relationships, as well as how others see us. Language used to understand and label illness experiences also is an important aspect of identity during and after treatment.

In cancer care, language and identity as "survivor" has been actively promoted and widely used. The National Coalition for Cancer Survivorship, formed in 1986 as a cancer advocacy group, chose the term "survivorship" to replace the words "cancer victim" and to indicate a more empowered notion of the cancer experience (National Coalition for Cancer Survivorship, 2018). The term "survivor" is used to represent living after a cancer diagnosis, regardless of how long a person lives. The term "survivor" is used by health-care professionals, researchers, and people recovering from cancer to refer not only to physical aspects, but also to the social, psychological, spiritual, and existential impact of cancer on one's life for the remainder of one's life (Twombly, 2004). Other life-threatening diseases have similarly adopted the term to indicate identity as survivor rather than victim. People who are reluctant to use the term "survivor" express hesitation indicating that the danger has passed, and people with high fears of cancer recurrence may be less likely to use the term "survivor" to describe themselves.

The term "patient" implies sick-role identity and active treatment. People may describe "patient" identity as connected to lower feelings of control and hope, and to more passivity, relinquished responsibility for the self and, instead, reliance on the medical establishment (Park, Zlateva, & Blank, 2009). Research indicates that survivor identity is reported as connected to active involvement in care such as wearing cancer-related items and talking about prevention, and survivor identity is associated with better psychological well-being than victim identity; self-identity after cancer also included references to "patient" and "person with cancer" (Park et al., 2009).

The language used to refer to people with a diagnosis also shapes beliefs and ideas about how identity is connected to diagnosis. Person-first language comes from a philosophy of putting individuals before their disability or diagnosis. The person-first movement in disability advocacy, autism advocacy, and other diagnoses recognizes people first and foremost as having individual abilities, interests, and needs, rather than being defined by disability or diagnoses. As we see in "survivorship" language in cancer and in person-first language in disability and diagnosis, the way we speak or write about someone influences the images and attitudes we form about them, leaving behind a positive or negative impression for others. By placing the person first, the disability or diagnosis is no longer *linguistically* identified as the primary, defining characteristic of an individual, but one of several aspects of the whole person.

RELATIONAL IDENTITY AND ILLNESS CHALLENGES

Another consideration for identity is the interconnection between health and illness behaviors and the intertwined identities of people in close relationships. Identity can influence and can be influenced by close relationships (Drigotas et al., 1999; Murray, Holmes, & Griffin, 2000). People change over time from many adaptations to situations where people mutually control and influence each other's behavior and identity (Rusbult et al., 2004). People in close relationships develop a relational identity (Cross & Morris, 2003), feel invested in and committed to the relationship (Rusbult, 1983), and include the partner within concepts of self (E. N. Aron & Aron, 1996).

Negative effects of illness can strain relational identity for some people more than others, and some illnesses (such as depression) pose more difficult challenges to relational identity. Independence, autonomy, and interconnectedness vary across close friendships and marriages. For example, an exploration of illness-related narratives in marriage indicates that people in some marriages need to be pampered and taken care of when an illness is present and need a great deal of attention when they are not feeling well (Walker & Dickson, 2004). More independent people in couples were autonomous and self-sufficient, wanting instead to be left alone and wanting to take care of their own emotional, medical, and physical needs when sick

(Walker & Dickson, 2004). People who need more pampering with lower-level illness might experience greater challenges to relational identity when their partner or close friend faces difficult diagnoses and prolonged treatment.

Relationship research provides evidence that some people are more strongly influenced by the ups and downs of close relationships than others. The success or failure of romantic relationships poses particular potential to shape self-esteem and well-being, but people are not equally impacted by the progress or pitfalls of their romantic relationships. For some people, self-worth is highly contingent on ongoing validation from the relationship and especially sensitive to everyday events as they occur. Researchers consider this *relationship-contingent self-esteem* to be an unhealthy form of self-esteem in which one's fundamental self-worth is tied strongly to relationship events (Knee et al., 2008). In general, when one's self-esteem is more contingent upon indications of success or failure within a specific domain, otherwise insignificant cues with either positive or negative valence have the potential to influence affect and fluctuations in self-esteem. As such, the primary feature of relationship-contingent self-esteem, that one's self-esteem is rooted in one's romantic relationship, means that indicators of relationship success or failure more strongly impact the self (Knee et al., 2008). This does not reflect mere dissatisfaction or disappointment with what happened, but rather an overall sense of the self as fundamentally a "good" or "bad" person as a result of relationship events. Thus, even minor fluctuations in relationship quality are tied to greater swings in affect and feelings of self-worth (Knee et al., 2008). Research also links relationship-contingent self-esteem with higher vulnerability to health-related risky behavior, including drinking to cope and drinking problems, in response to relationship difficulties (Rodriguez, Knee, & Neighbors, 2014). The extent to which people are more negatively influenced by the strains of illness is grounded, at least in part, by the development of social and emotional competence through which people learn during childhood to regulate and respond to stress and difficulties in social relationships (Luecken, Roubinov, & Tanaka, 2013).

Some illnesses pose particular difficulties to relational identity and to communication about the negative behaviors. People in close relationships sometimes unintentionally and subtly encourage negative behaviors such as disordered eating, substance abuse, and depression through their well-intentioned efforts to curtail this behavior (Duggan, Dailey, & Le Poire, 2008; Duggan & Kilmartin, 2016). Problems associated with depression may be especially salient among romantic partners due to the interdependence that characterizes intimate relationships (Kelley & Thibaut, 1978; Kelley et al., 1983a). Bodenmann and Randall (2013) conceptualize depression as a "we-disease," illustrating the relational nature of the depression experience. Attempting to understand the identity of the depressed person without understanding the person's close relationships may miss the broader picture; the relationship itself may be "sick" in addition to the individuals within that relationship (Mackinnon et al., 2012). Recognizing the systematic nature of depression involves explaining the interconnection between continued depression and the cycles of negativity and rejection manifest in interaction patterns in close relationships (Bodenmann & Randall, 2013; Ugazio, 2013).

Depressed individuals and partners might want to move beyond the depression, but at the same time their relational identity might become connected to nurturing behaviors during times of health crisis. Thus, people in close relationships might unwittingly reinforce the depressive behaviors they wish to curtail (Duggan & Le Poire Molineux, 2013; Duggan & Le Poire, 2006). Results from in-depth interviews of depressed individuals and their romantic partners suggest partners change their communication strategies over time such that they use more negative strategies before they label depression problematic, actively help and encourage depressed individuals more after the labeling, and revert to a less consistent sequence of positive and negative strategies once they become frustrated that their control strategies have proven unsuccessful (Duggan & Le Poire Molineux, 2013; Duggan & Le Poire, 2006).

Depression furnishes intense emotional experiences for couples that can spark negativity and rejection. In Sharabi, Delaney, and Knobloch's (2016) inductive, dyadic study of how depression affects romantic relationships, depressed couples describe in their own words the positive effect of enhanced intimacy, but they also described negative effects including negative emotional toll, challenges with romantic and sexual intimacy, communication challenges, isolation, lack of energy and motivation, dependence on the relationship, lack of understanding, and uncertainty. A dyadic framework for depression uses data to consider the extent to which partners agree on how the illness affects their relationship. A systematic view of depression emphasizes that romantic partners are interdependent such that both people share each other's experiences and can engage in patterns of interaction that can escalate or quell the cycle of depression. For example, criticism from a nondepressed partner might trigger self-blame and withdrawal from a depressed person, which could intensify the distance between them (Sharabi et al., 2016). A dyadic framework also addresses the roles individuals occupy within the relationship. For instance, a depressed individual's withdrawal and self-deprecation may position his or her partner in the role of guardian or protector. Realizing how the effects of depression are tied to people's illness status may be important for helping partners get the support they need from each other during treatment (Sharabi et al., 2016).

EMOTIONS AND ILLNESS CHALLENGES

In close relationships, people experience intense positive emotions, such as joy and love, and intense negative emotions, such as anger and fear (Berscheid, 1998). Close relationships are a fertile breeding ground for both positive and negative emotional experiences, and illness can be a catalyst for shifting emotional experiences. Emotions such as love, anger, sadness, and joy are felt more often in the context of relationships than alone, and other emotions such as guilt, shame, embarrassment, jealousy, and envy are inherently social (Planalp & Rosenberg, 2014). Emotional processes are central to human interactions and are tightly coupled with health and well-being in their own right (Butler & Sbarra, 2013). Social negativity with spouses, relatives, and friends is associated with higher anxiety and more frequent mood disorder episodes (Bertera, 2005).

Emotional experiences connected with illness and close relationships can be intense and complicated. People might worry they are burdening their family and close friends with their illness. People might fear that they become physically, emotionally, or financially dependent on family and friends. Illness diagnosis can increase anxiety for patients and for families and friends of patients, with potentially heightened, and often unanticipated, anxiety of dealing with longevity or mortality resulting from serious illness. Research on health and anxiety indicates high impact in concerns about long-term prognosis (Chan, 2011) as well as anxiety about diagnostic procedures (de Bie et al., 2011). Emotional reactions following a diagnosis or a turning point in illness trajectory can allow for adapting to new and potentially threatening information. Fear and sadness, and their psychopathological associates, anxiety and depression, can function as adaptive reactions to illness (Bowman, 2001).

The physical experiences of emotions can shift as a person makes sense of treatments manifest in the body. What feels highly intrusive in everyday interactions (e.g., chemotherapy treatments, needles probing the body) can become routine. The physical reaction to illness treatments can shape emotions; prescription drugs can intensify or numb emotional experiences. Emotional connections in close relationships can change when a partner is not prepared to physically or emotionally accompany a patient through an invasive or prolonged treatment. Friends might be willing to accompany a patient through treatment and might increase closeness. People who have experienced a particular diagnosis might accompany a patient through treatment or might provide support for the emotional turmoil of coping with illness. Support groups connect patients and families with others in similar situations who can share how they are coping. Counseling might be helpful in conversations about how to live fully and actively with a chronic medical condition.

Indirect cues such as nonverbal cues and stories of illness provide unique insights about changes in relationship processes during illness trajectories. Storytelling provides a context for making sense of the emotional tone and nuances of close relationships during illness trajectories. The ways in which people make meaning of "key events" in their lives and relationships through storytelling may reveal a great deal about their health and well-being, both as individuals (e.g., mental health), and within their relationships (e.g., relationship quality). Illness diagnosis and trajectory definitely would qualify as a key event. Research suggests that the construction of stories of key events and relationships that are successful in integrating themes of intimacy with a positive emotional frame are likely to foster psychological and relational well-being. Conversely, relationship stories that lack such integration can lack intimacy and dwell on negative emotions that may be indicative of depression and relational turmoil (Kellas et al., 2010).

The narrative construction of intimacy and affect in relationship stories is considered indicative of individuals' relationship quality, stability, and mental health. In one study of narratives, linguistic indicators of intimacy and affective tone of relationship story were positively associated with relationship quality and mental health (Frost, 2013). Concepts of narrative construction are also helpful in understanding the emotional attributes of health and illness contexts for close relationship processes. The intensity of emotions when receiving good medical news is similar to narrative analysis descriptions of "high-point experiences" in relationships, in which people feel a great sense of uplifting, joy, excitement, contentment, or some other highly positive emotional experience. Similarly, receiving bad medical news is similar to narrative analysis of "low-point experiences" in relationships, in which people felt extremely negative emotions, such as despair, disillusionment, terror, profound guilt, or shame (Frost, 2013).

The study of emotional attributes of health and illness contexts in close relationships will require further longitudinal study to provide cohesive understanding. Cross-sectional, laboratory, and traditional longitudinal designs all pose limitations in their ability to address the integrations of everyday family encounters, emotions, biological processes, and physical health. While emerging findings show promise in explaining how family settings get under our skin to influence health, the significance of this research in the eyes of the public and policymakers is clinical relevance, which requires incorporating clinical endpoints, or measures of how a patient feels, functions, or survives.

Research on family environments, emotions, and health has primarily focused on "snapshots" of family functioning through one-time, self–report measures, retrospective interviews, or behavioral observation. While more innovative designs that increase temporal resolutions such as multiple repeated assessments of families, and even intensive at-home observations of families, provide rich information about families, they can be burdensome on family schedules and routines. Initial research provides evidence for combining two-month diary protocol and measuring clinical endpoint (in this case, upper respiratory infection) (Robles et al., 2013). Communicative processes such as affection serve as a foundational force in any sort of human relationship, influencing such areas as relational closeness, stress, and depression (Hesse & Floyd, 2008). Research also points to the need to include multiple measures of stress-related biological processes (Granger et al., 2006) in understanding the interconnection between emotion, health and illness, and relational processes.

LONELINESS

One of the hardest things about being chronically ill is that people can find what a person is going through incomprehensible – if they believe that person *is* going through it; in that person's loneliness, their preoccupation with an enduring new reality, they want to be understood in a way that they cannot be understood (O'Rourke, 2013). Loneliness is a state of emotional distress accompanying perceived deficiencies in the quantity and/or quality of one's social relationships (Hawkley & Cacioppo, 2010). The melancholy emotion of loneliness arises from a desire for more social contact than is achieved; when people get less out of their social networks and social relationships than they desire, loneliness is ordinarily one of the consequents (Segrin, Burke, & Dunivan, 2012). The experience of loneliness is described as more closely associated with feelings of connectedness within various social relationships rather than sheer amount of contact within such relationships. Lonely people might seem to have extended social networks but do not feel closeness to the people they desire or in the forms they desire closeness. A lack of intimate social contacts is more likely to induce loneliness than a lack of regular social contacts for older adults (Green et al., 2001). Such intimate social contacts are important sources of social support in later life. Social support from an interpersonal communication perspective is understood as supportive behavior performed for an individual by others and is often assessed by an individual's perception of received support (Burleson, Metts, & Kirch, 2000; Goldsmith, 2004). Emotional support can be especially consequential, with significant physical and psychological health outcomes (Goldsmith, 2004).

Relationships can take on a wide range of qualities following illness diagnosis and throughout the trajectory of treatment, and some qualities can be detrimental in nature and could theoretically worsen loneliness. The illness experience can feel isolating or alienating and can reduce social and relational contacts. When people struggle with their own understanding of illness, reaching out to others can feel particularly challenging.

Loneliness tends to cluster within social networks. An investigation of relatives, friends, neighbors, and coworkers in social network assessments suggests that people are 52 percent more likely to be lonely if an immediate (i.e., one degree of separation) social network member is also lonely (Cacioppo, Fowler, & Christakis, 2009). Research indicates that loneliness has a moderate genetic component (Boomsma et al., 2007). Families are a unique type of social network in that they impart the social interaction and social learning effects of friendship networks, in addition to genetic and shared environment effects. Thus, it is not surprising that research provides evidence that loneliness clusters in families is found to predict poorer overall health and more self-reported physical symptoms in acute illness, particularly for older people (Segrin et al., 2012). Family role moderated the association between loneliness and physical symptoms such that the connection between loneliness and poorer health was strongest in the oldest family members including middle-aged parents and elderly grandparents; structural support from both friends and family was negatively associated with loneliness for all participants (Segrin et al., 2012).

Loneliness is an important contributor to human suffering, especially in elderly people, among whom prevalence of loneliness is higher. Both theoretical and empirical research provides evidence that the association between loneliness and pathways to poor health strengthens with age (Cacioppo, Hawkley, & Thisted, 2010). Loneliness is a common source of distress, suffering, and impaired quality of life in older people that has a unique and detrimental effect on physical and psychological health (Hawkley & Cacioppo, 2010). Studies on the aging population provide evidence that greater loneliness predicts increased systolic blood pressure (Hawkley et al., 2010), increased depression (Cacioppo et al., 2010), and poorer physical health (Cornwell & Waite, 2009) among older adults.

From the Health and Retirement Study, a longitudinal, nationally representative cohort study of older people, loneliness was associated with experiencing decline in activities of daily living (e.g., bathing, dressing, eating), difficulty performing upper extremity tasks (e.g., difficulty putting arms above shoulders), decline in mobility, increased difficulty in stair climbing, and increased risk of death (Perissinotto, Stijacic, & Covinsky, 2012). However, relationship research also using data from the Health and Retirement Study indicated that support from a spouse or partner and friends decreased loneliness, while strain from relational sources (spouse or partner, children, family, and friends) intensified loneliness; higher support and lower strain from various sources directly and indirectly improved well-being, with indirect effects mediated through reduced loneliness. In later life, various sources of support and strain engender distinct effects on loneliness and well-being, and loneliness serves as one of the psychological pathways linking support and strain to well-being (Chen & Feeley, 2014). Chen and Feeley (2014) found that social support decreased loneliness, but social strain intensified loneliness, suggesting that theories of loneliness take into account the deleterious impact of negative social interactions. As social support and social strain received from different sources exhibit distinct impacts on loneliness and well-being, future research on social relationships should differentiate support and strain from various sources rather than using a global measure consisting of support and strain that includes all possible sources.

COPING

Serious illness brings complications that require coping in close relationships. Facing the ongoing vulnerabilities of illness diagnosis and stressful events can challenge close relationships. The person with the diagnosis, and people in close relationships, find themselves needing to ask for help, to problem solve, to adjust to new needs, and to remain open to adapting and responding to what comes next. Couples and close friends vary in the degree to which they support and actively help one another during times of stress.

Traditionally, the coping literature largely focused on individual aspects of coping. For example, cognitive appraisal theory of stress and coping (Lazarus & Folkman, 1984) addresses the psychosocial effects of chronic illness. From this perspective, coping is a transactional process involving cognitions and behaviors that are directed toward altering the situation (problem-focused coping) or regulating emotions (emotion-focused coping). Whereas cognitive appraisal theory takes an individual perspective of examining how individuals are affected by their own reactions to illness, research on close relationships emphasizes the interdependence between marital partners and people in close relationships and requires considering the relational context in which coping occurs. More recent research on coping addresses dyadic, collective, and communal perspectives on coping.

A holistic understanding of coping includes emotion-focused, problem-focused, and relationship-focused coping (Badr, 2004). Badr (2004) highlights the importance of examining the ways in which spouses cope together in the face of a shared stressor. Within the context of spousal relationships, separating relationship-focused coping from emotion-focused coping and problem-focused coping can be difficult, because the lines separating what is good for one person from what is good for their spouse or what is good for the relationship become blurred (Badr, 2004). Because chronic illness is a shared stressor, one challenge for researchers is to account for the intersubjectivity of different people in their coping responses. People in close relationships who use similar coping strategies might reinforce one another, paving the way for better adjustment. Complementarity in coping expectations or strategies may buffer from the potential negative consequences of ways of coping. Research points to the idea that coping seems to be driven by the person who is sick. Some people focus on obtaining resources they need to cope, by soliciting network support and actively engaging their close relationship networks (Badr, 2004).

When one person has chronic illness, and the partner or good friend remains in good health, complications can occur. The person with the diagnosis and their spouse and close friends are affected by their own reactions to the elements of illness as well as how each of them cope. Relationship-focused coping includes active engagement, which is where partners are actively involved in decision-making and other problem-solving activities. Protective buffering involves the extent to which partners deny anxieties and concerns, put on a brave front, or defer to their partner to avoid disagreements. The distinction between active engagement and protective buffering mirrors the distinction between problem- and emotion-focused coping. The difference is that relationship-focused coping involves taking the partner's or close friend's emotions into consideration when making coping decisions (Badr, 2004).

The dramatic proliferation of coping research has spawned healthy debate and criticism and offered insight into the question of why some individuals fare better than others when encountering stressful events in their lives. Some of the additional considerations for coping include distinguishing between active and passive coping. Active coping focuses, for example, on trying to control pain or to function despite pain, while passive ways of coping refer to withdrawing and surrendering control over pain. Active coping strategies can include things like distraction or activity management (pacing), while passive coping can include things like rest or avoidance.

Like other theoretical attributes linking health and illness and relational processes, it is necessary to recognize the broader social and economic conditions within which coping strategies occur as well as the extent to which coping strategies are prosocial in encouraging positive, helpful behavior intended to promote acceptance or friendship. Research provides evidence for interactions between multiple ways of coping and the broader community conditions within which people live. Results of one examination of coping in single, inner-city African American and European American women suggest that when active and prosocial coping are linked they lead to a broad array of positive psychological and behavioral outcomes, and that active coping alone is no more advantageous than prosocial coping alone (Hobfoll & Schröder, 2001). Another study demonstrated community activism connected to coping; in comparison with non-activists, activists used more problem-focused coping and less emotion-focused coping, had greater knowledge of HIV treatment information sources, and had greater HIV social network integration (Brashers et al., 2002).

Coping connects to other attributes of the health and illness context in shaping relational processes. For example, in one study examining the impact of emotional distress and social relationships on health-related outcomes of parents living with HIV, active and passive coping styles were also interconnected by conflict with children and by social support (Leslie, Stein, & Rotheram-Borus, 2002).

Research on communal coping shifts to a broader understanding of coping as an interdependent process to actively work toward addressing a co-owned or shared problem. Communal coping involves pooling resources across multiple people and acting on "our" shared stressor or "our" problem rather than an individual problem to be managed alone (T. D. Afifi, Hutchinson, & Krouse, 2006). In their theoretical model of communal coping, Afifi and colleagues address risk and resiliency from a systems approach to provide a model of the interdependent nature of coping as transactional and fluid and addressing different levels of responsibility for stressors within groups (T. D. Afifi et al., 2006). A communal orientation involves perceptions and behaviors where individuals work as a collective unit to solve a mutually acknowledged and shared stressor (T. D. Afifi et al., 2006). In many instances, such as when one partner experiences a chronic illness, communal coping may not be occurring because only one person is directly affected by the stressor; other family members and close friends are reacting to this person's stress rather than experiencing a shared stressor (T. D. Afifi et al., 2006). That a relationship resides within a social infrastructure does not mean that communal coping exists; communal coping requires the perception of dual ownership and responsibility that is characteristic of communal coping (T. D. Afifi et al., 2006). A communal coping response, for example, could involve family members communicating about a health threat (e.g., family risk of disease), developing a shared appraisal of that threat, and engaging in cooperative action to address the threat (T. D. Afifi, Merrill, & Davis, 2016).

SOCIAL STRAIN

Diagnosis and illness trajectory can pose challenges and needs beyond what a relationship can accommodate. Investigations of social strain and health have acknowledged that social connections are not exclusively positive in nature, but instead function in a balance of both benefits and costs. Some relationships can accelerate health decline. Social strain, as characterized by greater interpersonal conflict, frequent criticisms, and excessive demands from significant members of one's social network, has the potential to act as a direct source of psychosocial distress (Newsom et al., 2005).

Research has also identified negative effects of strained relationships on physical health outcomes, particularly linking spousal conflict to increased risk of coronary heart disease and mortality (Umberson et al., 2006). In a longitudinal study of marriage, relational strain accelerated the typical decline in self-rated health that occurs over time, and this adverse effect of strained relationships was greater at older ages. Findings suggest a cumulative adversity in that marital strain seems to have a cumulative effect on health over time, and poorer health also increases vulnerability to marital strain with age (Umberson et al., 2006).

Close relationships that provide support can also embrace high strain. People can experience ambivalence in mixed and contradictory feelings toward a relationship. A person in a given relationship can feel loved, understood, or cared for, and also feel rejected, criticized, or ignored. This love–hate dynamic can be manifest within families and has been captured by the family solidarity–conflict model (Bengston, Rosenthal, & Burton, 1995). For example, among older adults, where the spouse is usually the preferred source of social support, the spousal relationship is also reported as the most negative relationship (Luescher & Pillemer, 1998). In another study of positive and negative social exchanges, psychological well-being, and health, partner support and strain and family support predicted well-being measures, and partner strain also predicted health problems (Walen & Lachman, 2000).

Other work shows that actually receiving social support (as opposed to perceiving available social support) can have negative effects and might strain interactions. A study of perceived and received affective and instrumental support on adaptation to chronic vision impairment in elderly adults provides evidence for a positive effect of affective support on well-being, but a negative effect of instrumental support (Reinhardt, Boerner, & Horowitz, 2006). Instrumental support receipt may be negative for people with chronic impairment as it may emphasize their inability to accomplish daily tasks. Social and economic considerations also impact social strain. For example, adverse effects of negative information on health were reported to be especially evident among respondents with less education. Levels of exposure to negative interaction were not greater among older adults with less education, but less educated elders may be differentially vulnerable to negative interactions due to depleted individual coping resources (Krause & Shaw, 2002).

STIGMA

As if being sick is not bad enough, some illnesses come with a social stigma that marks a person as different from others and that discredits or devalues individual identity. Stigma is a socialized, simplified, standardized image of the disgrace of a particular social group, and being marked as a person of a stigmatized group denotes the person through social construction of a devalued identity (Smith, 2007).

Stigma leaves people wanting to hide their illness or hide details of their life they feel might be negatively judged. People might blame the patient suffering from lung cancer for smoking, even though lung cancer can also be caused by environmental factors such as radon, occupational chemicals, and environmental tobacco smoke. People with mental illness might be treated as incompetent, irrational, or untrustworthy. Stigma results in an evaluative tendency to make moral judgments about the person and to use language indicating disgrace implying judgment about the "disgusting" person (Smith, 2011). Messages toward or about the person might imply blame or make attributions about a person's choice or control; labels indicate that people may be considered as if choosing their stigmatized condition, and empathy can be harder to evoke because of the notion of the person having control over their labeling condition (Smith, 2011).

In addition to stigmatizing attributions for illness, attributions for decisions about illness can be stigmatizing. Even if they are not perceived as having control over the illness itself, people can be stigmatized by the choices they make around how much intervention they received, where they are judged as not "fighting" hard enough if they forgo treatment or judged as selfish if they choose long-term treatments that are expensive and resource intensive, which "drain resources" from the health-care system. Stigma can also be associated with the relationship itself being perceived as marginalized, or in particular information perceived as marginalized when information exposed in illness treatment does not fit assumptions people make about the patient.

Consider HIV as an example of a stigmatized illness. People living with HIV experience higher rates of stigmatizing social interactions that may negatively impact psychological and physical health. They experience unsupportive social messages about their HIV, and depressive symptoms may function as an indirect mechanism through which unsupportive or stigmatizing messages predict poorer physical health. Furthermore, one study indicates ethnicity as a moderator in that the indirect effects between unsupportive social interactions, more depressive symptoms, and poorer health behaviors were significant for black men but not for white men (Fekete, Deichert, & Williams, 2014). Thus, depressive symptoms may be one pathway through which unsupportive social interactions are associated with physical health, and disconnecting unsupportive interactions may be particularly detrimental for black men living with HIV (Fekete et al., 2014).

Stigmatizing attributions reduce the nuances of illness and relational processes. Stigmatizing attributions include words that bring attention to the stigmatizing condition in the label and miss the particular nuances of the whole person. A more comprehensive understanding moves beyond the initial marks indicating group membership and addresses broad complexities. For example, the onset of serious mental illness might follow divorce, job loss, residential instability, or food insecurity, but the connections to these disruptive life events as connected to illness symptoms and stigma are seldom considered (Perry, 2014). The psychiatric perspective focuses on the impact of individual pathology on social interaction with new and existing network members (Knobloch & Knobloch-Fedders, 2010). Modified labeling theory argues that mental illness stigma leads to rejection by others and to maladaptive psychosocial responses that exacerbate social isolation and membership turnover. An additional, complementary mechanism of social network dynamics shifts the theoretical focus to the social impact of significant and disruptive life events.

This social isolation explanation suggests that social network turnover following the first major contact with mental health treatment has consequences for relationships, social networks, and well-being (Perry, 2014). Even if lost social ties are replaced with new social ties, replacement has implications for relationship duration and the presence of a greater number of newer relationships. Because intimacy, feelings of reciprocity, resource exchange, regular contacts, and shared history developed with relationship duration, unstable networks may be less resource rich than those that are more stable and established. Experiencing disruptive life events may subsequently increase vulnerability to psychiatric symptoms and stigmatization directly or through changes in relational ties.

Most research on stigma addresses perceptions of the illness, but relationship research poses additional considerations for moving past reductionist and stigmatized views of relationship choices. Among his other research in relationships that don't follow traditional social scripts, such as consensually nonmonogamous relationships, Lehmiller (2012) addresses perceived relationship marginalization and its association with physical and psychological health. Perceiving one's romantic relationship as socially marginalized (as lacking social approval or acceptance) has been linked to an array of worse relational outcomes, including a greater likelihood of breakup. Lehmiller's (2012) research provides evidence that individuals who perceive disapproval specifically because of their current romantic relationship tend to experience worse personal health as well. Perceived marginalization of one's relationship was associated with reporting more symptoms of poor physical health and lower self-esteem. Each of these associations was mediated by negative affect, suggesting that one possible reason marginalization may contribute to worse health is because perceived marginalization is stressful (Lehmiller, 2012). Moreover, perceived marginalization was directly associated with engagement in riskier health behaviors, including more cigarette smoking and less frequent condom use. The association between perceived marginalization and negative affect was moderated by perceived closeness to one's partner, suggesting that the relationship between marginalization and stress may become more pronounced as the partner becomes a more integral part of the self. Individuals who perceive their romantic relationships as socially marginalized (i.e., as the targets of disapproval by their social networks and/or society at large) tend to experience worse outcomes compared to those who see their relationships as garnering greater social acceptance (Lehmiller & Agnew, 2007). Lehmiller and colleagues' research moves beyond relationship outcomes to provide evidence that perception of social marginalization can predict personal health (and illness) (Lehmiller, 2012).

PERCEPTION AND USE OF TIME

Although research does not yet provide empirical evidence to address health and illness connected to relationships and perception of time, stories of health and illness address changes in perception and use of time. Time feels short when we face the devastation of a serious diagnosis. We never have enough time to "prepare" for the death of a close relationship. Time in treatment interrupts relationships with dizzying rounds of doctors' visits and hospital intakes. Relationship processes adapt to different facets of time. An initial sense of urgency often accompanies health-care delivery (Curtis, Tzannes, & Rudge, 2011). When a patient is "coding," which is a term indicating that a patient may be dying ("code blue" is the full term), there is little time to be polite (Duggan & Thompson, 2011). Instead, one must demand, yell, or command in ways that might not be tolerated in most relationships. Although such brusqueness is not unique to health care, health care is one of the few contexts in which death or severe disability is a potential consequence of time required for polite communication. Physicians become socialized to behave brusquely and abruptly, and these patterns continue in subsequent interactions that might not actually be as urgent. Within less urgent interactions, the provider is frequently instructing a patient about a treatment regimen, ultimately telling patients what to do and expecting them to follow these instructions (Duggan & Thompson, 2011). Family and close friends respond to the urgency of health-care delivery during times of crisis.

The urgency of initial diagnosis, and long courses of treatment, can change perception of time. The series of medical tests can come to feel less immediate and instead like one more part of a long-term treatment. Illness puts time constraints on relational processes. A spouse or close friend might respond to a presenting concern but then spends days, weeks, months, or years in an adapted relationship that includes treatment time, recovery time, healing time, building strength before beginning the process again, and slowing down. Illness progression shapes time and translates into loss of control over time.

SOCIAL CONTROL AND INFLUENCE

Being truly understood in the psychological and social experiences necessitates considering how people in close relationships mutually influence health and illness behavior and decisions about health and illness. Patient preferences and values cannot be disentangled from their close relationships. Given the myriad ways in which the lives of intimate partners are physically, socially, and emotionally interconnected (Kelley et al., 1983b), a close partner is arguably the most important and powerful source of influence in a person's life. Close relationships affect illness management. In relationship research, the mutual influence process includes positive processes such as health-promoting influence, as well as darker and more negative processes including behavioral resistance.

The chronic diseases that are leading causes of morbidity and mortality (i.e., heart disease, cancer, and diabetes) share common features such as being driven by behavior, influenced by the social environment, and negatively impacting close relationships. People who live with someone return home from an illness diagnosis or acute health event to daily life in which symptom management and lifestyle changes play out in a dyadic context of home life. Behavioral interventions designed to supplement medical treatment of chronic illness can impact the patient and people in close relationships, and not always for the better.

Some aspects of relationships may facilitate good health. Health-related social control, or the way that people in relationships attempt to influence and regulate each other's health behavior, may contribute to the health benefits of close relationships. Research suggests that one way in which social relationships may influence health is by changing health-related behaviors. First, social control operates indirectly when a person internalizes a sense of responsibility or obligation to a significant other and consequently avoids risky behaviors that might jeopardize performance of role obligations. Second, social control operates directly when a spouse actively prompts or persuades his or her partner to engage in health-enhancing behaviors, or conversely, deters or dissuades a person from engaging in health-compromising behaviors (Umberson, 1987).

In a study of spousal social control and the partner's behavior, affect, and relationship satisfaction during a weight-loss attempt, instrumental and reinforcing social control were associated with better health behavior, well-being, and relationship satisfaction at the start of the weight-loss attempt, but not over time (Novak & Webster, 2011). Influence tactics have been assessed under the umbrella of health-related social control. Researchers have noted the importance of distinguishing between different types of partner-influence strategies. Positive social control includes the use of modeling, positive reinforcement and logic, and negative social control includes expressions of negative emotions and attempts to make the target feel bad for his or her health behavior (Lewis & Butterfield, 2005). In another study, dyadic exchanges of support and control were investigated in heterosexual couples in which the husband had been recently treated or assessed for heart disease, and results indicated that social support and social control can help promote a healthy lifestyle (Franks et al., 2004).

Couple-oriented behavioral interventions for chronic illness can yield benefits for patients, particularly if couple-oriented interventions are tailored to couples' needs and delivered in ways that help couples apply new skills to challenges that they encounter in daily life (Martire, 2013). In addition to tailored messages, the relational dynamics in couples shape the perception of interventions and how interventions take shape in the relationship over time. Conflict can arise when someone feels controlled (e.g., saying to an overweight person *"You're going to eat that?"*) (Burke et al., 2012). A study examining conflict among couples found that mixed-weight couples, specifically couples including overweight women and healthy-weight men, reported greater conflict both generally and on a daily basis; lower conflict was associated with higher perceived support from the partner (Burke et al., 2012).

Spouses often monitor and seek to alter each other's health behavior, but such social control attempts sometimes provoke behavioral resistance and emotional distress. Expectations regarding spouses' roles in their partner's health may influence reactions to spousal social control, with resistance and hostility less likely to occur among people who believe spouses should be involved in their partner's health (Rook et al., 2011). In another study, wives' social control in their attempts to encourage appropriate health behavior among men with prostate cancer predicted poorer outcomes including greater psychological distress, less sleep, and more health-compromising behavior (e.g., smoking) (Helgeson et al., 2004).

COMPASSIONATE LOVE

In the vulnerability of illness, we may find we are less concerned with love as romance or with sexual attraction with intimate partners. Instead people find love connection through compassionate love. Compassionate love is defined as other-oriented cognitions, affect, and behavior (Fehr, Sprecher, & Underwood, 2009). Compassionate love is a self-giving, caring love that values the other highly and has the intention of giving life to the other (Fehr et al., 2009). Compassionate love is associated, but not synonymous with concepts such as empathy, perspective-taking, altruism, social support, volunteerism, attachment, and familial love. A cohesive collection on the scientific antecedents of compassionate love, and manifestations and consequences of compassionate love, can be found in Fehr, Sprecher, & Underwood's (2009) edited volume.

Compassionate love centers on the good of the other and has a nourishing quality. In this other-centered love a person tries to truly understand and accept the conditions and state of the recipient in order to become more fully alive (Underwood, 2009). Compassionate love can be seen in actions, expressions, and words, but at the core of the construct are motivation and discernment, facets of free choice and willingness to give (Underwood, 2009). The motivation behind the giving action is important in categorizing a behavior as compassionately loving in nature, as the ultimate focus is the giving of self for the good of the other; although expressed in the context of other kinds of love and altruistic behaviors, compassionate love reaches beyond other kinds of motivation and centers on the flourishing of another person (Underwood, 2009). Measures of depth and complexity of compassionate love include giving of the self with free choice for the other, accurate cognitive understanding of the situation, the other, and oneself, valuing the other at a fundamental level, openness and receptivity, and response of the heart or the core of one's being (Underwood, 2002).

In the scientific literature, compassionate love has often been overlooked by social scientists instead focused on other kinds of love, particularly romantic love (Aron, Fisher, & Strong, 2006; Felmlee & Sprecher, 2006). Emotion theorists who describe compassion focus on being moved by another's suffering and wanting to help. This definition of compassion misses the emotional and transcendent components which the word "love" adds (Underwood, 2002). Fehr and Sprecher present a measurement and validation of compassionate love that identify features laypeople regard as central or peripheral to compassionate love in their scale to measure compassionate love (Fehr & Sprecher, 2009; Sprecher & Fehr, 2005); they also discuss a program of research on conceptual, measurement, and relational issues pertaining to compassionate love (Fehr & Sprecher, 2009).

Compassionate love might help explain the health benefits associated with marriage in older adulthood. Marriage benefits in older adulthood are described as disproportionately large as compared to marriage benefits earlier in life, and these benefits may be attributed in part to the powerful role spouses play in promoting each other's well-being (Rauer, Sabey, & Jensen, 2014). Conceptual research proposes that spouses' compassionate love motivates them to tend to their partner's health, such that compassionate love enables individuals to adapt to the physical, emotional, and psychological changes associated with their own and their partner's aging. These concepts are explored in one study focusing on health benefits among a population of higher-functioning older adults (Rauer et al., 2014). In that study, feeling compassionate love was linked to better health for wives; partner effects, however, painted a more complicated picture, with the receipt of compassionate love appearing to undermine health (Rauer et al., 2014).

The seeds of caregiving necessary when a loved one goes through a long-term illness are planted earlier in the relationship. Sprecher and Fehr's (2005) definition of compassionate love is an enduring attitude that includes an orientation toward supporting, helping, or understanding another person, particularly when that person is perceived to be suffering or in need. These authors have found that this orientation for a person was linked with providing more support for that person (Sprecher & Fehr, 2005; Sprecher & Fehr, 2006).

Fehr and Sprecher (2009) suggested that although the provision of compassionate love is associated with a number of positive benefits to the self, individuals report even more positive outcomes when they report being the recipient of compassionate love. However, while help can be supportive when it communicates caring, it can simultaneously imply an inferiority–superiority relationship. If compassionate love activates feelings of inferiority in the recipient, it may unintentionally undermine that person's health. This may help explain why providing support is more beneficial than receiving it, as there is no such ambivalence for the support provider. What is needed is a way to also capture the conditions under which people are sensitive to being the beneficiaries of compassionate love and how those conditions can translate into expected outcomes (Perlman & Sanchez-Aragon, 2008).

Relatively fewer studies address compassionate love in older adulthood, as compared to studies of compassionate love in younger populations (Neff & Karney, 2009; Sprecher & Fehr, 2005; Sprecher & Fehr, 2006). For several reasons, the period of older adulthood represents an ideal window into the nature and potential health benefits of compassionate love. For example, Marks and Song (2009) suggest that older adults are more concerned with caring for others than are younger adults because the older adults have more time and energy to devote to others. In addition, many marriages in older adulthood may be longer term, and thus compassionate love has had years or even decades to deepen. Couples who have been together a long time should be fairly accurate at identifying each other's needs and responding accordingly (Neff & Karney, 2009). Also, many of the roles and responsibilities that may have precluded spouses attending to each other are reduced in older adulthood (e.g., work, parenthood), and spouses have an easier time putting each other first. Health declines in older adulthood present more opportunities for spouses to demonstrate their compassionate love for each other. The few studies that have looked at compassionate love in older adulthood have focused on families in which partners are suffering from terminal illnesses and cognitive impairments (Ott, Sanders, & Kelber, 2007; Roberts, Wise, & DuBenske, 2009). Slatcher's (2010) conceptual model linking marriage to physical health would suggest that we would find more links between couples' compassionate love and their health even in a more normative population of older adults.

TRUST AND FORGIVENESS

In the challenges of uncertainty, need to renegotiate established roles, and upheaval of daily routines, people in close relationships also find positive relational constructs connected to the illness experience. In addition to compassionate love, people describe positive attributes and positive actions including manifestations of trust and forgiveness.

Attitudes of trust reflect people's abstract, positive expectations that they can count on partners to care for them and be responsive to their needs, now and in the future (Holmes & Rempel, 1989). Trust is related to adjustment and vitality and ongoing close relationships (Rempel, Holmes, & Zanna, 1985). Trust has been argued to emerge and develop in situations where an individual's direct, automatic responses are at odds with the needs of the partner and relationship (Holmes & Rempel, 1989; Kelley, 1983). Theories of close relationships suggest that trust is "afforded" by diagnostic situations. The concept of affordance describes what an interpersonal situation activates and "makes possible" for interacting individuals (Kelley et al., 2003).

In the context of illness, a close relationship may have developed in interpersonally "easy," non-diagnostic situations, where the needs of both people are compatible. Trustworthiness is particularly relevant in situations that test mutually incompatible interests. A serious illness poses an example of a diagnostic interaction for trust. People in close relationships may come into the interaction with trusting expectations, where they feel relatively secure in knowing they can rely on the partner or close friend to be responsive to their needs. People in close relationships with low trust, in contrast, likely face serious diagnosis with insecurity and anxiety about how the situation connects to their relationship. Given that partners in low-trust relationships may have negative expectations regarding one another's pro-relationship motives and behaviors, they will be somewhat more preoccupied with the possibility of bad outcomes. They may, for instance, think that their partner will not consider their needs, may not understand their feelings, or may not offer emotional support (Weber, Johnson, & Corrigan, 2004), thus worrying about possible negative outcomes. Individuals with anxious-avoidant attachment style not only exhibit lower levels of trust but also engage in ruminative worry more often than more trusting, securely attached individuals (Collins & Read, 1990; Mikulincer, 1998). In addition to navigating relationship changes after initial diagnosis in serious illness, people face ongoing challenges where emerging concerns about the illness are incompatible with the desires of the partner or close friend.

Relationship research provides evidence that the positive effects of trust are manifold. In a five-wave longitudinal data set, researchers found that trust was positively related to physical health. Participants reported fewer health problems when they trusted their partners more (Schneider et al., 2011). More importantly, symptoms of anxiety and depression mediated the effect of trust on self-reported health. That is, the researchers found that strong trust inhibits anxiety and depression, which in turn promotes physical health. Conversely, they found that weak trust promotes anxiety and depression, which in turn is harmful to physical health (Schneider et al., 2011). Their results of lagged analysis show that earlier levels of trust predict later symptoms of anxiety and depression symptoms, in turn predicting changes in physical health symptoms over time (Schneider et al., 2011). Trust plays a key role in promoting intimacy, forgiveness, and willingness to sacrifice (Rusbult et al., 2004).

Illness might also prompt forgiveness over past relational regressions and may predict better health. In studies of interpersonal conflict, such as betrayal within a committed relationship, individuals who describe themselves as more forgiving (trait forgiveness) or who express forgiveness about a particular incident (state forgiveness) also measured as having lower blood pressure (Lawler-Row et al., 2011) and better self-reported health on a variety of negative measures, such as physical symptoms of illness, depression, and stress (Lawler-Row et al., 2011).

Initially, researchers described the association between forgiveness and health as resting upon well-studied correlations between anger and/or hostility and physiological responses, primarily blood pressure and heart rate, related to health. Forgiveness and anger (also measured as hostility or aggression) are inversely related; one could logically deduce that the expected benefits of forgiveness connect to decreased anger and better health. However, the correlation between forgiveness and anger does not necessarily mean that the health benefits of forgiveness are uniquely tied to anger reduction. As forgiveness occurs in a relational context, focusing on the role of forgiveness in maintaining meaningful and satisfying relationships may prove to be a more fruitful explanatory concept than anger for understanding the link between forgiveness and health, and one that capitalizes on the potential positive effects of forgiveness on health.

Individuals differ in their propensity to forgive, and the context of forgiveness is an important consideration. Both Fincham and Beach (2007) and Kluwer and Karremans (2009) question the generality of forgiveness effects estimated from a single, generally serious, recalled betrayal offence. Although the latent variable of forgiveness related more strongly to state forgiveness, the researchers also found that a substantial part of the variance in trait forgiveness is explained by also considering latent variables (Fincham & Beach, 2007; Kluwer & Karremans, 2009).

DISCLOSURE

Furthermore, dealing with an illness changes the *disclosure boundaries* for communication in close relationships, as disclosing illness may make individuals feel embarrassed, uncomfortable, or exposed (Petronio, 2002). Illness shifts boundaries for sharing private information. Illness shifts expectations and rules for how information is shared, for who has access to information, and under what circumstances private information is shared. An illness crisis can function as a catalyst for shifting privacy rules, and patients and their families may be surprised at what they are willing to disclose or withhold. Family and friends may also function as informal health-care advocates such that they too consider themselves to be part of the disclosure and health-care decision-making (Petronio et al., 2004). However, patients may have different expectations for particular friends and family members with regard to who has access to which parts of their private health information. Disclosure about health information poses a communicative dilemma, where the interconnection among multiple social relationships may sacrifice trust and cross boundaries even with mindfulness of ways to extend the health-care interaction to include friends and family. Patients themselves might not want to know all the details of their illness (Schofield et al., 2003).

Making choices about sharing health information in a serious illness involves initial disclosure patterns, but considering illness as a trajectory means that disclosure about health and illness information is an ongoing process where decisions have to be made about sharing updated information and changes in information, not simply the initial diagnosis (Greene, 2009). Disclosure considerations involve acute, life-threatening, and contagious conditions on one hand, but many people living with a chronic health and illness condition make choices about providing information to others regarding their condition on an ongoing basis (Checton & Greene, 2012). Uncertainty is an ongoing feature of disclosure decisions as people report uncertainty about whether to disclose, or how to disclose, or when to avoid disclosing health information (Greene, 2009). In considering disclosure about health information in close relationships, people consider aspects of uncertainty including information assessment (prognosis and symptom uncertainty), uncertainty about support in close relationships, and communication efficacy in disclosure patterns (Checton & Greene, 2012).

Ongoing relationships also involve everyday choices and discussions about disclosure of private health and illness information. A study of personal relationships investigated how individuals seek and disclose information related to testing for sexually transmitted infections in sexual relationships (Dillow & LaBelle, 2014) based on the theory of motivated information management (W. A. Afifi & Morse, 2009). The theory of motivated information management posits that the information management process begins with an individual become aware that the level of certainty that he or she has about an important issue is lesser or greater than the amount that is desired (W. A. Afifi & Weiner, 2004). In the original model, this discrepancy between current and desired levels of uncertainty was thought to produce anxiety, which then motivates the remainder of the information management process (W. A. Afifi & Weiner, 2004). More recently, however, Afifi and Morse (2009) revised the theory of motivated information management, in part, by replacing anxiety with the more general concept of emotion, as uncertainty discrepancy may result in a variety of emotions, including, but not limited to, anxiety (W. A. Afifi & Morse, 2009; Brashers, 2001). The experience of emotion in response to the uncertainty discrepancy mediated assessments made in evaluating information and making decisions about seeking information and sharing information (Dillow & LaBelle, 2014). Efficacy emerged as a mediator of seekers' negative emotional responses and indirect information seeking and of providers' outcome expectancies and indirect information provision (Dillow & LaBelle, 2014).

Disclosure about health and illness information is an ongoing process that involves a complex web of disclosure decisions. Sometimes revealing private health and illness information can be helpful, and other times stories of disclosure illustrate painful consequences of intentional or unintentional disclosures. The process of disclosure connects to a final theoretical consideration of health and illness in close relationships: the communicative process.

COMMUNICATIVE PROCESS AND EVERYDAY CONVERSATION

Communication and everyday events. Just because someone faces serious illness, conversation and communication with that person does not become limited to the illness, to treatment, or to adjustment to symptoms. Everyday conversation remains quite important throughout an illness trajectory. Finding a new normal means recognizing illness, but within ordinary conversations and shared time. Some aspects most central to our core identity are not the aspects of ourselves we share explicitly in "difficult conversations," but what unfolds in small moments and in conversation about everyday life.

For example, relational regulation theory (Lakey & Orehek, 2011) predicts that the correlation between perceived support and mental health emerges through ordinary conversation and shared activities rather than through conversations about illness-related stress and how to cope with it. Observing the conversations and activities of others also helps regulate mental health (Lakey et al., 2014). Relational regulation theory provides an alternative to the idea that perceived support reflects the receipt of specific supportive actions that prompt adaptive coping and appraisal. Everyday conversation in close relationships might provide a communicative model through which people regulate their emotions and responses through ordinary conversations and shared activities, which produce both mental health and perceived support (Lakey & Orehek, 2011). Thus, communication provides the possibility for regulating affect on a moment-to-moment basis through ordinary, yet consequential, conversations and shared activities rather than by talking about stress and how to cope with it (Lakey et al., 2014). Although ordinary, these interactions potentially have important influences on affect. For example, conversations about football or celebrities might be ordinary in that they occur daily, but such conversations might consistently elicit emotional well-being in a recipient; similarly, shared activities also play an important role (Lakey et al., 2014). Then, perceived support is not seen as the cause of affect; instead, affect and perceived support emerge in tandem from specific kinds of social interaction in that people can infer support from everyday conversations. This idea is consistent with other research on social support in that perceived support is not primarily based on the receipt of specific supportive actions (Goldsmith, 2004; Uchino, 2009). Connecting communication about everyday events as helpful in emotions and responses brings a holistic quality to communication in that the everyday interplay of close relationships connects to health (Bylund & Duck, 2004).

Communication and resilience. Afifi and colleagues' (2016) theory of resilience and relational load brings a recent advancement that bridges communicative, perceptual, and physiological aspects of stress within the context of social relationships to explain personal/relational risk, resilience and thriving during stressful experiences. The theory of resilience and relational load examines how relational partners and family members' communal orientation and maintenance of their relationship on a daily basis influence their communication during stressful experiences, as well as their appraisals of the stress (T. D. Afifi et al., 2016). The theory addresses how communication patterns and appraisals influence personal and relational health and adaptation and how the wear and tear of chronic stress can deplete emotional, psychological, and relational resources (T. D. Afifi et al., 2016). The theory poses that positive relationship maintenance serves as the primary mechanism underlying stress and resilience in close relationships. Specifically, the pro-social, daily verbal and nonverbal behaviors, perceptions, and actions allow relational partners and family members to become resilient and to thrive (T. D. Afifi et al., 2016). Initial development of the theory emerged from coding couples' conversations about their financial uncertainty and stress and indicated that "unified couples" uplifted each other, were unified in combatting hardship, were present emotionally and communicatively, and blamed outside forces (T. D. Afifi et al., 2016). "Thriving" couples also talked about growing and learning positively from hardship; "at-risk" couples quickly became stuck in intractable cycles of conflict; "pragmatic" couples focused on how to solve the problem (T. D. Afifi et al., 2016). The theory assumes that when people validate their relational partners and family members on an ongoing basis, they accumulate positive emotional reserves or emotional capital, which helps safeguard their relationships. Couples or family members who lack emotional reserves are likely to engage in more threatening appraisals and conflict behaviors when they are stressed, which depletes cognitive, emotional, and relational resources and exacerbates stress. If the depletion continues over time, it can wear at the relationship through the relational load that makes the individuals and the relational system more susceptible to poor mental, physical, and relational health (T. D. Afifi et al., 2016).

As I close this chapter, reconsider the opening passages on illness as the hub around which the new life revolves and on challenged assumptions that we can be the architect of our own life. Those passages, and the books from which they came, provide narrative illustrations of people who are shifting conceptualization of their lives to make sense of illness diagnosis. The attributes described in this chapter give a sense of the theoretical and empirical relationship research. Through combinations of attributes, we can better understand the stories of illness as they connect to changes in relationship processes.

PART II Health and Illness, the Body, and Relational Processes

4　Relationships as Buffering or Exacerbating Health and Illness Outcomes

TYPE 2 DIABETES EMBEDDED WITHIN SOCIETAL SYSTEMS

Type 2 diabetes was once known as adult-onset diabetes. Now that term is outdated, as diabetes is increasingly a disease that begins in childhood. The prevalence of diabetes in the United States doubled in the last decade among black children and tripled among American Indian children. Black and Hispanic children have eight times the risk of developing the disease compared to others. Faced with these numbers, public health experts and art educators have created a novel approach that brings agency to teenagers in giving voice and agency to diabetes not just as a medical problem related to poor diet and lack of exercise but as a social justice problem tied to stress, poverty, violence, and limited access to healthy and affordable foods (O'Connor, 2018). The campaign called "The Bigger Picture" teaches young artists that diabetes is not simply a consequence of individual lifestyle choices but of broader, dysfunctional systems that constrain and shape behavior; the forces that reduce costs of obesogenic food, incentivize its marketing to people of color, unequally allocate physical activity opportunities, and perpetuate poverty and stress – all in ways that disproportionately focus diabetes risk within vulnerable populations. The Bigger Picture directs attention to the structural causes of the diabetes epidemic in youth, particularly people of color, and taps into adolescents' deeply held values of social justice, resistance to manipulation, and desire to protect their families and communities. The Bigger Picture drives youth to find a voice and sense of agency in effecting change. Youth wrote poems that synthesize their knowledge with lived experience, which reflect their life as primary text, and feature the youth poets themselves, often with their family members, with their own homes and neighborhoods as backdrops (Schillinger & Huey, 2018; Schillinger et al., 2017). For video content see www.thebiggerpictureproject.org.

– O'Connor, 2018

– Schillinger & Huey, 2018

– Schillinger et al., 2017

DISABILITY AND SOCIETAL EXPECTATIONS OF LIMITATIONS

> *"When you are disabled, the two things people think you can't do are fight and have sex. So I've got a black belt and I'm really good at shagging." Mat Fraser, a multi-disciplinary performer, explores connections between disability, entertainment, and sexuality.*
>
> *Disabled people's sexuality has been suppressed, exploited, and at times, destroyed over centuries. Images of disability and sexuality tend to be absent, where disabled people are presented as asexual, or else perverse and hypersexual. Disabled people are rendered impotent and sexless by disability and seen as unattractive and vulnerable to mockery and exploitation.*

– Quarmby, 2015. "Disabled and Fighting for a Sex Life."

Note that "disabled people" is as used in the quoted article and retained for the purpose of illustrating how language communicatively constitutes reality. One of the key movements of the disability advocacy community is "person first" language (person with a disability).

SOCIETAL CONDITIONS AND ENVIRONMENTAL FACTORS

These examples of type 2 diabetes and physical disability give a brief glimpse into the complexities of health and illness and disability as interconnected with broader contexts of relationships, which co-occur within extensive considerations of social networks and societal-level attributions, bias, and other distortions. Public discourse around type 2 diabetes might be interpreted as shame and blame, the idea that people who develop the disease knowingly make bad or maladaptive choices; considering diabetes as a social and environmental problem positions the crisis around neighborhoods awash in fast food chains, liquor stores, billboards advertising junk food, and limited incomes (Schillinger & Huey, 2018). Public discourse around disability at worst focuses on deviance and dependence. Conversely, public discourse around disability sometimes focuses on the societal-level concerns that shift the assumed problem from the person to the society and allows for recognizing difference. Public discourse around disability and sexual pleasure seems to be a missing discourse, a stark contrast from more general sexualized images of sexual pleasure as part of authentic, abiding satisfaction in feeling alive. Both diabetes and physical disability can be used as exemplary illustrations of how the social construction of health and illness is interconnected with social conditions and environmental factors such that people attribute stigmatized attributions that systematically distort the problems.

In this chapter, I synthesize empirical literature linking relationship characteristics with health and illness outcomes. Prior research indicates that features of relationships can either buffer against or, on the contrary, can further exacerbate the negative consequences of a chronic disease or a health crisis. Relationship characteristics are associated with exacerbating or buffering against physical health including such biomedical markers as blood pressure, ulcers, LDL cholesterol levels, and cortisol levels. Relationship characteristics are associated with exacerbating or buffering against mental health including depression and anxiety. This chapter provides an overview of empirical research linking relationships with physical and mental health outcomes.

Human behavior plays a meaningful role in most of the leading causes of death. Social scientific research on human behavior has the potential to enhance health outcomes by addressing the health-promoting and health-damaging behaviors (Kaplan, 2009). Across social scientific disciplines, research focuses on the interplay among biological dispositions, behavior, and the social context (Kaplan, 2009). Empirical research across many disciplines provides evidence that high-quality relationships and strong social networks are correlated with good physical and mental health. Research in psychology, family studies, sociology, communication, and epidemiology provides empirical evidence that connects the quantity and quality of relationships with physical and mental health and with survival. The empirical and theoretical literature is based on prospective correlational research where studies control for additional factors such as sex, age, ethnicity, and socioeconomic status that could influence both the nature of social networks and health (Cohen & Janicki-Deverts, 2009). Note that the associations cannot be considered causal, as there are still many psychosocial, environmental, and biological factors that could account for a correlation between a social factor and health and illness outcomes (Cohen & Janicki-Deverts, 2009).

Epidemiologists interested in how social conditions might influence health developed the idea that one of the most fundamental conditions that protected people exposed to what appeared to be overwhelming insults was the protective mechanisms in maintaining close personal relationships with other people and the degree to which people were embedded or socially integrated into their communities (Cassel, 1976). This research does not always focus on any specific disease or illness but instead on the degree to which social conditions and social connections influence resistance. This focus on close relationships as protective mechanisms was developed alongside scientific evidence for psychological stresses and influences in diseases. Social conditions can influence health in a variety of ways across the life span and can connect with diagnoses of disabilities and changes in physical and mental functioning at different points in time (Berkman, 2000). Social conditions can influence health and illness alongside specific agents that cause disease and a host of other factors that contribute to the onset of course of disease. Focus on the social conditions does not negate the biomedical explanatory frameworks but provides ample evidence for a need to address multiple levels including both the biomedical mechanisms and social conditions associated with health and illness. Ongoing research across disciplines provides evidence that disease and illness recovery among patients with similar severity in symptoms is highly variable. Social integration and strong relationships can buffer against or, on the contrary, negative relationships can further exacerbate the negative consequences of a chronic disease or a health crisis.

For example, in their quantitative synthesis of research on social integration and mortality, House, Landis, and Umberson (1988) found a robust association between low levels of social integration and risk for early death. More recently, Holt-Lunstad, Smith, and Layton (2010) conducted a qualitative benchmarking analysis comparing the association between social integration and mortality with the magnitude of other well-known public health risks such as light to moderate smoking, excessive alcohol use, lack of physical exercise, and obesity; the connection between social integration and mortality, as indicated in effect sizes, rivaled the observed effect for these other significant public health risks and provided evidence for the clarity in association between people's relationships and their survival.

SOCIAL NETWORKS AND HEALTH AND ILLNESS

The French sociologist Emile Durkheim's (1858–1917) contribution as a macro-analytical framework to the study of the relationship between society and health provided an initial explanation for understanding how social integration and cohesion influence mortality (Berkman et al., 2000). In his analysis of suicide, Durkheim proposed that patterns of one of the most psychologically intimate and seemingly individual acts rests not on psychological foundations but upon patterns of social facts that explain changing patterns of aggregate tendency towards suicide (Berkman et al., 2000). Durkheim examined the social patterns of suicide in observations of countries and other geographic units and showed how social groups have very stable rates of suicide year after year. Durkheim then theorized that the underlying reasons for suicide rates connect to the level of social integration of the group. This way of examining suicide was particularly relevant because it described large-scale suicide crises of an economic or political nature that often occurred during times of rapid social change and turbulence (Berkman et al., 2000). In such situations, social control and norms are weakened because the regulatory function of integration shifts with the societal turbulence. Rapid social change serves to deregulate values, beliefs, and general norms, and the erosion of society's capacity for integration can trigger suicide (Berkman et al., 2000). This theoretical orientation can extend to other outcomes including violence and homicides and cardiovascular disease and has served as a foundation for current leaders in social connections to health and illness (Berkman et al., 2000).

Social networks and social integration are now considered critical components of understanding mortality and morbidity, and researchers widely accept that social relationships and affiliation at the societal level have powerful effects on physical and mental health. Conceptual models and empirical evidence continue to become more sophisticated theoretically and empirically. Social network theories rest on the assumption that social structure and the network itself are responsible for determining individual behavior and attitudes by shaping the flow of resources that then determine access to opportunities and constraints on behavior (Berkman et al., 2000). By assessing actual ties between network members, researchers can empirically test community ties and how community is defined. For example, community ties can be defined in terms of neighborhood, kinship, friendship, institutional affiliation, or other characteristics (Berkman et al., 2000).

In their seminal study linking social relationships to mortality, Berkman and Syme (1979) linked the questions about the extent of people's social connections to overall mortality and found that people who were less socially integrated also had higher mortality rates, even controlling for alternative explanations such as poorer initial health status. Much subsequent research has provided compelling empirical and theoretical evidence linking social networks to better social support and better physical health outcomes. Both observational evidence and experimental evidence reveal the importance of social networks and the support they provide in shaping health outcomes from the onset of disease to functioning and mortality (Ertel, Glymour, & Berkman, 2009). Social networks broadly refer to aspects of the social environment that have to do with social relationships, including close relationships, to more extended community ties and social engagement, participation, and social integration (Ertel et al., 2009). More specifically regarding measurement, social networks refer to the structure of social ties and the web of relations that surround an individual including size, density, and homogeneity (Ertel et al., 2009). Social networks have powerful effects on physical and mental health, but the interpretations and measures vary across studies. Social networks include the web of social relationships that surround an individual and the characteristics of the links or ties among people. Network models describe the structure of one or more networks of relations within a system or people, including range or size (the number of network members), density (the extent to which members are connected to each other), boundedness (the degree to which people are defined on the basis of traditional structures such as kin, work, or neighborhood), and homogeneity (the extent to which individuals are similar to each other in a network) (Burt, 1982). Characteristics of individual ties related to network structure include frequency of contact, multiplexity in the number of types of transactions or support flowing through ties, duration in length of time an individual knows another, and reciprocity in the extent to which exchanges are bidirectional (Burt, 1982).

In conceptual work linking social networks to health, Lisa Berkman has been a leader in developing research and articulating pathways by which social networks may influence physical and mental health status (Berkman, 2004). She acknowledges the qualitative aspects of social relations in the provision of social support or, conversely, in documenting detrimental aspects of relationships, but she also elaborates on the structural aspects of social networks (Berkman, 2004). Berkman and her colleagues' research provides theoretical and empirical evidence for social networks as embedded in a macro-social environment in which large-scale social forces influence network structure, which in turn influences a cascading causal process beginning with the macro-social to psychobiological processes to affect health (Berkman, 2004). In this framework, social networks are embedded in a larger social and cultural context in which upstream forces are seen to condition network structure.

In addition to close relationships that provide social support over time, Berkman and colleagues address extended ties characterized by people a person may not know well but who help get things done. These low-intimacy relationships include community contacts and the potential for effective extended contacts in negotiating the broader health-care systems. Thus, Berkman and her colleagues in their research on social networks give serious consideration of the larger macro-social context in which networks form and are sustained. Networks may operate at the biobehavioral level through at least four primary pathways: provision of social support, social influence, social engagement and attachment, and access to resources and material goods (Berkman, 2004). These psychosocial and behavioral processes may influence more proximate pathways to health status including (1) direct physiological responses, (2) psychological states including self-esteem, self-efficacy, and depression, (3) health-damaging behaviors such as using tobacco or high-risk sexual activity, and health-promoting behavior such as exercise and using health services appropriately, and (4) exposure to infectious disease agents such as HIV, other sexually transmitted diseases and infections, or tuberculosis (Berkman, 2004).

Although many observational studies and small-scale studies reveal the importance of social networks and the support they provide in shaping health outcomes, large-scale interventions aimed at reducing social isolation, changing social network structure, and improving social support indicate weak effects on the health outcomes they were designed to impact (Ertel et al., 2009). In their analysis of the literature connecting social networks and support to cardiovascular and cerebrovascular disease, Ertel, Glymour, and Berkman (2009) employ life-course models of health and provide evidence for patterns of social networks across the life span and where potential windows of opportunity exist for intervening upon social networks to promote health. They find that social networks are relatively stable across the life course and possible points at which they are more likely to change include marriage, divorce, and the aftermath of disease (Ertel et al., 2009).

Although the particular people in the social networks may change, the networks remain stable, but the researchers highlight important points that can serve as critical periods for social network shifts. Long-term correlations point to a surprising degree of stability across many years, but researchers suggest the stability masks potentially important year-to-year changes (Ertel et al., 2009). Marriage, parenthood, and divorce are transition periods that may affect social networks. Changes during the years before marriage and in the early years of marriage may affect social networks. Social ties and contacts shift during romantic relationships, with more contact and social support from the partners' friends and family and with married individuals having larger networks (Kalmijn, 2003; Milardo, 1987). The transition to parenthood is associated with increased contact with family members and with the view that social networks may become more homogenous, including family and other parents with young children during early years of parenthood (Ertel et al., 2009). Separation or divorce is associated in the short term with a reduction in network size and frequency of contact with network members, but does not appear to have effect generally on social integration; this indicates some aspects of social integration may be negatively affected but other aspects may be positively affected (Ertel et al., 2009). Retirement is another transition period where social contacts and group membership opportunities embedded in the workplace may be lost but where people have more time and energy to devote to developing different social networks and participating in social activities (Ertel et al., 2009). Changes in educational settings, in residency, and in employment may be important for people who need different types of support.

Although network size may remain stable, life changes might indicate decreases in certain aspects of relationships and increases in other aspects of relationships. For example, widowed individuals may be less likely to have a confidant but may receive more social support from relatives or friends compared to married individuals (Ha, 2008). The increased contact and support after widowhood are observed to remain elevated until three years after the loss of a spouse, at which point they begin to decrease to their pre-widowhood levels (Guiaux, van Tilburg, & van Groenou, 2007).

Health and illness status changes may shape social integration and may differ across chronic disease (Ertel et al., 2009). The Longitudinal Aging Study Amsterdam indicated that the presence of chronic disease (i.e., cardiac disease, peripheral vascular disease, stroke, diabetes, lung disease, cancer, arthritis) was not associated with social network size or emotional support, but stroke and arthritis were associated with higher instrumental support, and lung disease and arthritis were associated with greater feelings of loneliness (Penninx et al., 1999). However, these measures of social support miss the potential aspects of changes in support and assistance in how social networks are manifest. As friends also become more elderly and frailer, the reciprocal support and assistance may shift to more one-sided relationships in which support and assistance are largely received, and this may have important psychological and health consequences (Ertel et al., 2009). Close relationships with friends are most likely to be destabilized or threatened in older people as people become frailer and need to move to another location, so the frequent contact with close friends likely decreases in ways that are important relationship processes but are not captured by measures of social networks (Ertel et al., 2009). Over the life span people compensate for losses, but in the oldest people structural isolation and illness may compromise the ability to compensate for close relationship loss (Ertel et al., 2009). The composite measures of social networks may not capture the lived experiences of close relationships across health and illness trajectories. Cognitive function and cognitive outcomes can connect to social integration. Examination of the effect of social ties and social support on cognitive function and cognitive change six months after stroke provided evidence that emotional support may promote cognitive resilience, while social ties provide cognitive reserve that protects against impaired cognition after stroke (Glymour et al., 2008). Relationship transitions require individuals to adapt to a changing environment, and adaptation can be connected to stress and psychological reactivity.

SOCIAL AND ECONOMIC CONDITIONS AND RELATIONSHIP STAGES AS CONTEXTS

Social and economic conditions coexist with social networks and social integration. The ability to offer and receive social support and to be connected to resources coexists with social conditions. For example, oppressive social conditions, lower-status positions in society, and challenges of parenthood and family responsibilities pose particular trials to marriages (Orbuch et al., 2002). Results from the Early Years of Marriage Project provide evidence for objective social and economic conditions in accounts for divorce over time (Orbuch et al., 2002). Terri Orbuch and her colleagues provide evidence that race, gender, and time act as context in which to understand the quality and impact of structure and the perception of interaction in predicting divorce. Both race and education predicted the risk of divorce over a fourteen-year period, and perceived interactional processes were connected to the contexts of race and gender (Orbuch et al., 2002). Their framework cuts across sociological and psychological theories in their contention that both structural and interactive factors can independently predict divorce (Orbuch & Eyster, 1997; Peterson, Orbuch, & Brown, 2014). Further, Orbuch and colleagues propose and find evidence that interpersonal processes can act as mediators of social conditions and that both structural and interactive factors may differ by race and gender (Orbuch et al., 2002). Orbuch and her colleagues provide evidence that social conditions can set the stage for divorce and can be mediated by interactional processes, and that social conditions can also act as contexts in which to understand the quality and impact of the interactional variables under investigation (Orbuch et al., 2002). Perceived styles of interaction can shape positive or negative marital consequences differently in various groups and for the same group at different points in the marital trajectory (Orbuch et al., 2002).

Styles of interaction can have different effects on men and women, on people from different educational strata, on people from different races, and on people at different points in their life course or their marriage (Orbuch et al., 2002). In addition to social and economic conditions, these researchers examined patterns of marital well-being over the first seven years of marriage and whether factors connected to early marital well-being during year one impacted marital well-being over time (Brown et al., 2013). After accounting for differences in early marital conditions, having a child before marriage was significant in predicting marital well-being over time for husbands (Brown et al., 2013). Divorced parents affected the rate of change for wives. The findings from the Early Years of Marriage project suggest that as couples settle into their marriages, social and economic risk factors have fewer consequences on marital well-being (Brown et al., 2013). When considering that marriage is one of the primary forms of social support connected to health processes, understanding the additional social and economic conditions that shape marriage allows for better explaining how support processes in illness might be constrained by social and economic conditions.

Relationship stages in addition to marriage changes can connect to health and illness outcomes, as described in Loving and Sbarra's (2015) chapter on relationships and health. Early relationships can shape physiological responses in that experiences in relationships can shape how people perceive their environment, which in turn results in biological responses. Studies of the biological pre-determinants and consequences of relationship initiation can shed light on the health-protective effects of close relationship processes. Evidence for the connection between relationship initiation and health includes research showing that when women are fertile they are more attracted to short-term (as opposed to long-term) mates who display traits such as facial symmetry indicative of greater genetic fitness (Gangestad et al., 2007). The effects of relationship initiation include physical and psychological domains, as falling in love alters physiological outcomes including chronic and acute cortisol production (Loving, Crockett, & Paxson, 2009). Relationship initiation may promote physical health and increased affectionate behaviors (Guerrero & Andersen, 1994), and affectionate behaviors are a defining feature of most high-quality relationships (Call, Sprecher, & Schwartz, 1995).

Meta-analysis provides evidence that the link between social support and mortality from all causes remains predictive across age and sex (Holt-Lunstad et al., 2010). Of the pathways by which social support may influence health, indicators of inflammation functions as a biomarker of the pathway linking social support to health and illness. Inflammation can predict the development and course of chronic health conditions including heart disease. Ethnicity and race may influence links between social support and markers of inflammation because markers of inflammation connect to one's sensitivity to social resources such as social support, as indicated in a 2016 study of c-reactive proteins (Uchino et al., 2016). The researchers in this study did not find an overall link between social support and c-reactive protein levels, but they did find that the association between c-reactive protein levels was moderated by ethnicity and race, primarily in African American people (Uchino et al., 2016). These results suggest the importance of considering how ethnicity and race may inform models on the complex biological mechanisms linking social support to health and illness (Uchino et al., 2016).

Studies demonstrate that socioeconomic status is related to health such that demonstrated socioeconomic disparities exist among and across a wide range of diseases. The role of social support and integration for understanding socioeconomic disparities is documented in self-rated health behaviors and hypertension (Gorman & Sivaganesan, 2007). Research provides evidence that social support and social integration are connected to effects of socioeconomic status on health in that many aspects of social integration are directly related to self-rated health and hypertension, but that these measures do not mediate the relationship between socioeconomic status and health (Gorman & Sivaganesan, 2007). However, interaction tests show substantial evidence that measures of social integration buffer some of the negative effects of low socioeconomic status, particularly the negative influence of not working on self-rated health (Gorman & Sivaganesan, 2007). In addition, findings indicate potential evidence of help-seeking behavior among adults who did not finish high school or who report financial barriers to medical care (Gorman & Sivaganesan, 2007).

Marital transitions remain a focus in connecting health behaviors and health indicators with relationship processes. Historically, marriage has been associated with lower mortality and transitions into marriage were generally accompanied by improved health status, while divorce has been associated with increased mortality. Recent research provides evidence in postmenopausal women that women's transitions into marriage or marriage-like relationships were associated with poorer (not better) health outcomes (Kutob et al., 2017). Specifically, women's transitions into marriage, or marriage-like relationships, were accompanied by increases in body mass index relative to remaining unmarried (Kutob et al., 2017). Contrary to historical research, divorce or separation was associated with a reduction in body mass index and in waist circumference, changes that were accompanied by improvements in diet quality and physical activity relative to women who remained married (Kutob et al., 2017).

Recent research also suggests that a macro-level approach can be helpful in understanding how demographic patterns and social policies shape interdependence in families (Dykstra & Hagestad, 2016). Interdependence as a social-psychological and communicative construct is addressed in foundations of understanding close relationship definitions, processes, and theories. Dykstra & Hagestad (2016) illustrate how demographic changes, such as increased life spans, create different opportunities for interdependence for men and women. The researchers also draw attention to the role of national policies where legislation shapes interdependence (Dykstra & Hagestad, 2016). For example, legislation can mandate generational interdependence by implementing legal obligations to provide support; legislation can block generational interdependence when grandparents are not granted the right to raise grandchildren when parents cannot provide adequate care; immigration laws can enable or block visits that enable or limit the provision of care; legislation generates and lightens generational interdependence through laws supporting parents of young children, thus indicating less reliance on grandparents caring for the young children (Dykstra & Hagestad, 2016). Considering interdependence connected to legislation poses implications for social and economic conditions through implications for childless men and women, and through questioning the primacy assigned to kinship ties in health care and long-term support policies (Dykstra & Hagestad, 2016).

The concept of interconnected or linked lives across generations moves considerations of social and psychological processes to the broader contexts of social influences in broader shared relationships. Transitions in one family member affect trajectories of close others (Dykstra & Hagestad, 2016), and macro-level understanding of interdependence considers broader societal-level social control manifest both in formal laws and regulations and in the size and composition of family networks and the duration of ties for men, for women, and for people in different social and economic conditions (Dykstra & Hagestad, 2016). For example, as women live longer, role engagements involve more women in later life, which shape the parent–child as well as the grandparent–grandchild relationships (Dykstra & Hagestad, 2016). Women's cross-generational ties in longer durations have received little attention in the life-course literature or on the implications for age and gender (Dykstra & Hagestad, 2016). When considering how health and illness trajectories also connect to macro-level interdependence, researchers and practitioners will need to address implications for caregivers, for models of care, and for social and communicative implications of this cross-generational interdependence.

BIOLOGICAL SYSTEMS AND HEALTH OUTCOMES

Two broad outcome types indicating relevant biological systems and health outcomes are (1) physiological biomarkers such as autonomic, neuroendocrine, and immune activity implicated in a range of physical health outcomes, and (2) objective disease outcomes including physical and mental illnesses (Loving & Sbarra, 2015). Physiological biomarkers include some assessment of autonomic, neuroendocrine, or immune functioning (Gouin et al., 2010; Kiecolt-Glaser et al., 2005). Measures indicate sensory and motor nerves that mark processes in body systems that regulate activity. For example, regulation of the digestive tract, energy mobilization, energy conservation, and metabolism are connected to fight-or-flight response during threat or danger. Heightened heart rate, organ activity indicating preparation for physical exertion, hormone changes, and increased sugar levels can be used as biomarkers (Loving & Sbarra, 2015).

Cardiovascular outcomes account for much of the research in the romantic relationships and health context. Scientists report that individuals who had recently lost a spouse were at increased risk for mortality from coronary heart disease. Over time, these findings became more nuanced and addressed that social isolation, not just the loss of an intimate romantic partner, was associated with mortality risk. Common biomarkers in research on cardiovascular disease include heart rate and blood pressure (both systolic and diastolic blood pressure), which serve as indirect markers of autonomic activity as well as sympathetically influenced endocrine activity. Cardiac output and vascular reactance are also used as markers of cardiovascular functioning and indicate something about the manner in which the body is responding physiologically (Loving & Sbarra, 2015). Endocrine measures are used as biomarkers indicative of the release of hormones that serve to coordinate metabolic and behavioral responses during stress. Cortisol is especially important for maintaining normal metabolic function but also is very important during stress response because it enhances the responses of the sympathetic nervous system and increases the release of glucose and stored fats for energy (Loving & Sbarra, 2015). Neuroendocrine responses can be directly assessed. Cortisol can be measured in saliva in addition to measuring cortisol in blood and urine (Loving & Sbarra, 2015). Some researchers argue that alpha-amylase, an enzyme found in saliva, may provide a marker of sympathetic nervous system activity and may be a reliable marker of general autonomic activity (Loving & Sbarra, 2015). Oxytocin and vasopressin are peptide hormones associated with relationship quality and behaviors capable of influencing immune functioning including inflammation and wound healing and with hypothesized roles in relationship development and maintenance as documented in animal models (Loving & Sbarra, 2015). Biomarkers are helpful because of their downstream role in physical effects such as immunity. However, multiple counter-regulatory mechanisms involved in physiological responses make it challenging to know how biomarkers translate into real-world morbidity or mortality (Loving & Sbarra, 2015). Research provides evidence for the link between inflammation and morbidity and mortality indicative of the helpfulness in measuring immune functioning.

Close relationships are associated with physical and mental outcomes. Physical disease outcomes include cardiovascular disease outcomes as specific diseases that affect the heart or the blood vessel system such as coronary heart disease and congestive heart failure. The major outcomes of cardiovascular disease include angina pectoris or pain resulting from decreased blood flow to the heart, myocardial infection or heart attack resulting from interrupted blood to the heart, and stroke or disturbance of blood supply to the brain. Ultrasound can measure thickness of artery walls, which permits noninvasive assessment of early-stage thickening of artery walls.

In addition to myocardial measures, other malignant processes include unregulated cell growth in cancer and pain, and relationship research links perceptions of social support, social network size, and marital status with cancer survival (Pinquart & Duberstein, 2010). In the pain literature, positive relationship processes including caretaking behaviors by a spouse can sometime unintentionally maintain and sometimes exacerbate the experience of chronic pain (Loving & Sbarra, 2015). Mental health and illness outcomes in the research literature include measures found in the *Diagnostic and Statistical Manual of Mental Disorders* as well as self-reports of anxiety and mental health challenges that do not reach the threshold for diagnosis or have not been formally diagnosed. Diagnosed mental health problems reflect considerable functional impairment. Among mental disorders, the most commonly studied in the context of relationships are mood disorders such as depressive disorders and anxiety disorders including post-traumatic stress disorder (Loving & Sbarra, 2015). Much of the research on health and illness outcomes associated with close relationships focuses on communication and behavior dynamics in established relationships, particularly conflict and support processes (Loving & Sbarra, 2015). Although the bodies of work on conflict and support are summarized in other reviews and therefore only briefly considered here, identifying the implications for health and illness in close relationships requires consideration of both conflict and support processes.

SOCIAL SUPPORT AS BEHAVIORAL PATHWAY LINKING SOCIAL PROCESSES AND HEALTH

Positive aspects of relationships such as perceived social support are associated with lower risk of disease morbidity and mortality. People who lack emotional support also indicate increased mortality risk that is not accounted for by the severity of disease, comorbidity, or age, gender, or race (Berkman, 2000). However, even strong relationships that can be major sources of support are not uniformly positive and can add to the feeling of distress during a person's time of need. For example, in a study measuring independent effects of both positive and negative exchanges on both positive and negative affect in older adults, negative exchanges such as ineffective information, feeling frustrated, and feeling let down by the support provider indicated potent and long-lasting effects (Newsom et al., 2003). Acknowledging the strengths and challenges of intended support and for both positive and negative aspects of relationships poses important implications for theory and interventions.

The concept of social support and its association to physical health yields mixed results. As a leader in the research linking social ties, relationship processes, and health, Bert Uchino has produced work examining how social relationships influence health at multiple levels of analysis. The strongest evidence that social support is related to health or disease comes from studies of large populations demonstrating that social support or social networks are protective against all-cause mortality (Uchino, 2004). Research provides evidence that social support is negatively associated with cardiovascular death, and correlational evidence suggests the potential for social support to protect against recurrent events and death after being diagnosed with a disease or illness (Uchino, 2004). However, research involving the predictive relationship between social support or social networks and incidence of disease (especially measured in cardiovascular disease), has produced inconclusive and inconsistent results (Uchino, 2004). Similarly, studies of the connection between social support or social networks and cancer and other manifestations of disease or illness have been similarly conflicting (Uchino, 2004). Inconsistencies in connecting social support or social networks to physical health may result from a number of factors. Social support or social network features are measured differently across studies. The association between social support and health may be bidirectional such that intended social support can help in some circumstances but can be counterproductive in other circumstances. The effects of social support may vary by characteristics such as age, sex, socioeconomic status, cultural setting, disease, or illness progression (Uchino, 2004).

Uchino and his colleagues examine the social (i.e., types of social interactions), cognitive (i.e., how these interactions are interpreted or construed), and physiological (i.e., cardiovascular, endocrine, and immune) processes associated with social relationships and with close relationships (Uchino, Cacioppo, & Kiecolt-Glaser, 1996;

Uchino, 2004; Uchino, 2009). With regard to social support, Uchino and his colleagues' program of research indicates that perceptions of supportive relationships predict reduced cardiovascular reactivity during stress (Smith et al., 2011; Uchino & Garvey, 1997), lower blood pressure in older adults (Uchino et al., 1995; Uchino et al., 1999; Uchino, Kiecolt-Glaser, & Cacioppo, 1992), and lower ambulatory blood pressure during daily life (Bowen et al., 2013). Understanding the links between social support and physical health necessitates distinguishing between perceived and received social support. Individuals who perceive support to be available may not actually seek social support as a first coping option, but knowing support is available may alleviate stress by acting as a potential safety net (Uchino & Reblin, 2009). Similarly, not all functions or types of social support are necessarily beneficial to health. Perceived support has been more consistently related to beneficial health outcomes than has received support (Uchino, 2004). Emotional support appears to be mostly beneficial, but people who depend on a high degree of tangible support and aid tend to have higher mortality (Uchino & Reblin, 2009). Studies do not provide evidence that these people receiving tangible aid are more physically impaired as measured by initial health status or limitation in activities of daily living (Uchino & Reblin, 2009). Negative psychological effects of dependence and increased conflict during support processes remain under investigation as mechanisms through which social support might function to enhance health or, on the contrary, might be connected to poorer health.

Broader theoretical explanation can be found in Uchino's general model for examining the health-related consequences of social relationships that incorporates both positive and negative aspects of social support (Uchino, 2009; Uchino et al., 2001). A unique feature of Uchino's model is the specification of ambivalent relationships that are viewed as relatively high in both positivity and negativity. For example, overbearing parents, volatile romance, "out of touch" friends, and emotionally charged friendships can be high in both positivity and negativity (Fingerman, Hay, & Birditt, 2004). Despite the positivity in such relationships, the co-occurrence of negativity and emotional volatility may be uniquely associated with worse health outcomes. This may be because ambivalent ties require heightened vigilance during social interactions or may be frustrating and ineffective sources of support during times of need (Uchino, 2009; Uchino et al., 2001). Perceptions of closeness in ambivalent ties might exacerbate the interpersonal stress with such network ties. People with ambivalent ties engage in more negative behaviors (e.g., criticism) and less emotionally supportive behaviors and thus appear stress-enhancing (Reblin, Uchino, & Smith, 2010).

Ambivalent ties are also not an isolated feature of most individuals' social networks. They comprise almost 50 percent of important network members and hence have ample opportunity to influence health-related outcomes (Campo et al., 2009). Uchino and his colleagues suggest that ambivalent ties are related to worse outcomes compared to other relationship types (e.g., primarily positive or primarily negative), such as increased cardiovascular reactivity at both conscious and less conscious levels of processing (Carlisle et al., 2012; Holt-Lunstad et al., 2007), higher ambulatory blood pressure during daily life (Holt-Lunstad, Birmingham, & Light, 2015; Holt-Lunstad et al., 2003; Uchino, 2013; Uchino et al., 2012), increased inflammation (Uchino et al., 2013), faster cellular aging (Uchino et al., 2012), and greater coronary calcification (Uchino, Smith, & Berg, 2014). In proposing stronger bridges between relationship science and health, Uchino (Uchino, 2013; Uchino et al., 2012) suggests that relationship positivity, negativity, and ambivalence influence biological processes and physical health outcomes, but that the antecedent processes, contexts, and mechanisms such as the experience of emotions by which ambivalent ties can be health-relevant need further explication.

Ambivalence may be manifest in behavioral patterns as indicated in Uchino's work, but combinations of support and anxiety may also be manifest in other forms. In receiving a difficult diagnosis such as breast cancer, people describe challenges in emotional impact, worries about treatment, concerns about disruptions in day-to-day life, and anxiety and distress in how the diagnosis relates to life demands (Borstelmann et al., 2015). A recent study indicated that partner support was not necessarily associated with being in a stable relationship. Among young women diagnosed with breast cancer and in a partnered or significant relationship, 20 percent were categorized as unsupported (Borstelmann et al., 2015). Women in unsupported-partnered relationships had higher odds of anxiety symptoms compared with women in a supported-partnered relationship (Borstelmann et al., 2015). Young age and being financially insecure were both independently associated with anxiety (Borstelmann et al., 2015). Younger age and inability to rely on partner support increases vulnerability, as does struggling with finances.

DISPARITIES IN HEALTH AND ILLNESS AND DISPARITIES IN HEALTH CARE

So far this chapter has addressed relationship characteristics associated with health and illness outcomes. In order to understand the connection between relationship characteristics and health and illness outcomes, we must also address the social, economic, organizational, and interpersonal contexts in which health care and social influence take place. Health disparities become worse with each step down the socioeconomic ladder. Adults with lower incomes, less education, and less prestigious jobs are at greater risk for chronic disease, disability, and premature mortality. Income limits access to health care, but the connection between lower socioeconomic status and poor health exists in countries even with universal health-care access, suggesting that access to health care is not the sole mechanism; further evidence suggests that lower socioeconomic status is connected to higher levels of stress hormones (Cohen, Doyle, & Baum, 2006). Both stress and depression are higher among people with lower incomes and less education (Adler & Rehkopf, 2008).

Psychological stress and depression are associated with impairing the ability of the cellular immune system to control viral latency.

Across a broad spectrum of mental and physical illnesses, people who are members of socially disadvantaged groups experience poorer physical and mental health than people from socially advantaged groups. The global impact of income inequality on health discrepancies is documented in both mental and physical health and is a persistent social problem across at least 126 countries, which is 94.4 percent of the world's population (Dorling, Mitchell, & Pearce, 2007). Health disparities or health inequalities is the social problem of variations in the mental or physical well-being of people of different social groups that specifically result from inequitable economic, political, social, and psychological processes. Although genetic and biological factors play important roles in mental and physical health, research on health disparities provides strong evidence for social factors. Disparities are observed in health and in the provision of health care.

Health-care disparities are inequalities in access to and/or the quality of medical care among people in different social groups (Penner et al., 2013). Health-care disparities exist when members of socially disadvantaged groups experience poorer health than members of socially advantaged groups as connected to receiving poorer health care (Penner et al., 2013). Much of this section focuses on disparities among members of racial or ethnic minorities because health disparities are a focus of much of the research on disparities in receiving health care (Shavers et al., 2012). However, race and ethnicity are not the only group characteristics linked to health-care disparities, and race and ethnicity is often interconnected to other attributes also associated with discrimination and with health disparities. For example, people who have physical disabilities, people who have lower socioeconomic status, people who are members of certain religions, people who are gay, lesbian, bisexual, or transgendered all experience health-care disparities. Research in discrimination provides strong evidence that perceived and actual discrimination directly affects the physical and mental health of members of target groups. The aim of this section on health disparities is to summarize research on how social-psychological and communicative processes can produce health-care disparities. Addressing social-psychological and communicative processes as connected to health-care disparities positions health care within a broader social and economic framework but still keeps the focus on close relationship implications central to this volume. The focus on generalizable psychological and communicative processes should apply to other forms of bias beyond those involving race or ethnicity.

BIAS IN HEALTH AND ILLNESS DISPARITIES

Research shows that throughout the world people who are racial or ethnic minorities typically receive poorer health care than people who are members of the racial or ethnic majority groups. In the United States, the health status of people who self-identify as black and/or African or Afro-Caribbean American is worse than the health status of people who self-identify as white (National Center for Health Statistics, 2015). Racial minority patients receive less appropriate health care in general medicine and in the treatment of specific diseases. These disparities cut across specific mental and physical diseases and across health-care settings (Institute of Medicine, 2003). In the United States, issues around health-care disparities have received more attention in both the medical and social-psychological literatures than in other countries, and social psychologists have a long-standing interest in racial bias research (Penner et al., 2013). Research in the United States provides strong evidence that minority patients face issues about whether their race or ethnicity affects the kind of health care they receive. Wide differences exist between racial and ethnic groups in access to health care and availability of health insurance; in addition, medical research shows that racial and ethnic minority patients tend to receive lower-quality health care than non-minorities, even when they have the same type of health insurance (Institute of Medicine, 2003). The organization and delivery structure of health-care systems pose barriers to minority patients' ability to access care. Policies and practices that might be designed to keep costs down can hurt minority patients. For example, financial incentives to physicians to limit the number of expensive tests or procedures may differentially affect patients who are least educated about their treatment options and are least likely to push their doctor for additional health-care services (Institute of Medicine, 2003). In addition, health-care plans may not cover professional interpreters or translation services for patients whose first language is not English.

Health-care providers' biases, prejudices, and uncertainty when treating people from minority groups can contribute to health-care disparities. Health-care providers' attitudes and beliefs may influence the quality of patient care, even when providers are not consciously aware they are treating minority patients differently (Institute of Medicine, 2003). Privately financed health care and health insurance does not fully account for health and health-care disparities. Unequal treatment is well documented in the United States, but health-care disparities also exist in countries with government-supported health-care systems, such as Canada, Israel, New Zealand, Sweden, Serbia, and many Latin American countries. Health-care disparities among racial and ethnic minorities and majorities represent a ubiquitous multinational problem (Penner et al., 2013). Racial biases and discrimination covary with other factors. For example, in many countries socioeconomic status strongly covaries with race such that people who are racial minorities on average have lower socioeconomic status than people who are racial majorities (Penner et al., 2013). People with lower socioeconomic status might not be able to take time off work to seek medical care or to afford health insurance or copayments. Socioeconomic status is important in that the root of chronic illnesses like diabetes and hypertension cannot be distinguished from stresses in lifestyle. Statistically controlling for socioeconomic status does not eliminate health-care disparities (Cooper et al., 2012). Socioeconomic status is a cause of health-care disparities but not a sufficient explanation for racial health-care disparities reported throughout the world

(Penner et al., 2013). Language proficiency and language barriers faced by immigrants also play a role in health-care disparities among people who belong to racial minority groups (Penner et al., 2013). Cultural misunderstandings can exist beyond the language problems such that patients' understanding of their illness may be different from the provider's perspective. Without language and cultural understanding, the diagnosis and treatment plan may not be well suited to patients' needs.

Health literacy, or the degree to which people have the capacity to obtain, process, and understand health information and services they need, and to make well-informed health-care decisions, also provides additional challenges. The jargon and complexities of medical information and the unfamiliar terms pose difficulty and challenges. People with low literacy or low health literacy may experience such intimidation and discouragement that they do not disclose their limited understanding and may be reluctant to seek health care. In the United States, low health literacy often exists alongside race (Cooper, Hill, & Powe, 2002). When controlling for health literacy, the size of health-care disparities decreases, but disparities still remain.

Research provides evidence for intersectionality of discrimination attributes. In other words, the co-occurrence of multiple forms of discrimination is well documented. The prevalence and deleterious health effects of racial discrimination among adults has been well documented. Theoretical and empirical evidence connected to bullying and discrimination in youth is also documented. Research using latent class analysis illustrates the intersections of discrimination attributes and bullying among youth (Garnett et al., 2014). Compared to the low-discrimination class, individuals in the sexual orientation discrimination class and the intersectional class had higher odds of engaging in deliberate self-harm; individuals in the intersectional class also had higher odds of suicidal ideation; all of the discrimination latent classes had significantly higher depressive symptoms compared to the low-discrimination class (Garnett et al., 2014).

Black patients also tend to receive more life-prolonging care and less comfort-directed care at the end of life than white patients. Life-prolonging care includes such care as resuscitation, intensive care admission, and feeding tubes, while comfort-directed care includes hospice care. A multi-institutional prospective longitudinal cohort study of white and black advanced cancer patients indicated that communication goals were important in understanding health-care interventions (Mack et al., 2010). End-of-life discussions between physicians and their white patients were associated with less life-prolonging end-of-life care; more black patients than white patients received life-prolonging care, despite similar rates of end-of-life dis-cussions (Mack et al., 2010). End-of-life discussions were associated with the attainment of some communication goals among black patients, including placement of "do not resuscitate" orders, but these communicative goals were not consistently associated with end-of-life care received by black patients (Mack et al., 2010). For example, black patients with "do not resuscitate" orders were no less likely than black patients without these orders to receive life-prolonging care. Results indicate that end-of-life discussions and communication goals appear to assist white patients in receiving less life-prolonging care at the end of life (Mack et al., 2010). However, black patients tend to receive life-extending measures even when they have stated a clear pre-ference for symptom-directed care (Mack et al., 2010). These findings raise concerns that black patients receive inferior end of life care, a possibility underscored by black–white disparities in other aspects of health care.

MULTIPLE-LEVEL PROCESSES IN HEALTH-CARE DISPARITIES

Health-care disparities at the societal level include increased stress due to difficult social environments, to widespread discrimination, and to difficulty accessing high-quality medical care (Institute of

Medicine, 2003). At the societal level, widespread biases and discrimination are related to historical, societal, economic, and structural factors that result in certain groups such as racial and ethnic minority groups experiencing persistent and widespread unfair treatment and institutionalized discrimination on a variety of realms (Penner et al., 2013). Feelings of being the target of discrimination may serve as a life stressor in addition to challenging social and institutional constraints that prevent some people from receiving the same quality of health care as people living in resource-rich neighborhoods.

Intrapersonal thoughts and feelings that operate within the person can translate into health-care disparities through both explicit and implicit processes. For example, race-related thoughts and feelings of minority patients and non-minority physicians about past racial discrimination may affect the kind of medical care they seek, what they think of the care they receive, the health behaviors in which they engage, and their reactions to interactions with health-care providers (Penner et al., 2013). Race bias and stereotyping among physicians may affect their diagnosis and treatment decisions and their reactions to racial minority patients (Penner et al., 2013). Interpersonal processes in the medical interactions between patients from one ethnic or racial group and physicians from another racial group concern what patients and physicians do and say during the interaction and how they react to each other's words and actions. This is an especially important aspect of racial health-care disparities in the United States and across the world because racial minority patients are much more likely to engage in racially discordant medical interactions (e.g., black patient with a white physician) (Haider, Sriram, & Cooper, 2011). People from racial minority groups are also dramatically underrepresented in medical school and medical practice (Nunez-Smith et al., 2012). Black patients report higher-quality care and greater satisfaction with the interaction when the physician is black than when the physician is white (Haider et al., 2011). Racial minorities may experience negative perceptions of physicians and negative reactions to the interaction.

The social and historical racism and racial discrimination that are part of the past and sometimes the present cannot be dismissed from understanding the potential mistrust in medical interactions between black patients and white physicians. In the United States and Europe, the theory of polygenism, that human races were separate biological species, was part of scientific theory until as recently as the early twentieth century (Byrd & Clayton, 2002). Blacks, Latinos, and other socially disadvantaged racial minority groups were also frequently used as participants in dangerous medical experiments without their willing consent and with little regard to their welfare (Byrd & Clayton, 2002). The minority patients' negative perceptions of physicians may be at least connected to mistrust of general medical care that is rooted in harsh and potentially tragic historical realities (Earnshaw et al., 2013). Mistrust can be a rational response to a system that has ill-served racial minorities in the past.

INTERGROUP ORIENTATION AND RACE

Social categorization and social identity (Tajfel & Turner, 1979) also set a foundation for an intergroup context and theory for what racial minority patients feel and think about their medical care and their health care-related behavior and for what majority group physicians think and feel about racial minority patients. In racially discordant interactions, physicians and patients who may only be minimally acquainted with each other prior to the interaction react to each other in an exchange that involves considerable dialogue and vulnerability and uncertainty, and the interaction may represent a type of intergroup contact (Penner et al., 2013). Intergroup encounters are experiences where people are likely to behave (or to be perceived to behave) in terms of their social group membership more than as individuals. According to intergroup theories, social categorization and social identity serve as a process of categorization and application of social categories to evaluations, perceptions, and treatment of others. Minority group members are particularly vigilant about cues to bias from outgroup members, as their identity as a member of a racial minority group that has been the target of prejudice and discrimination is salient (Penner et al., 2013).

Expectations of prejudice or discrimination among minority patients plays an important role in intergroup encounters, particularly in medicine, where they worry they will be the target of prejudice or that they will confirm negative stereotypes associated with their racial groups (Penner et al., 2013). One source of racial minority patients' possible negative reactions to the health-care system may be expectations they will experience stereotyping, prejudice, or discrimination in their medical care. This stereotype threat through activation can trigger stereotype-confirming behavior that may have detrimental effects on the responses of racial minorities to health-care interventions that might reinforce these stereotypes (Penner et al., 2013). For example, some black patients could be reluctant to participate in classes that provide health information (e.g., cancer screening, diabetes care, prenatal care) because they fear (even subconsciously) that this would reinforce stereotypes about their intellectual abilities and educational achievements (Penner et al., 2013). In the context of provider–patient interactions, identity as a member of a racial minority group that has been the target of prejudice and discrimination is highly salient. Perceptions of general discrimination, including experiences of bias outside the medical encounter and in everyday life, can also affect reactions to individual medical interactions. In a sample of black patients at an inner-city health-care clinic, over half of the patients reported they had experienced discrimination or unfair treatment in the past in at least one social domain including jobs, education, medical treatment, job applications, police encounters, housing, and dealing with neighbors (Penner et al., 2013). In a follow-up mail survey, black patients who reported experiencing high levels of past discrimination expressed significantly less satisfaction with their medical interaction with the physician they had just seen, compared with black patients who reported relatively little past discrimination (Penner et al., 2013).

Within the medical profession, explicit expressions of racial bias are especially rare and behavior that indicates bias in medical care is widely and vigorously condemned (Penner et al., 2010). However, evidence of more subtle, often unintentional, contemporary race bias is likely manifest (Penner et al., 2013). Physicians' implicit indications of preferences for white patients relative to black patients can be manifest in subtle behaviors as well as in physicians making more aggressive and appropriate treatment recommendations for a white patient than for a black patient (Penner et al., 2013). For example, discourse analysis of transcribed discussions of clinical trials with matched socioeconomic samples of black and white patients provided evidence that physicians overall used more words in the discussions with white patients and said more words specifically about clinical trials (1,867 vs. 1,090 words); furthermore, physicians spoke more about the purpose of the study and about risks to white than black patients (Eggly et al., 2015). A similar study indicated that black cancer patients were less likely than white cancer patients to receive important general information in oncology settings. Specifically, black cancer patients asked fewer questions than white patients, and fewer of the questions they did ask were direct questions that place the burden on the physician to respond (e.g., "Will I lose my hair if I have chemotherapy?") (Eggly et al., 2011). The differences in the nature of the interpersonal exchanges in racially discordant physician–patient interactions may stem from implicit bias (Penner et al., 2013). This is consistent with Cooper et al.'s (2012) research indicating that higher implicit physician attitude bias was associated with less positive affect and poorer ratings of interpersonal care from black patients. A communication-based intervention intended to help individuate racial minority cancer patients in the eyes of their oncologists includes providing minority patients with a list of questions they might ask their non-minority oncologists during discussions of their treatment, and patients are given advice on asking more questions about their specific treatment (Eggly et al., 2013). The intervention is intended to activate more individuated impressions of minority patients during the interactions. The intended result is that treatment decisions will be more likely based on the particular characteristics of the individual patient than stereotypes about the group to which the patient belongs.

INTERGROUP COMMUNICATION AND HEALTH DISPARITIES FOR PEOPLE WITH DISABILITIES

People with disabilities have more health problems (U.S. Census Bureau, 2001), are in poorer health (U.S. Census Bureau, 2001), are at an increased risk for preventable secondary health conditions that arise from their disability (U.S. Department of Health and Human Services, 2000), and utilize more health-care services than the non-disabled (D. C. Thomas, 1999). Similarly, people with disabilities in the United States report that they are less likely to avail themselves of preventive health services (U.S. Department of Health and Human Services, 2000), and are less likely to receive health behavior counseling and wellness counseling than able-bodied individuals.

These biased attitudes, then, negatively impact the quality of health care that people with disabilities receive. For example, women with disabilities are less likely to be screened for breast cancer (Schootman & Jeffe, 2003). Health-care professionals are frequently ignorant of sexuality and maternity issues as they relate to people with disabilities (Frank, 2000). They also lack knowledge in other areas (e.g., availability of assistive aid and devices) and are poorly prepared to make appropriate referrals to other physicians and specialists. In interactions with health providers, people with disabilities report challenges including failures to accommodate communication needs, erroneous perceptions of the underlying condition or of the role of assistive technology, and assumptions about how the disability affects daily living (Cumella & Martin, 2004). For people with disabilities, everyday encounters with family, friends and health-care providers may feel defined in terms of group membership. Able-bodied individuals in encounters with people with disabilities may communicate with a person with a disability as if the disability frames the interaction. Similarly, people with disabilities may interpret communicative behaviors through the lens of group membership affiliated with a disability group. An intergroup understanding helps explain the challenges people with disabilities describe about navigating relationships and interpersonal encounters, such that people respond to the disability more than responding to individual attributes (Duggan, Robinson, & Thompson, 2012).

Disability shapes and is shaped by communication. Physical or mental disability serves as a social identity whereby perception of the disability rather than unique individual features are seen as salient. Intergroup communication exchanges can occur when either individual perceives the disability as a salient feature, or where communicative messages indicate the salience of the disability (Duggan et al., 2012). Disability has a wide range of meaning and manifestations. Disability may necessitate a physical adaptation (e.g., using a guide dog for blindness), may be a cognitive issue (e.g., requiring adaptation to default models of teaching or learning), may involve a developmental diagnosis (e.g., delays in child development), or may involve an acquired need for adaptation as part of the aging process (e.g., following a stroke or hearing-loss event, or transitioning into needing a walker or wheelchair). Disability is not a neutral term, but instead reflects a complicated, socially constructed concept fraught with value-laden assumptions (Canary, 2008). In intergroup terms, able-bodied people may treat a person who happens to have a disability as if the limitation is central to the identity of the person, rather than responding to the many individual features also unique to the person with a disability (Duggan et al., 2012).

DISABILITY SALIENCE IN CLOSE RELATIONSHIPS

The salience of disability is evident in close relationships. Many people with disabilities describe a sense of estrangement within their families and articulate ways that their sense of self-acceptance is related to how friends and family members react to their disability. Parents often do not understand the nature of their children's disabilities but continue to try to do so; they also indicate that a perplexing aspect of their children with disabilities is that the same children are in many ways not disabled (Canary, 2008). These parents note that one manifestation of the puzzling nature of their children's disabilities is a lack of communication about disability within the family as a whole, such that the disability is not something to discuss with other children even though it may be the focus of negative evaluations and teasing. Mothers of children with cerebral palsy also describe worrying about the child, particularly about how their relationships and the child's other relationships are affected by lack of communication outside the family (Power, McManus, & Fourie, 2009). Similarly, mothers describe strong emotional investment in the child's communicative progress and making sacrifices; the communication challenges may be seen as more important than physical problems. The focus on disability rather than ability can shape existing relationships and pose hardships in forming new relationships. For example, children with disabilities are often ignored socially, and loneliness and isolation are recurring themes in the literature. Spouses of aphasia patients, who lose language ability following brain injury, may compensate by speaking for their spouse (Croteau & Le Dorze, 2006). This overprotection is associated with an over-controlling caregiving style, negative affect, and resentment (Thompson et al., 2002). Social isolation and loneliness are common experiences for people with disabilities. This may result from problems with communication, difficulties in developing friendships and maintaining social relationship, and/or a tendency to rely on staff as friends (Ballin & Balandin, 2007).

COMMUNICATION ACCOMMODATION AND HEALTH DISPARITIES

An intergroup perspective suggests that a focus on relationship and emotional needs may be helpful in shifting from an intergroup orientation to responding to interpersonal characteristics (Watson & Gallois, 1998). In turn, the extent to which patients are able to interact with health professionals as *individuals,* rather than as only professionals, is a key determinant of satisfaction with the interaction. Patients describing satisfactory conversations indicate that their health professionals view them in abstract, positive terms, suggesting low intergroup bias (Watson & Gallois, 2002). Paying attention to disability means acknowledging the limitations of humanity, where people with disabilities show some limits more clearly and know them better than most, and are at once vulnerable, adaptable, and strong (Ferris, 2009).

Adapting communication to people with disabilities can be seen as a tension between dominant group discourse used as control management to keep "others" in place (Braithwaite & Eckstein, 2003) or, in contrast, empowering exchanges by emphasizing "person first" language and discourse about the person as a whole. Communication accommodation theory describes and explains the ways people modify their verbal and nonverbal communication based on the situation (Giles, Reid, & Harwood, 2010). Communication messages are shaped and defined by social identity, and communication accommodation theory explains speech in encounters between people with and without disabilities (Fox & Giles, 1997). Consequently, a person may behave in ways that reduce the communicative differences in interactions and adopt or imitate some of the other person's communicative behaviors. Behaviors associated with increased likelihood of acceptance by high-status individuals are described as convergence, achieved through similarity in verbal and nonverbal styles or messages. However, when a person interacts with someone believed to be of a lower social status, that person may desire to maintain or increase communicative differences between them. Instead of adopting the communicative partner's behaviors, the person may behave in ways that are different so they are not judged as being similar to the partner. If that person's communicative partner is of a lower social status (such as being a member of a group that is not socially desirable), the person may behave differently from the conversational partner to maintain or increase the social distance between them. Sometimes people accommodate or adjust their linguistic and nonverbal behavior in face-to-face conversations as a conscious strategy to gain approval from or influence the other communicant and sometimes accommodation occurs without a person's conscious awareness (Giles, Coupland, & Coupland, 1991; Giles et al., 2010).

Divergence emphasizes differentiation between the communication of the individuals (Williams, 1999) and is described as demonstrating differences from the "other." Physicians, for instance, who use different language from patients with disabilities, particularly by attributing "sickness" instead of using the patient label of "disability," would be diverging. Maintenance can occur when individuals resist change in communication.

Physicians who believe that there is nothing that they can do if a cure is not possible may under-accommodate to patients with disabilities by indicating uneasiness, avoidance, and low rapport. Conversely, physicians may intentionally display smiling, leaning forward, and using a wide range of vocal inflection, behaviors sometimes described as "faking good," in attempts to be socially appropriate (Thomas et al., 2003). These otherwise positive behaviors may extend beyond the boundaries of expected accommodation, and instead may result in over-accommodation through pity; this can leave individuals feeling "infantilized" (Duggan et al., 2011).

Communication *toward* and *about* people with disabilities can shape outcomes, including social identity, health consequences, and access to care. Outcomes of communication are evident across types of disability and across the life span of people with disabilities. Individuals who face disability as a result of a traumatic brain injury report losing friends, and they engage in more task-oriented than social conversation (Kilov, Togher, & Grant, 2009). Individuals who develop hearing impairment also may face challenges in terms of perceptions of their success in conversations and may miss specific content in their attempts to repair conversation breakdown (Lind, Hickson, & Erber, 2006). In the co-construction of identity, what it means to be disabled is created not just in the narratives told by the persons with disabilities themselves. There is co-constructions with significant others, with personnel working with them, and with societal-level systems (Antelius, 2009).

In a much more positive light, intergroup explanations provide potential for envisioning disability as a cornerstone example for bringing theory development to social application through individual, social, and community opportunities to understand and respond to intergroup messages in ways that build empowerment and vitality. Independent living provides a social structure resulting from in-group members' initiatives and determination to positively reframe and refocus the potential predicament, essentially bringing social structure that illustrates the theoretical construct of group vitality. The philosophy of independent living replaces the concepts of integration and rehabilitation with a paradigm developed by people with disabilities (Independent Living Institute, 2005). Invoking an intergroup lens, independent living could be called creative reframing that promotes group vitality. Today, independent living attracts people whose daily lives depend on some assistance, and provides social and physical structure to take initiative individually and collectively to advocate and promote better solutions. It also allows for political positing to promote the equal rights of participation, options, freedoms, control, and self-determination that able-bodied individuals take for granted. Many centers for independent living are organized and run by people with disabilities, and a primary foundation is peer support to develop coping and intervention strategies. Affiliated individuals work with local and regional leaders to build infrastructure that addresses necessary modifications, to increase awareness of disability as a natural part of the human condition, and to promote equal opportunities for people with disabilities. Thus, independent living provides a model for understanding that intergroup communication need not be negative, and in fact can be a cornerstone for vitality. Instead, understanding intergroup communication offers an opportunity to recognize the ways messages are inherently laden with assumptions, and the ways we can be more mindful of the implications of our messages.

5 Reconsidering Embodiment and Language for Illness

COMPLEX INTERRELATIONSHIP OF MIND AND BODY

Romantic love provides us with a window into the complex interrelationship between our minds and bodies ... On the physical level, we trade bits of ourselves when we make love to our partner, absorbing one another's energy and identity. Rejection from a lover generates a painful physical manifestation in every molecule of our being. A scorned lover describes their pain as crushing, crippling – the feeling of being emotionally punched in the stomach. Just as love has the power to create a sensation of physical pain, so too can it heal the physical body in the most astounding of ways.

Healthy romantic and compassionate love allows space for the brain to expand, heal and evolve. We stand up tall, radiate warmth and move around our world with the grace and poise that only a person in the grips of love can exude. When love hurts, fear and pain force us to close the doors of compassion, as we hunker down and physically shield ourselves in an act of emotional self-preservation. Our bodies constrict; we avoid eye contact; and we disappear into the dark thoughts and insecurities within.

– Ottenstein, 2015. "The Mind-Body Connection on Love."

WHAT THE BODY KNOWS, BUT MEDICINE CANNOT NAME

I remember that soon after my mother died I developed a case of frozen shoulder, technically called adhesive capsulitis, in my left shoulder. It causes stiffness and pain in the shoulder joint and often occurs for no known reason. My doctor had told me that because my shoulder was "frozen," there must be adhesions, or scar tissue that were freezing up my shoulder joint. And probably my body lacked something called synovial fluid, needed to lubricate the shoulder joint. I asked him what caused this to happen. He could not say, because medicine does not really understand why it happens. He referred me for physical therapy.

I like to understand why things happen the way they do, and he could not tell me. But I was in pain. I could not sleep in my usual position. I couldn't reach for something on a shelf without feeling pain. So I made an appointment for a physical therapy evaluation for treatment. As I lay on the examining table, the physical therapist came in, smiled, introduced herself and explained what she was going to do. As soon as she put her warm hands on my shoulder, tears welled up in my eyes. I was surprised and embarrassed and turned my head away from her gaze so that she would not see. I suspect she noticed. She continued examining me, and I found that I enjoyed it. It felt like a massage, something I am not used to having. She recommended that I come in three times a week, and I had to arrange my schedule to do that. She did various exercises with me that I was advised to do at home. As I followed her instructions, I thought and felt a great deal about my mother, with whom I had a complex and ambivalent relationship. I stretched and cried, cried and stretched, wrote about what I was feeling, and after a few months I was better. The pain of my loss had lodged itself in my body, and a woman's warm touch started to release it. It also probably released some oxytocin in me, the hormone of love and attachment. As I mourned her loss over several months, I realized something. I had had a hard time crying for my mother, whom I loved very much but whom I was angry with too. When there are difficulties in mourning a loss, somatic or psychological difficulties may present themselves. The therapist's warm touch on my shoulder was lubrication for my soul, needed for me to let go and feel the loss, complicated and ambivalent as it was.

– Farber, 2013. "The Mind-Body Connection: Why We All Need to Be Touched."

The idea of physical connection through romantic love and sex, and of rejection from love as physical pain, exists in poetry and song and in notions of feeling love in the heart, as the first illustration above indicates. But the illustration also indicates the power of healing in the physical body, with an image of love as giving space for the brain to heal and expand, a contrast to the restrictive and hurtful physical feeling when we feel rejection in romantic love. As indicated in this passage, romantic love as connected to (or rejected from) physical sensation, including sex, taps into a sort of knowing, a "physical manifestation in every molecule of our being." The first illustration is consistent with popular notions of the physical sense of romantic love. The second illustration indicates more mystery, a knowing that exists in the body, but where we do not yet have language or understanding to connect what happens in the body with theoretical or empirical constructs. The second illustration of holding pain in the physical body is resonant with the conceptualization I propose in this chapter, where embodiment encompasses complexities that exceed the understanding for which we have language.

In this chapter, I reconsider theoretical foundations for the concept of embodiment to show how the experience of the physical and emotional notions in the body connect to health and illness in close relationships and how language shapes conceptualization and understanding of health and illness. I illustrate how research on illness in medicine and relationship science sometimes reveals dualism and body alienation in the concepts of self and body and in the language of illness and disease. Dualism is observed in biomedical illness diagnosis and treatment that focuses on symptoms such that the body is conceived and described in language implying a material object to which the self happens to be attached. I illustrate how the relational and embodied experiences of people living with illness or disability indicate a more fundamental intertwining of body and self than biomedical language currently indicates.

THE PHYSICAL BODY IN PERSONAL RELATIONSHIPS

Close relationship processes involve both the body and the mind; stories of how we "feel" in our emotional state and in our body illustrate an instinctive knowledge of the intimate and dynamic relationship between our feelings and our thoughts, and what happens in the body. This connection between mind and body, between what we feel in our physical selves and how we make sense of relationships, leaves much that has not yet been addressed in research. When we consider illness as inherently manifest in the body, we introduce yet another element to the physical self as interconnected to relationships during illness trajectories and experiences.

A special issue on mind–body connections in *Personal Relationships* in 2011 brought together empirical contributions by researchers from a wide variety of disciplinary backgrounds to high-light research in this domain. The editors of the special issue on mind–body connections, Timothy Loving and Lorne Campbell, outline how close relationship scholars are in a prime position to contribute to a holistic understanding of the mechanisms underlying the reciprocal association between close relationships and physical and psychologi-cal functioning (Loving & Campbell, 2011). The science to provide evidence for pathways linking close relationship process and the phy-sical body does not yet provide a cohesive picture.

I begin by addressing the strengths of what close relationship researchers have to offer as addressed in social science. As the editors of the special issue note, research investigating mind–body connec-tions in the context of close relationships represents a particularly robust example of the benefits of interdisciplinary research for expanding the field of close relationships in novel and exciting direc-tions (Loving & Campbell, 2011). The articles feature the interdisci-plinary nature of the work on mind–body connections in personal relationships as allowing cross-fertilization of ideas. The editors refer back to the general idea that the personal relationships context in studying mind–body interactions can be traced back to René Descartes' theory of mind–body dualism and the six passions, "most of which can be easily stirred in interpersonal contexts" (Loving & Campbell, 2011). Over three centuries later, research in close relation-ships regularly integrates biological, physiological, or neurological measures through particular biomarkers such as cortisol and mea-sures of brain activity through functional magnetic resonance imaging (fMRI). Close relationship researchers have added a level of sophisti-cation to the empirical agenda in theoretical frameworks, methodolo-gical paradigms, and statistical tools contributing to the study of mind-body connections (Loving & Campbell, 2011).

This chapter takes an intentional theoretical leap beyond cur-rent conceptualizations and measures in proposing that the physical body serves as a more holistic way of knowing and processing than currently addressed in relationship theories or empirical measures. To the extent that this "advances in personal relationships" series proposes stretching beyond what we already know, this chapter proposes a broader consideration of embodiment in order that "what the body knows" can be addressed as one mechanism underlying the reciprocal association between close relationships and physical and psychological functioning.

EMBODIMENT: A BROADER CONCEPTION THAN THE PHYSICAL BODY

The foundation of this chapter rests in the tenant that the physical body "holds" and enables the experience of illness just as the physical body enables touch and sexual expressiveness. The language used to talk about health and illness and to talk about relationships holds consequences and opportunities for understanding. This chapter explicates the concept of embodiment in health and illness and in close relationships and illustrates the need for a broader and more holistic understanding that integrates biomarkers and brain activity but that also considers how the body holds information that is not captured in current measures. This chapter describes ideas about the philosophy of illness and outlines how manifestations of the physical body serve as a different disruption to life and to relationships than other experienced disruptions. Based on ideas of illness experiences in the body, I explain how illness as experienced in our bodies can displace our assumptions about ourselves and our close relationships.

By illness, I intend to refer to a serious, chronic, and life-changing ill-health. A cold or infection does not pose the same implications for the physical body as a serious illness. The experience of illness onset is tied to recognizing a disease or physiological dysfunction. The illness experience includes making meaning of one's symptoms and bodily changes including pain, as well as navigating the health-care system. Moreover, the social experience of illness includes sense-making around engaging with social attitudes toward illness and disability, and negotiating close relationships with bodily changes connected to illness and choices in treatment.

Embodiment, the experience of living in a body, is a fundamental characteristic of human experience. A foundational assumption in explicating embodiment in this chapter is that the experiences within the body in perceiving and interacting in the world cannot be disentangled from cognitive knowledge or understanding. Consistent with philosopher Maurice Merleau-Ponty's (1964) emphasis on the *body* as the primary site of knowing the world, this chapter describes illness as an example of embodiment such that the body, and that which it perceives, cannot be disentangled from each other. As a social science volume, I do not intend to describe the richer complications of whether philosophy is intended to prepare us for illness and ultimately for death. Questions of meaning, priorities, values, and personal quest connected to illness are well documented in medical anthropology, qualitative health-care research, medical sociology, philosophy, and health psychology. Addressing embodiment in this chapter provides broader context for experiences of *being* in a body in close relationships, how those experiences shift with illness, and how the potential dualism between self and body poses complications for the social science of relationships.

UNDERSTANDING ILLNESS AS LIVED EXPERIENCE

The lived experience of illness is broader than the physiological processes of disease and dysfunction that fall within the domain of medical science. Although language to distinguish between illness and disease poses different consequences and opportunities, the physical embodiment of illness cannot be fully disentangled from the measures of symptoms and objectification of disease progression.

Illness is an intense lived experience that holds meaning more broadly than the measureable systems and functions of the body. Stories and poetry about illness provide glimpses into the intensity of the illness experience and how illness can challenge and shatter the values and beliefs assumed to be stable before the illness experience. Illness can be physically and emotionally draining. Illness can challenge our concept of self and abilities. Illness can challenge our beliefs and assumptions about our closest relationships. Illness requires us to adapt to physical restrictions, to experiences of pain, to being probed and prodded and touched in ways considered extremely invasive outside the context of medicine. Illness brings questions of mortality to the forefront. Illness can require sustained labor, attention, life changes, and ongoing emotional adjustment. Illness can challenge assumptions of the self. Conversely, a person can have a chronic illness or disability and not consider himself or herself to be physically ill.

Questions of lived experience. Considering illness as a lived experience connects the social science questions posed so far in this volume with questions about how physical and emotional embodiment of illness are different from other intense life experiences or from other major changes to close relationships. In addition, considering illness as a lived experience invites us to consider how social scientific questions fit with the social dimensions of philosophical questions (Carel, 2016).

Illness is a qualitatively complex experience that shapes the experience of being in the world and of being embodied as we interact in the world. Illness can be a philosophical tool for considering profoundly complex questions posed by the lived experience of illness such as the belief that a longer life is better than a shorter one; that is, whether the value of life depends on its duration (Carel, 2009). A common initial reaction to illness diagnosis is a sense of meaninglessness and despair. Challenges of illness can prompt philosophical tools about human existence that normally go unnoticed; a tacit sense of bodily certainty only comes to our attention when it is disrupted and replaced by bodily doubt (Carel, 2013). As such, illness can function as a philosophical tool for challenging previously held beliefs and shedding light on the structure and meaning of human existence and experience as connected to the body. Illness can prompt a person to reflect on questions of vulnerability, morbidity, and mortality and to be more open to questions in the future (Carel, 2015).

The embodied existence and experiences of illness can reveal dimensions of human life sometimes overlooked by broadening the spectrum of embodied experience into the pathological domain and in the process shedding light on assumptions about longevity, capability, and autonomy (Carel, 2014; Carel & Kidd, 2014). Illness as lived experience poses a form of philosophical question that is uninvited and unanticipated and can feel threatening. Philosophical methods have been used to study illness for decades, but considering illness as physical manifestation of understanding reverses the questions already asked; to that end, illness modifies, and thus sheds light on, normal experience, revealing its ordinary and therefore overlooked structure (Carel, 2014; Carel & Kidd, 2014).

Experiencing illness also alters how we think about ethical and moral issues including our inner compass for engaging in everyday life and how we companion people who are close to us through their trajectories with serious illness. People who are close to us do things to address physical aspects of illness that would provoke reasonable disgust in everyday interactions. In illness, people engage with the physical body in close relationships in ways that would otherwise be taboo and uncomfortable.

Meaning-making in the body. Over the years, people come to "know" their body's peculiarities, to understand the body's needs and language. Though there are many changes that occur in a body over the life course, such as during adolescence, pregnancy, menopause, and aging, and these have identity implications, people have a sense of "knowing one's body" (Corbin, 2003). The self becomes the vehicle through which people experience sensations anchored in meaning (Corbin, 2003). Through sensations in the body, people know how their own body reacts to stress, how much they can do before becoming fatigued, and what happens when they eat too much or play too hard (Corbin, 2003). People learn to trust their body's language, or at least to engage in the body with what people learn as normative experience over time. When something is wrong, people talk about a change in sensations or appearance, such as "having difficulty climbing stairs" or "not feeling good." The word "symptoms" is an outsider's labeling of what people are interpreting: a medical interpretation, a bio-based language of what is happening in a body (DiGiacomo, 1992). Illness challenges the feelings of trusting in the body as well as the host of assumptions and planning that depend on trusting the body and knowing what to expect in the body.

What happens in the body connects to the self. People rarely say "my body had a heart attack" or "my body has cancer," but instead "I had a heart attack" or "I have cancer" (Corbin, 2003). Body and self are described as a unit until the body acts, functions, appears, experiences, or emotes differently from how the person has become accustomed to and learned to trust (Corbin, 2003). With illness onset, people describe themselves as more than their body, and this language indicates the person recognizes a split between the body and identity. In other words, with illness onset, people experience bodily doubt.

Bodily doubt. The embodied experience of illness gives physical experience to the breakdown in being able to trust the body, bringing doubt to previous tacit beliefs about bodily abilities and signals and how the body serves as a vehicle for sense-making. Bodily doubt is not just a disturbance of beliefs but a disruption in one's most fundamental sense of being in the world (Carel, 2016). The body feels a physical sense of uncertainty and anxiety, causing one to detach from the physical and social environments and instead to focus on the body. With serious illness, a radical bodily doubt can profoundly change the structure of one's experiences (Carel, 2016). A person can experience bodily doubt about a specific behavior (such as walking up a flight of stairs) without questioning seemingly related behaviors (such as ability to balance). Bodily doubt can invade the sense of normalcy and give way to feeling exposed and threatened and vulnerable. Bodily doubt is different from questioning bodily failures such as tripping or feeling exhausted at the end of a week of working, or failing to learn a dance move. Bodily doubt instead is an experience of more serious embodied doubt about body capabilities and sensations normally taken for granted (Carel, 2016). Bodily doubt is making meaning of doubt itself as experienced in the body, and the doubt is different from irrational or disconnected doubt such as in anxiety disorders. Bodily doubt is appropriate for the situation of explanation and expression of illness. Bodily doubt is the experience of vulnerability as the unpredictability in assumptions.

Bodily doubt can be considered part of serious illness and an indication of the transition from health (bodily capacity and trust in listening to the body) to illness, bringing questions of doubt and hesitation consistent with changed content in experiences. The body's taken-for-granted capacities become explicit achievements. The body becomes understood in terms of limits and this may lead to loss of spontaneity and changed meaning of routine tasks.

EMBODIMENT OF ILLNESS SENSATIONS

Illness is manifest in the body. With illness, sensations of the body are not anchored in the meaning that used to be familiar. The healthy body might be considered *transparent* in that it does not pose ongoing questions but is interpreted as neutral and tacit and taken for granted (Carel, 2016). The transparent healthy body makes sense as a whole; we do not experience the healthy body as explicitly the focus of our attention. The sensations experienced in the body are not the focus of everyday careful observation. The healthy body is essentially characterized by absence of careful thematic attention to experience; the healthy body can be understood with silence, as the vehicle through which we experience everyday functioning but not as the focus of attention to the experience. Although people have narrower experiences with the healthy body as explicit attention such as during exercise or sex, the body functions as the background for moment-to-moment attentiveness and toward the goal or action, such as completing the race or connecting intimately with our sexual partner. The body is not absent but functions as the vehicle for experience rather than the explicit focus of the experience.

When something goes wrong with the body (e.g., a headache, pain, difficulty walking, excessive shortness of breath, or change in appearance on a part of the body), the experience shifts focus such that the malfunction or distinction becomes the focus of attention (Carel, 2016). With serious illness, the harmony between the body and the lived experience is disrupted, and the continuity between everyday interpretation and the body (or some part of the body) feels discontinuous. The bodily disruption modifies one's tacit sense of trust in one's body. Small injuries and small changes in bodily functions are experienced as frustrating or painful but also as benign, but an experience of serious illness that interferes with everyday functioning over time can radically modify self-understanding (Carel, 2016). Serious illness brings embodiment to the forefront and changes a person's habits, abilities to plan or pursue goals, and sense of restricted freedom in the physical self (Carel, 2016).

TIME AND SPACE OF ILLNESS

Illness as an embodied experience is manifest in temporal experiences and spatial relations. The body serves as the medium for experiences of space and time and for unifying sensory experiences to create meaning.

Time. In health, time is scheduled, but it is scheduled around what people want to do with their lives. *Clock time* is open for people to carry out activities as chosen. People can put off an activity because they perceive time will continue to be available (Corbin, 2003). *Historical time* is the story of one's body over time, including developmental changes and wear and tear the body experiences over the years. Historical time also includes family medical history and the genetic factors that are passed down over generations (Corbin, 2003). *Biographical time* includes experiences derived over a lifetime of living the memories and emotions experienced within the body (Corbin, 2003). People sense a biographical continuity about life, past, present, and future. The body has predictable rhythms over the course of the day when it feels tired, hungry, or more energetic.

In illness, clock time is scheduled around time that is free from pain and from fatigue between treatments rather than scheduled around activities of life. Carrying out medical regimens can involve a need to carefully attend to clock time. The amount of time necessary to attend to activities of daily living can take much longer because of associated disabilities and limitations, and the extra time invested in necessary activities can cut into leisure time and more pleasurable creative time (Corbin, 2003). During illness, time is sometimes perceived as closing in; a person might not be certain how much biological time is left and what that time that remains will be like. Time can become more precious and not taken for granted (Corbin, 2003). Time can feel prolonged when confined to bed or to a hospital. Time can pass too quickly when a person is having difficulty attending to the next need. Historical time in illness takes on additional dimensions of the medical history such that illness disrupts biographical time. Comparing the body of the present and the future to the body of the past can lead to a profound sense of loss (Corbin, 2003). Body rhythms can be unpredictable and turned upside down by medical treatment.

As many cancer narratives illustrate, getting the "bad news" divided life into "before" and "after" cancer diagnosis, a time of blissful ignorance of the body, and then a time of fear and vigilance. People may experience ongoing worries about whether the cancer will reappear, possibly in the form of another cancer. Time in medical treatment is not linear or cyclical, but overlapping and unfolding in varying rhythms. Symptoms, diagnosis, illness progression, treatment, and prognosis may repeat rhythms and reoccurrence.

Space. In health, space is not bounded. A person can move through space with ease that is taken for granted. In illness, space can feel bounded and constrained. With illness and disability, spatial arrangements are very important (Corbin, 2003). Sitting up can be a chore, and reaching things can feel like a major accomplishment. Objects need to be within reach, and spaces need to be left open to move through. Sometimes objects are strategically placed so that a person can sit or hold onto the object for assistance.

Consider a person with Parkinson's disease as an example of changes in experiences with space. A person with Parkinson's disease sometimes experiences freezing or motor block, which is a brief inability to start movement or to continue rhythmic movement such as writing or walking. A person with Parkinson's disease might experience a leg feeling stuck or frozen in space, and it can take tremendous concentration to get the leg moving again. The stuck or frozen movement is sometimes also associated with spatial perception such that they bump into obstructions such as doorways; they may widen their base of support and change their gait and take shorter steps when approaching a doorway. People may prefer more space on one side of their body than on the other.

BODY ALIENATION

> Following intermittent abdominal pains and weight loss, my wife was diagnosed with an ovarian cyst, then appendicitis. The original appendectomy was a keyhole procedure and expectation was that she would need to take three days off work. But the operation resulted in a postoperative abscesses, and further surgery to deal with them revealed a tumor and perforated gut that required the removal of two sections of intestine and left a 30cm long incision. That incision became infected and eventually required a vacuum drain during which she was tethered by tubing that ran from her abdomen to an external pump. Infections eventually required seven further procedures to re-open and clean the wound, one of which had to be performed without anesthesia. For several weeks, my partner had an unfamiliar view of the pink and meaty inside of her body. Worse was the smell of infection from the wound and struggling not to assume this meant her body was rotting from the inside out. The pump was the size of a couple of large bricks, and it sucked and wheezed noisily. The pump was constant, noisy, painful, and unwanted, but at the same time was more intimately part of her body than any person around her. It would be a two-month stay in the hospital and a total of 16 weeks before the wound completely closed.
>
> That is not my body; my body is even less me.

– Scully, 2013. "Body Alienation and the Moral Sense of Self."

The passage above indicates a clear sense of body alienation, where we do not understand the self anymore in what we see in our body. In explicating illness as embodiment and considering a holistic view of embodiment, we gain a sense of the concept of bodily doubt. The body alienation experienced in illness can give rise to different estrangement and detachment, to a sense of differentiation between the self and the body. The connection between the body and the self can change in striking and unanticipated ways. The physical and cognitive effort for dealing with the illness and surgeries and physical consequences can give way to a dualism between the body and the self. With illness, people can experience an alienation from what is happening to their bodies. The inherent sense of self as person and embodied agent can become dualities, and language and nonverbal symbols further differentiate between integrated self and symbols indicating differentiation from identity. Medical symbols remove individual identity. For example, consider the backless open gowns patients wear and the symbolic nature of perceiving the self as near naked in the backless gown but in conversation with a surgeon who was a complete stranger just hour earlier.

Serious illness modifies one's entire interaction with objects and with the environment, with one's way of being in the world (Carel, 2014). Consider how even an acute flu disrupts everyday life and what we take for granted in a day. Tacit assumptions fall into abeyance in the case of serious sudden illness; feelings of missing out, being useless, and feeling weak and nauseous expose the underlying sense of participation, purposefulness, and potency that has been disturbed. Although distancing can also occur in bereavement, moving, or divorce, I argue that the physical embodiment and bodily doubt in illness is a different sort of embodied process. Carel (2014) suggests that philosophical methods have been used to study illness for several decades, but she reverses the relationship between philosophical methods and illness and suggests that illness has a philosophical role; she suggests that illness modifies, and thus sheds light on, normal experience, revealing its ordinary and therefore overlooked structure. Consistent with the idea that illness modifies experience, I suggest that illness changes not only the individual understanding of experiences but also the relational understanding of how close relationships are inherently connected to understanding.

One response to the physical experience of illness is to distance oneself from physicality, to see the body as alien, as some secondary experience to the lived body. In illness, the patient's body causes disruption to the sense of self, to the agency of the person (Scully, 2013). Although people still retain the capability of making decisions about treatment or care, self-concept can lurch and shift along with the shifts of the body during the radical instability and invasiveness of medical treatment (Scully, 2013). During treatment, people may lose sense of the physical self. Incisions and technology turn the body into what can feel like a science experiment, into alien terrain. In the medical world, surgery is taken for granted as an intervention into the body. The intrusion into the body integrity and impact on personal identity is not part of the medical conversation. Biomedicine turns body and self into strangers (Scully, 2013).

In health, the body is often conceived as a material object to which the self happens to be attached, but the experiences of individuals living with an illness cannot be accounted for without conceptualizing a more fundamental intertwining of body and self and considering processes and consequences for body alienation during illness. In body alienation, people experience the dualism of the self and body. A dualism, like a dichotomy, is the sense of two different elements, which may live together in an uneasy truce but are frequently in conflict. They are essentially foreign to each other. This sense of dualism is different from duality, or from its parallel term, polarity, in which two harmonious elements essentially belonging together are yet indistinguishable and may exist in creative tension.

DUALITY BETWEEN BIOLOGICAL AND LIVED BODY

In medicine, aspects of the biological body become something to be measured. The science underlying medicine relies on measuring the body as an objective set of systems in order to address a biomedical problem. The experience of illness includes recognizing that something in the body is in question and participating in medical processes where some part(s) of the body are measured as objective indication. Objectification of the measured body brings a dualistic understanding of body and self, or of a rift between biological and lived body. The objectification of the body includes two aspects of dualism. Both aspects of dualism can limit generativity. Awareness of the embodied aspects of the self as experienced in relationships and in illness allows for a more generative opportunity for understanding.

One aspect of dualism is experiencing body as pre-reflective, invisible, or as vehicle of lived experience, in contrast to body as objectified, observed, and measured as object in third-person observation (Merleau-Ponty, 1964). In this lived body/measured body dualism, the person experiences the two different elements of body as vehicle for experience through which people understand the world as unified with body and body as distanced and objectified in order to receive accurate medical inquiry, diagnosis, and treatment. In considering embodiment, I first consider the lived body/measured body aspect of dualism, which is consistent with philosophical explanations of phenomenology of body and phenomenology of body as articulated also in medical anthropology, medical sociology, and medical humanities.

Another aspect of dualism is the body alienation where people disconnect more dramatically from the experiences of the physical body and psychosocial and emotional sense-making, such as described following trauma where the dialogue between the physical body and the psycho-emotional interior landscape becomes disconnected. This aspect of dualism is consistent with the healing and treatment of trauma victims where people try to leave trauma behind but their bodies hold emotions and feelings associated with traumatic experiences (van der Kolk, 2014). In the subsequent section, I describe the second aspect of dualism as articulated in the trauma literature and pose implications for illness and medical intervention as trauma.

BODY AS OBJECTIVELY MEASURED

The duality of the body as lived experience in contrast to body as objectified and measured is illustrated in modern medical treatment. Modern medicine relies on viewing the body as physical object. Health-care professionals are taught to focus on a particular organ or function in order to understand it as a medical object. Medical technology provides objective and sophisticated measures of the body. Internal examination blurs the experience of what is foreign about the body. For example, examining one's intestines gives rise to the passivity of the patient with regard to the body (Carel, 2014).

The body as object is a necessary process of measurement in medical care, but this process means the patient becomes the recipient of reports about his or her own body. For example, the patient sees X-rays as an image of measuring the bone as object or the patient sees a CT scan to measure and illustrate a tumor. Health-care professionals describe to the patient what the health-care professionals see of the patient's body. The patient is not able to access this information experientially through the body (Carel, 2014). These objectifying experiences of measurement may also lead to a sense of alienation from one's body, as to treating the body as an aberrant object over which one has little control; the ill body becomes unloved, feared, and alien (Carel, 2014). The process of measurement and receiving information functions as objectification in addition to the third-party interpretation of the body. Information from tests and measures of dysfunction in the body are *sent to* the health-care professional, but the information is *about* the patient. Thus, the objective measures as process and content fall outside the patient's primary experience. The patient's information becomes content under the ownership of the health-care professionals.

However, people cannot sustain an abstract view of their own body; we cannot actually view ourselves objectively in any sustained sense, and it is unrealistic to expect that of others (Carel, 2014). For the patient, the objective measurements of aspects of the body are just one part of the illness experience. Patients experience the health-care interventions as happening to their body, but still perceive overall illness experiences as happening through their body. The lack of ability to completely reduce the body to objective measures is the subject of ongoing literature and research in medicine and reveals the struggles with integrating biomedical competence with humanistic aspects of understanding people (Gawande, 2014). Ongoing understanding of challenges with health-care provision based in biology and in the body as objectively measured can be understood as challenges of duality when health-care professionals, for example, apologize for cold hands when touching the part of the body being measured (Carel, 2014).

Language also indicates the experience of the physical world as less welcoming, as difficult and full of obstacles for a person with serious illness (Carel, 2014). For example, experiences with "far," "difficult," and "heavy" change their meaning as people become less able to move with ease through distances and spaces they used to take for granted (Carel, 2014). Language indicating "conquering" or "kicking" cancer or other illness is consistent with the dualism of understanding the body as objectively measured but also with the lack of completion of this duality.

PHYSICAL BODY AS DISCONNECTED FROM PSYCHO-EMOTIONAL SENSATIONS

The second potential form of dualism, as identified in the literature on bodily knowing and trauma, is an experience of body alienation where people disconnect the physical body from the psychosocial and emotional sense-making. To understand the second aspect of dualism I illustrate using examples following trauma where people disconnect the sensations experienced in the body from the emotions and feelings associated with traumatic experiences (van der Kolk, 2014). Based on examples from the trauma literature, I propose that the experiences of medical intervention actually function as trauma because of the physical intrusion and strangeness of surgeries, cancer chemotherapies, and other medical interventions.

Drawing on research and examples from combat veterans and on victims of accidents and crimes, Van der Kolk (2014) proposes a neurological process whereby people who experience painful traumatic histories disconnect understanding from embodied experience. For people who survived trauma, neurological processes to monitor for danger remain over-activated such that the slightest sign of danger, whether real or misperceived, can trigger stress responses, intense unpleasant emotions, and overwhelming sensations (van der Kolk, 2014). The body–psycho-emotional connection over time can become muffled. In response to trauma, people may learn to shut down the brain areas that transmit the visceral feeling and emotions that accompany and define terror, but those same brain areas are also responsible for registering the experience of the entire range of emotions and sensations that form the foundation of our self-awareness, our sense of who we are (van der Kolk, 2014). The body adapts to trauma by disassociating from experience so that the intensity of the overwhelming sense of fear and terror and physiological arousal are not constantly activated. From feeling they are regularly in imminent danger, people who experience trauma shut down sensations and feelings through freezing and dissociation (van der Kolk, 2014).

LANGUAGE AND BODY ALIENATION

People in close relationships with survivors of trauma can experience challenges in connecting with the person who experienced the trauma, and closeness and vulnerability may trigger the psycho-emotional disconnect as also manifest in language. Trauma can decrease the ability to accurately detect subtle emotional shifts in close relationships or can leave the person with a heightened sense of tuning into and responding to even the subtlest emotional shifts (van der

Kolk, 2014). People in close relationships can provide friendship and love that give safe space for rebuilding capacity for the person who experienced trauma to reintegrate embodied experience with psycho-emotional sensations. Language can help give more subtle sense of meaning and can reframe to give shared sense of meaning.

The line between duality and dualism, between polarity and dichotomy, sometimes seems hazy. Everyday language reveals some of the challenges with language and the potential consequences of language to label the dualism experienced during illness. One might argue that to speak of my body as an object or possession of the self – "I have a body," "my body," the body as "it" – does not necessarily signal a problem of dualistic division or alienation. This is simply everyday language for distinguishing the parts that are essentially "me." It is possible that language can describe a feeling in the body. But our ordinary language still betrays the potential dualistic threat. It is far easier, for example, to speak of "the personality" as identical with the self than it is to speak of the body and the self as one. People describe being as a personality, as a core identity. People do not have language that seems "natural" for "I am a body." If people experience person-ality (mind, spirit, emotions) as disoriented, then people have lan-guage for describing the "I" aspects of such disorientation. However, we do not have ordinary language for the body as inherently connected to the everyday self. Ordinary language betrays the problem.

In addition to manifestations and language limitations about the embodied self, there is also a physiology of the self–body dualism illustrated in the ways medical language is used to describe health and illness. Medical language describes manifestations of the body that are intended to be measured. However, when considering the broader experience of illness people can know they are unwell but not have symptoms that indicate the root of the ailment. Body aliena-tion can be experienced as self-alienation in a variety of ways that might not be relevant to the medical experience. Body alienation might not translate into a need for therapy or psychiatry or to psycho-somatic illnesses. Body alienation might instead be experienced in not feeling "right" about being in the body. Consider, for example, the language limitations in describing gender as binary or in describing sexuality as binary. In the oversimplification, we miss the opportunity for fluidity, for emergence, for understanding the bodily experience differently from how we have language to do so.

In the alienated body, language and experience can be detached from the potential depth of feelings. The alienated body might feel narrow and controlling, machine-like in its observation and calculation, restricted to language that exists and is used in a known context. To that end, rational explanations for the body might be privileged over emotions. Language might indicate such dichotomized thinking in disassociating measured body from experiential body. The complexities of the person might give way to seeking simpler conceptual explanations for what the body knows, or once knew, as multilayered identity with complexities functioning as a whole instead of needing to be understood in their singular function. Our conceptual worlds become populated with dichotomies – me/not me, male/female, masculine/feminine, good/bad, right/wrong. If the mind is alienated from the body, so also is the body from the mind.

The depersonalization and language limitations can constrict the most intimate aspects of self that might otherwise come into play in close relationships. Consider living in a body that does not feel consistent with gendered language, and how that experience then translates into the restricted descriptions for sexuality that inevitably follow. The body becomes a physical object possessed and used by the self and as experienced with the breadth of language available. Both the experiential self and language to engage in relationships with the fully experienced self then miss the sense of unity with the spontaneous rhythms of the body. The experiential body and the language lacking can translate into missing the sense of full participation in the body's stresses and pains, its joys and delights. More characteristic instead is the sense of body as machine.

When the body is experienced as a thing (an object), then language similarly restricts the body to its mechanic processes. We reject the body as outside the self when we experience the physical aspects as different from, as distinct from, the self. We instead conceptualize the manifestation of difference as the problem. Conceptualizations of difference might include the bad knee that gets in the way of walking, the cancer that invades the cells, or the illness that intrudes on how we consider the self. Conceptualizations of difference might also include attributed aspects of identity that feel "wrong," or queer, or not fitting, or outside the self, such as identifying as a different (or neutral) gender, identifying as sexually fluid, or understanding the self differently from how society attributes. Illness as experienced in the physical self might prompt alienation in recognizing other points of difference. Language to describe the illness can simplify experience as symptoms and body as just the carrier of symptoms.

The problem of this dualistic alienation is further complicated by the fact that an oppressed or rejected body may be understood as a nemesis. The rejected body seeks revenge as we "conquer" the cancer or as we reject the fuller dimensions of the self for which we do not have language. This bodily rejection and alienation is described in the trauma literature, but in moving to that literature note that the intention is to build from existing research, not to suggest that trauma is the accurate representation of this restricted sense of self.

TRAUMA AND BODY ALIENATION

Being able to feel safe with other people is one of the important aspects of mental health. Safe relational connections are fundamental to meaningful and satisfying lives. People evolve mechanisms for detecting danger by attuning to emotional shifts in people around them. In people who survive trauma, the parts of the brain that have evolved to monitor for danger remain over-activated and detect even the smallest indications or the slightest signs of danger; real or misperceived indications can trigger acute stress response accompanied by unpleasant emotions and overwhelming sensations (van der Kolk, 2014). These post-traumatic reactions make it difficult for trauma survivors to connect with other people, since closeness can trigger the sense of danger (van der Kolk, 2014). Yet, the experience of trauma can disrupt the ability to accurately read others and can cause people to misperceive danger where it does not exist (van der Kolk, 2014). The experience of trauma can interrupt the ability to see and interpret socioemotional signals.

With the dualism of body alienation, Van der Kolk (2014) proposes that after trauma people lose the body-based feelings and experience disruption in ability to know what they feel or to trust their gut feelings. Mistrust instead can trigger people with history of trauma to misperceive threat and to feel chronically unsafe inside their own bodies. The history of trauma instead brings some form of numbing awareness of what is played out inside; people learn to hide from themselves. Depersonalization can be manifest as a lost sense of agency (van der Kolk, 2014). He proposes paths to recovery by actively rebuilding and reestablishing ownership over the body and the mind, ownership of the self. This means feeling free to know what you feel and to feel what you feel without becoming overwhelmed, enraged, ashamed, or collapsed. Processes of reengaging body with socioemotional sensations involve connecting with images, thoughts, sounds, or physical sensations that remind the person of the trauma and practicing being fully present and aware of the experience as sensation (van der Kolk, 2014).

ACTIVE AND PASSIVE BODILY DEFENSE RESPONSES

Neurobiology provides evidence for active and passive defense responses to threat. When people are threatened by physical injury, death, or social exclusion, the brain has well-established responses, immediate and sequential, to promote safety (Corrigan, Wilson, & Fay, 2014). Persistence and ongoing need for defense responses can promote responses that are too easily activated, prolonged, blocked, or ineffective and can trigger the clinical expression of post-traumatic stress disorder (Corrigan, 2014). The hypothesis that people activate defense-response systems originally developed for surviving physical threats but activated by social threats has been supported by fMRI imaging studies (Corrigan, 2014). Physiological responses of distressing social events can result in intrusive memories, avoidance, and hyperarousal (Carleton et al., 2011). Active defense-or-fight responses can include verbal hectoring and abuse, sarcasm, unwarranted criticism, swearing, name-calling, snarling, scowling, and shouting (Carleton et al., 2011). Flight might be expressed through alcohol or drug use, removal from a situation of conflict, social withdrawal, avoidance of any unpredictable interpersonal situations, or an urge to hide rather than flee (Carleton et al., 2011). People may describe their experience as "panic" when they feel terror in situations from which they feel unable to extricate themselves, such as on a crowded bus, on a boat, on a stage, or in an unprecedented social situation (Corrigan, 2014). This may represent a preflight "freeze" rather than the acute separation distress of abandonment and helplessness in panic (Corrigan, 2014). Turning away from an interaction that could have been pleasurable or from relationships that could bring closeness when they feel threatening are behavioral effects postulated to involve the avoidant defenses (Corrigan, 2014). Humiliation may instigate an acute high-arousal phase of cringing and embarrassment and then a more protracted phase of shame that is lower in arousal (Corrigan, 2014). Shame can be the consequence of misattunement and loss but can also arise from defeat in agonistic encounters that require submission (Corrigan, 2014). In addition to emotional blocking and defense responses, manifestations of dissociation may include physical defense responses such as immobility, freezing, or diminished perception of pain (Paulsen & Lanius, 2014).

Trauma may fragment the self. Cognitive dissociation from the past occurs in having trouble integrating memories, their sense of identity, and aspects of their consciousness into a continuous whole; people may find many parts of their experience alien, as if belonging to someone else (Spiegel, 2009). As with cognitive dissociation from past trauma, people may dissociate the physical experience such that the body holds information that no longer connects to the overall sense of self. Trauma compromises the brain area that communicates the physical, embodied feeling of being alive (van der Kolk, 2014). The physiological changes that follow trauma include a recalibration of the brain's alarm system, an increase in stress hormone activity, and alterations in the system that filters relevant information from irrelevant (van der Kolk, 2014). Similarly, the fragmented self may manifest in trouble allowing the full self to engage and in repeating the same problematic patterns and experiences.

In addition to cognitive behavioral therapy to address the fragmented self, sensory integration experiences focus on physical opportunities for integration. For example, recent therapies address integration of psychological and emotional processes of the brain with neural perspectives such as eye movement desensitization and reprocessing (EMDR) procedures. During EMDR therapy the client attends to emotionally disturbing material in brief sequential doses while simultaneously focusing on an external stimulus. Therapist-directed lateral eye movements are the most commonly used external stimulus but there is a variety of other stimuli including hand-tapping and audio stimulation. The idea of the treatment is to address information processing that is blocked as a defensive and survival strategy (Paulsen & Lanius, 2014). The dissociative response may occur in nonclinical populations exposed to everyday stressors as a hardwired, normal underlying neurobiological mechanism (Paulsen & Lanius, 2014).

Safe embodiment is a concept at the core of treating traumatic stress syndromes and dissociation. A key component in neurobiological treatments is not the reprocessing of the adverse experiences that occurred in life, but the development of brain mechanisms for a state of core compassion toward the self, a state of calmness, security, and safety that may not have developed in infancy or that has been interrupted through trauma (Corrigan et al., 2014). The intention of the word "safe" is freedom from danger as well as a condition that includes minimal activation of defense responses and minimal vigilance for threat, and that these states are experienced in the body mindfully. This state would include positive predisposition for affiliative behavior and nonjudgmental awareness of the self in the moment (Corrigan et al., 2014). The idea is that the experiences of belonging, safety, mindful awareness, and compassion for self and others create and restore the body state of security displaced by trauma, abuse, or neglect (Corrigan et al., 2014) or, as proposed in the following section, the body state of security may be displaced by invasive medical procedures. Whatever the treatment modality, the ability to recognize, and perhaps induce, a state of nurturing compassion, which can then be directed toward the parts of the self that hold the trauma-based feelings and memories, holds great potential.

INVASIVE MEDICAL PROCEDURES AS TRAUMA EXPERIENCES

The experience of medicine can also function as trauma inducing and can function as trauma in disconnecting physical body from socioemotional understanding. First consider the strangeness of surgical intervention and the necessity of disconnecting understanding from embodied experience. The patient first receives anesthesia to medically promote pain control. In everyday language, anesthetics can slow breathing, can relax a patient, can make a patient sleepy or forgetful, can make a patient unconsciousness for surgery, and can block a specific group of nerves in order to avoid a patient experiencing pain during a medical procedure. Anesthesia functions to prompt a temporary disconnect between bodily experience and perception of pain. During surgery, some part of the body is opened; parts of the body are removed or modified, sometimes with major changes to organs most associated with feelings, including the heart and the brain. During chemotherapy treatments for cancer, invasive chemical substances are inserted into (or otherwise taken into) the body with drugs that are, by definition, destructive to some cells or tissues. A host of other medical interventions intentionally invade the body and require patients to come to terms with disconnecting the invasive experience with perception of the invasion into the body. Although in modern medicine we have an intended goal in separating physical body from experience and disassociation from experience, the invasive process into the body cannot be overlooked. Physical invasion into the body can be considered a traumatic event.

IMPLICATIONS

A holistic understanding of the body as a vehicle for health and social information opens the door to articulating how the body exists as a pathway between close relationships and the experiences and sense-making of health and illness. Recognizing the body as holding physical, emotional, and relational information allows the potential to integrate rather than constrain and contain embodied understanding. An array of theoretical pathways may be manifest in a holistic understanding of the body. Interventions that address the emotional and relational embodiment can allow a different sense of self-perception and attentiveness to addressing what the body holds. Discussions of post-traumatic stress and body alienation tend to focus on people who have survived war, victims of terrorist bombings, or survivors of terrible accidents (van der Kolk, 2014). Manifestations of trauma and medical intrusions may be manifest in what the body holds more broadly than the current research indicates. Integrating a holistic sense of embodiment allows for recognizing a more systematic explanatory framework connecting health and illness with close relationship processes.

6 Relationship Theories Applied to Illness Transitions

Amber Miller, a 26-year-old college student in Oklahoma City, was waiting to tell Josh about her type one diabetes. They had been dating for a month. So when he didn't hear from her for a month while she was recovering from a diabetic coma, he expected the worst.

"Josh thought I broke up with him because none of my family told him about the coma and he didn't hear from me for a month," Miller said. "I was like, 'Oh yeah, I was in a coma.' – The classic coma excuse."

In Miller's case, it turned out okay, even with the misunderstanding – the couple eventually married. But that's not always the case, which is why the question of disclosure remains a hot topic in the chronically ill community. Some choose to be upfront from the get-go, others wait until things head in the direction of exclusive dating.

Disclosure becomes even more nerve-wracking if the chronic illness is contagious, like Nate Butler's HIV. The 51-year-old Denver native has had the disease for nearly 25 years and has dated both HIV-positive and negative men and women since then. And while it's unlikely he would spread the disease through protected sex, he's had a decent number of people turn him down. He usually tells the person about his HIV after he sees that it's going to be more than a platonic relationship. Even waiting two or three dates is too long for some people, who accuse him of wasting their time.

Butler has been dating an HIV-negative woman for three months now, though he thinks dating someone with HIV would be simpler. He's been on many HIV dating sites in hopes to avoid the nuisances of dating an HIV-negative person, namely disclosure and condoms.

"Most of us HIV-positive people know the online dating drill completely," said Butler, who owns a small business. "If we like each other, someone's flying out on an expensive date weekend. In most cases, sex happens more quickly, probably due to not having had it as frequently as they would like to. You don't have to have the disclosure talk. Then it turns into a joke. 'Oh by the way, did I remind you I'm HIV positive? Oh, you too? Good.'"

– Fortenbury, 2013. "Love in the Time of Chronic Illness: When Should You Disclose Medical Conditions to a Date? When Is Illness Too Much for a Relationship to Survive?"

DISCLOSURE AND RELATIONSHIP INSTABILITY

This story from *The Atlantic* magazine directly addresses disclosure challenges about private illness information in the context of dating with a chronic illness. People with chronic illness face dilemmas about when and how to share about their illness. People also face dilemmas about whether they would want to date a chronically ill person, about whether getting into the complications of chronic illness will be too much, or whether they will find the challenges too difficult over time.

This story indirectly addresses relational instability or turbulence in the uncertainty of negotiating intimacy and closeness in dating. This story also indirectly addresses interdependence in the mutual psychological and behavioral processes in romantic relationships. Disclosure, relational turbulence, and interdependence are three of the most important processes in navigating close relationships. Disclosure of private information is the key communication process through which people get to know each other. Relational instability or turbulence erupts because the process of navigating close relationships involves uncertainty and vulnerability. Interdependence in psychological and behavioral processes may be understood as the theoretical explanation for interconnections inherent in navigating close relationships.

In this chapter, I illustrate the current strengths and limitations of applying relationship theories to health and illness transitions by focusing on three theories: *interdependence theory* (as reviewed in Arriaga, 2013; Thibaut & Kelley, 1959) *communication privacy management theory* (Petronio, 2002), and *relational turbulence theory* (and its antecedent, the relational turbulence model) (Solomon & Knobloch, 2001). I outline theoretical assumptions for these three exemplary relationship theories to show strengths and limitations of understanding health and illness trajectories through relationship theories. In these illustrations and applications, we can see how these exemplary relationship theories can account for illness as a relational transition, as a point of recalibrating disclosure about private information, as a point of turbulence, or as a relational stressor. I illustrate examples of relationship theories that explain how interactions are constrained or enhanced by the contexts in which they take place. The strengths of these exemplary relationship theories reside in their dyadic explanations for co-negotiating vulnerable or uncertain information. The limitations of these exemplary theories lie in the scope of what they address and indicate the potential for richer explanations by considering interconnectivity between illness trajectories and relational processes as a broader system and over time.

EACH THEORY AS DYADIC

The three theories outlined in this chapter for the purpose of applying them to illness contexts are all dyadic theories, which means they all assume a social and interconnected explanatory framework involving multiple people. To that end, all three theories emphasize the interpersonal or interactional features of relationships as coproduced by two people. Instead of focusing on each individual person or on trends over time within a population of individuals, the three theories each explain relationship processes occurring between people as meaningful.

Interdependence theory, which comes from the field of social psychology, holds particular strengths in explaining the science of what is truly social about situations and how situations influence social behavior (for review see Reis & Arriaga, 2015). Interdependence theory is inherently dyadic because it provides a conceptual framework for understanding how people in relationships affect each other and how behavior in specific interactions influences the general course of a relationship (Holmes, 2002; Kelley, 1979). Interdependence theory is meaningful for explaining close relationships in that a defining characteristic of close relationships is that people share interactions over some period of time. The foundation of interdependence is that people are connected in ways that shape and are shaped by another person; interdependence functions as a cornerstone relational process.

Similarly, relational turbulence theory is dyadic in that the theory identifies specific *relationship* qualities that exacerbate the experience of negative emotions, promote negative cognitions, and complicate communication between partners (Solomon, 2016). Relational turbulence is manifest in more frequent experiences of conflict, more frequent and intense negative emotions, and heightened relationship thinking. Relational turbulence theory addresses contexts where relationships are in transition, such as transitioning from courtship to serious involvement. The dyadic focus rests in the experience of relational uncertainty and experience of interdependence as people in close relationships grapple with life changes. A defining characteristic of grappling with relationship changes is that people are connected such that next steps in negotiation occur within the relationship.

Finally, communication privacy management theory is dyadic in that people cannot negotiate privacy rules alone but address the shared boundaries of information together (Petronio, 2002). The rule-based system of disclosing private information depends on controlling the level of accessibility of the private information. Disclosure involves some understanding of privacy rules at the dyadic level such that people have similar expectations for privacy management. A distressing sense of boundary turbulence can arise when people do not share the same understanding of the privacy rules. Interconnection occurs in co-ownership of shared information. Dyadic processes include negotiating links among information and how to coordinate ownership of knowledge and information. The rule-based disclosures between people essentially rest in recognizing the "owner" of the information as the person who is vulnerable in the information being shared. The theory addresses how sharing information involves coordinating information when an additional owner or stakeholder of the information is involved; the theory addresses how people are then bound to the rules of privacy maintenance.

This chapter provides an overview of the three theories and is not intended to elucidate in depth the nuances of the theories (that can be found elsewhere in the tests of the theories) but instead to show how dyadic relationship theories address particular sets of components of health and illness trajectories in close relationships. Each theory provides rich implications for ongoing application to many contexts, and interested readers can find large bodies of excellent research on each of the three theories.

In this volume, the overall application of dyadic relationship theories is intended to serve as a foundation for explaining interconnecting relationship frameworks with health and illness trajectories, not to serve as extensive applications of each nuance of the theory. The overall application provides a broad way of considering the systematic co-generative processes of close relationships and health and illness trajectories, which advances understanding differently from applying an individual theory. Co-generative theoretical processes of close relationships and health and illness trajectories are then considered in the subsequent section of this volume.

INTERDEPENDENCE THEORY

Interdependence theory indicates how distinct interaction processes and different levels of analysis help people solve problems as a function of the people in the relationship and the environment (Reis & Arriaga 2015; Thibaut & Kelley, 1959). Interdependence theory is a classic social and behavioral science theory, originally proposed over fifty years ago to account for dyadic behavior among individuals who influence each other in social interactions (Thibaut & Kelley, 1959). Interdependence theory provides a framework for understanding interaction among people in close relationships.

Theoretical assumptions. Interdependence theory provides a functional explanation for the extent to which people in close relationships influence each other and shape the general course of their relationship (Kelley, 1979). In close relationships, the essence of interdependence is about how a change in one person affects the state of another person. The interdependence process addresses how people in interactions influence each other's experiences, or how people mutually influence each other's thoughts, emotions, motives, behavior, and outcomes (Van Lange & Balliet, 2015). The concept of interdependence is very broad and poses implications for a wide variety of topics. Interdependence theory in close relationships stems from Thibaut and Kelley's (1959) book on the social psychology of groups and later Kelley and Thibaut's (1978) volume on interdependence as a theory in interpersonal relations. The theory articulates a formal analysis of the objective properties of a situation from a taxonomy of situations. The theory provides a conceptualization of psychological processes in terms of transformations, including motives, cognitions, and affect (what people make of the situation), as well as behavior and social interaction resulting from both the objective properties of the situation and what people make of it (Van Lange & Balliet, 2015). The differences among people in their transformational tendencies were later conceptualized in terms of dispositions, relationship-specific motives, and social norms (Rusbult & Van Lange, 2003). The theory continued to be developed and tested in conceptualizing phenomena as diverse as altruism, attribution, coordination, conflict, cooperation, competition, delay of gratification, exchange, investments, fairness, justice, love, power, pro-social behavior, trust, sacrifice, self-presentation, stereotyping, and hostility and aggression in the context of dyads, as well as a myriad of group applications, environmental issues, organizational issues, and political issues (Rusbult & Van Lange, 2003; Van Lange & Joireman, 2008). A collaborative application of interdependence theory in interpersonal situations across contexts resulted in adding the dimensions of temporal structure and information availability to the core dimensions of the theory (Kelley et al., 2003).

Interdependence theory grew out of the two previous classic theories of social exchange theory and game theory and explained how people represent and consider situations of interdependence with respect to choosing among potential courses of action. Interdependence theory addresses how cognition and emotion interact with individual differences to address how people influence each other's preferences, motives, and actions (Reis & Arriaga, 2015). As a relational theory, interdependence theory addresses commitment to the relationship such that people are dependent on the relationship, and the experience of dependence shapes reactions to new situations. For example, in committed relationships, people are willing to sacrifice when outcomes are non-correspondent. Commitment represents a long-term orientation, including feelings of attachment to a partner or close friend and desire to maintain the relationship even when people face challenges (Rusbult & Buunk, 1993).

Interdependence theory provides a functional analysis in assuming that interpersonal behavior is ultimately driven by securing interpersonal ties that are personally adaptive in functioning to maximize odds of having fulfilling experiences and minimizing the odds of having harmful or aversive experiences (Arriaga, 2013). As a social exchange theory, the assumption is that interactions with others are affectively evaluated in terms of personal benefit over cost incurred from the overall positive and negative experiences each person experiences as a result of joint action in a *given situation*. The given situation considers benefits and costs without concern for the interaction partner (Kelley & Thibaut, 1978). Outcomes from the experience are scaled by valence (positive, negative, or neutral) that reflects how an interaction subjectively feels rather than tangible or objective rewards or costs (Arriaga, 2013). Functionality and benefit must be measured over a broad time frame, as actions can be costly in the short term but ultimately beneficial for the relationship. Benefits or outcomes can include major concepts including perceived security, satisfaction, overall acceptance, understanding, achieving desired goals, emotion regulation, and feelings of valuing the relationship (Arriaga, 2013). People do not need to be consciously or explicitly aware of the benefits their behavior poses for the relationship in order for the behavior to be adaptive or to make sense over time (Holmes, 2004).

Analyzing interactions includes identifying specific situations that trigger each individual, expectations and knowledge structures, abilities and behavior tendencies, and general interaction motives (Holmes, 2004). Applying interdependence theory includes considering matrices of how individual characteristics filter perceptions of a partner's behavior and how these perceptions of a partner's behavior predict interaction behavior, changes in the situation, and whether broader influences are established from the interaction (Arriaga, 2013).

Two key assumptions of interdependence theory are that (1) features of situations are found in their interpersonal core, and (2) social situations are best understood by considering people's dependence on each other to attain desired outcomes (Reis & Arriaga, 2015). In other words, the first assumption is that behavior is a function of the interaction between the person and the environment. The second assumption considers the nature and extent to which people are dependent on each other and is based on repeating behavior that is reinforced or rewarded but also takes into account the co-acting behavior of another person or group (Reis & Arriaga, 2015). The foundational assumptions bring an inherently dyadic understanding to social-psychological theories that may otherwise explain behavior in terms of individual needs or goals. Interdependence theory begins with situational explanation such that interpersonal interactions become the fundamental unit of analysis instead of the individual or the population (Reis & Arriaga, 2015). Outcomes are considered by considering complexity and diversity of human needs and values beyond what can be understood as maximized outcome for an individual person in an encounter.

Interdependence theory articulates interpersonal situations according to six properties that define patterns of interdependence. These properties are the degree to which individuals' interests correspond or conflict; the extent to which outcomes depend on one's own actions or on the actions of others; whether co-participants have mutual or asymmetric power over each other's outcomes; whether the task requires coordination or exchange to produce a desired result; whether the situation involves interaction over time; and whether or not substantial uncertainty exists about the likely result of particular actions (Reis & Arriaga, 2015). Properties can be combined, and alternatives consistent with the theory should have logical and discernable implications for interaction (Reis & Arriaga, 2015).

Interdependence theory distinguishes a given situation where direct and immediate outcomes are likely to follow from an *effective situation* that re-conceptualizes sets of outcomes over time that take into account the immediate and long-term impact of actions for both the self and the relational partner (Kelley & Thibaut, 1978; Reis & Arriaga, 2015). Thus, a broader understanding of self-interest and outcomes includes making inferences about how a partner will likely feel about each possible alternative that a person might pursue. People make choices that consider the self but also consider the self in relationship to another person, taking into account aspects such as their partner's interests, long-term relational goals, social norms, and strategic considerations (Kelley & Thibaut, 1978; Reis & Arriaga, 2015). Underlying motivational processes are understood in terms of longer-term outcomes. Individual differences are considered in terms of situations that provide opportunities for traits, motives, values, preferences, beliefs, and feelings to be revealed in behavior (Van Lange & Balliet, 2015). Conceptualizations of self-interest might run counterintuitively to immediate self-interest but might offer benefit for the self in the long run. For example, contributing to the well-being of another person or delaying gratification to further a long-term goal could contribute to longer-term or broader needs, values, or goals over time (Reis & Arriaga, 2015).

Interdependence theory is best understood by considering situation-by-person analysis: situation structure combined with psychological and social factors residing within each partner, as well as emerging from the specific pairing of two partners, that matter just as much as situation structure (Reis & Arriaga, 2015). In close relationships, people come to interactions with individual expectations and shared expectations and ideas about what they expect to occur in an interaction based on their shared history and on their individual experiences (Arriaga, 2013).

Interdependence in close relationships. Person factors of interdependence studied extensively in close relationships include trust and commitment. Trust reflects expectation that a person in a close relationship will be caring and responsive to an individual's needs (Holmes & Rempel, 1989). Trust is conceptually similar to feelings of intimacy (Reis, Clark, & Holmes, 2004). Commitment is a subjective sense that the relationship will continue even when confronted with challenges (Rusbult, 1983). People who experience high commitment in close relationships feel attached or tied to their partner and anticipate their future as being in the relationship (Arriaga & Agnew, 2001). People who are highly dependent on their partner come to feel committed and anticipate that the relationship will continue (Rusbult, Agnew, & Arriaga, 2011). Commitment remains even in abusive relationships, where partners who feel high commitment downplay or minimize descriptions of the partner's aggression (Agnew, Arriaga, & Wilson, 2008; Arriaga et al., 2007). Trust and commitment often co-occur but are not necessarily linearly related. For example, when romantic partners synchronize their goals for high closeness and intimacy they also describe high commitment and high trust (Murray & Holmes, 2009). Conversely, people in close relationships might remain committed but feel their partner is not responsive to their needs, or people might infer high commitment in their partner and thus trust their partner but might feel much lower commitment themselves.

Most people seek a satisfying romantic relationship, and that requires establishing a deep and intimate connection with another person. (I will leave the explanations for people seeking unsatisfying relationships to another author.) However, people vary with regard to how closely intertwined they want to be with their romantic partner. Some people want to be relatively independent, and other people want to be very closely intertwined (Arriaga, 2013). One motive in a romantic relationship is to have a partner whose desired connection level is in sync with one's own desired connection level. Relationship characteristics where one person desires more closeness than the other can leave the person who wants more closeness feeling emotionally vulnerable. Some people, such as anxiously attached individuals, are prone to feeling more vulnerable and anxious than other people; other people, such as avoidantly attached people, more easily feel smothered and constrained in relationships. Interdependence processes interconnect with personal motives and desires for connection with partners along with person factors including trust and commitment.

Situation structures shape how people respond and tailor their behavior based on the situation at hand. Situations also activate specific person factors and characteristics (Reis, 2008). Feeling more dependent than the partner can activate concerns about control and vulnerability. People may register such situations faster and more strongly if their person factors trigger concerns about being taken advantage of, or hurt, by their partner (Arriaga, 2013). Feeling less dependent than the partner may activate dominance and controlling behaviors. Situations of non-correspondence may be particularly anxiety provoking for people who are low in self-esteem or who are anxiously attached.

Mental events can also combine with person characteristics and situation structure. People might engage in elaborate, thoughtful process that specifically takes into account personal, relational, and social considerations (Arriaga, 2013). More often, responses instead are enacted because of habits between people in close relationships. To that end, people do things because they act out of awareness in an instantaneous manner with little cognitive effort. People in highly committed relationships might not pay attention to issues that once required greater attention and thought (Arriaga, 2013). Perceptions of relationships can become automated, and the way couples handle a situation unfolds in a relatively automatic response guided by person and situation variables but also by their own relationship history. Situations can still strongly activate thoughts and emotions and alert consequences for one's outcomes and needs (Berscheid, 1983). People become more aware of their interaction motives when they want to change their relationship through professional intervention (e.g., therapy), self-help resources, or self-generated efforts (Arriaga, 2013). Situations that provoke dependence pose higher consequences and higher stakes than patterned interactions that fit the couple's relationship history. Unfamiliar situations also elicit increased cognitive activity and affect. Interdependence occurs in that each person's *behavior* directly affects the other person.

Interdependence theory versus statistical modeling. Interdependence theory is primarily a relational theory, and applications in relationship contexts provide nuanced and sophisticated understanding and adaptation of the theory. Applications of interdependence theory are tested through the actor–partner interdependence model (APIM; Kenny & Kashy, 2011; Spain, Jackson, & Edmonds, 2012) in order to analyze dyadic data. Researchers have found the APIM to be very useful in the study of dyadic relationships, but the conceptual scope of interdependence theory extends beyond what can necessarily be measured through the APIM.

The appeal of the APIM as a statistical tool is that it allows for the statistical measurement of the influence of a person's own causal variable on his or her own outcome variable, which is called the actor effect, and on the outcome variable of the partner, which is called the partner effect. These two effects can be measured while proper statistical allowances are made for the non-independence in the two persons' responses. The statistical analysis is broadly based on interdependence theory (Kelley et al., 2003) in that the general APIM accounts for patterns consistent with individual and joint effects.

The term "partner" in the APIM refers to the other person in the dyad and could include a romantic partner, a close friend, a parent, or any other person that makes sense as a dyadic influence in a given study. Tests of the APIM consider and measure the possibility that each couple member influences his or her own outcome (actor effect) (Kenny & Kashy, 2011). This type of influence suggests each partner is responsible for some part of an outcome with little influence from the partner. In addition, each couple member influences his or her partner's outcomes; this influence suggests that health and behavior are determined by partners. Together the outcomes are also determined by a joint effect, the health and behavior determined both by individual actions and the actions of the partner.

Interdependence constructs in predicting health behavior change. To that end, the language of interdependence theory in health and illness contexts considers dyadic influences and determinants of couple behavior. However, the statistical models of interdependence miss the nuances of the causal interchain sequences of time unfolding such that a sequence of behavior meshes with another person in a close relationship.

In explaining health behavior change among couples, interdependence theory serves as a lens to understand the extent to which couple members are jointly motivated to actively engage in health-enhancing behaviors (Lewis et al., 2006). Marriage is consistently linked to better health, and application of interdependence theory considers dyadic processes and couple dynamics that predict the adoption and integration of risk-reducing health habits (Lewis et al., 2006). Couples' interdependence can transform motivation from acting in the best interest of the self (person centered) to selfless actions that are best for continuing the relationship (relationship centered), including enhanced motivation for couples to act cooperatively in adopting health-enhancing behavior change (Lewis et al., 2006). The negative and positive outcomes that partners experience when they interact can be motives, preferences, emotions, or behavior.

Structural characteristics within couples' relationships can function in a variety of ways, some of which may be more beneficial to the relationship or to achieving behavior changes to prevent health problems (Lewis et al., 2006). One spouse's health and behavior are determined by his or her own actions and those of his or her partner; in addition, both partners experience mutual joint effects where each spouse's health and behavior are determined by both their own actions and those of their partner. Spouses may or may not enact the exact same behavior to be mutually influential. For example, couples may work together to decrease cancer risk when one partner has been diagnosed with a condition that signals an increased cancer risk (Lewis et al., 2004). One spouse may need to increase physical activity to reduce risk of colorectal cancer. The diagnosis may spur that person's physical activity (actor effect) and also prompt the spouse to be more physically active in support (partner effect). Alternatively, one spouse's efforts to support physical activity for the other spouse may entail creating opportunities for work schedules for physical activity rather than engaging in the physical activity themselves, and this in conjunction with perceived risk may facilitate both people being more physically active (joint effect). In addition, if one partner enjoys companionship while walking and creates opportunities for them to be physically active together, then both may be more physically active (mutual joint effects) (Lewis et al., 2006). As this example illustrates, spouses can engage so that both people participate in the same way in the health behavior (exercise); spouses can work together to enact different behavior so that one of them can engage in the health behavior; or spouses can enact different behaviors so both of them enact different behaviors (Lewis et al., 2006).

Given the potential variety of interdependent structures, couples may either foster health-enhancing behaviors (as described above) or, on the contrary, they may undermine health-enhancing efforts they perceive as interfering with their own goals. Transformation of motivation is a key construct from interdependence theory that may explain how patterns of interdependence arise, when spouses may accommodate to work together, and why marital relationships can influence health outcomes. Transformation of motivation shifts the focus from a primarily self-centered orientation or motivation to a relationship-enhancing orientation. Transformation of motivation occurs when people ascribe health events as meaningful for the relationship or for their spouse (or close friend); events are interpreted as significant for the spouse rather than simply for oneself (Rusbult & Van Lange, 2003). This relational explanation of motivation for health behavior change differs from the individual or cognitive-based social influence models. Transformation of motivation addresses the emotional and cognitive implications of a health threat and its impact on the relationship or on the partner (or close friend) (Lewis et al., 2006). Furthermore, one couple member's preferences for particular outcomes can be quite similar or different from the other person's preferences, and lower degrees of correspondence in their interests in similar outcomes can predict higher conflict. Decisions and cooperation in choices may be most difficult when people want different outcomes.

Interdependence and coping with life-threatening illness. Life-threatening illness brings high levels of stress for the individual with the diagnosis and the relational partner and close friends. When we conceptualize interdependence in terms of people in a dyad or in a close relationship in which they mutually influence each other, the impact of illness cannot be fully understood independent of the relationship (Fife et al., 2013). Interdependence theory applied to coping suggests that patterns that are adaptive or maladaptive develop and are sustained by connected interaction patterns of partners or close friends within the dyadic relationship. In response to life-threatening illness, the romantic partners and close friends connected to the person with the diagnosis also face fear, uncertainty, and high levels of disruption and distress within relationships (Fife et al., 2013). The treatment trajectory of life-threatening illness includes multiple turning points that can introduce distress for the recipient of care and the caregivers and close friends.

Dyadic coping serves as an application of interdependent behaviors in the context of life-threatening illness. In a study of people receiving cancer treatment by bone marrow or stem-cell transplantation, dyadic interdependence and dyadic adjustment over the course of treatment were predicted by care recipient behavior and the behavior of people in their network of close friends (Fife et al., 2013). The study suggests that the mental health of the caregiver and coping for the family are connected to supportive coping interventions. The high level of threat inherent in bone marrow transplant treatment for the person receiving care and for dyadic coping were associated with the adaptation of committed partners as indicated by the quality of adjustment within their relationship (Fife et al., 2013). As also indicated in other studies of dyadic coping, the bone marrow transplant trajectory is characterized by critical events that occur as the patient progresses through the treatment process. The ongoing nature of treatment requires understanding that the data are longitudinal so that changes throughout the treatment trajectory can be evaluated (Fife et al., 2013). This study indicated that caregivers consistently experienced higher levels of distress than patients, and this result indicates the potential benefit of intervention aimed at partners in addition to support provided to patients. Findings point to the need to promote ongoing adaptive partner-related coping that cannot be fully anticipated by couples (Fife et al., 2013). The mutual impact of partner behavior and patient behavior provides evidence for addressing ongoing behavior within interdependent relationships.

Communication theories address the role of messages specific to negotiating relationship features and trajectories. For example, communication privacy management theory addresses how people make decisions about revealing and concealing private information in particular relationships and how they coordinate rules for sharing private information within and beyond the relationship (Petronio, 2002). Relational turbulence theory poses a perspective on communication during transitions in particular personal relationships and how emotions and cognitive appraisals can disrupt the exchange of messages between people in close relationships (Solomon, 2016).

COMMUNICATION PRIVACY MANAGEMENT THEORY

Communication privacy management theory is an evidence-based theory about the way people make decisions about revealing and concealing private information derived from social-behavioral research investigating how people manage private information (Petronio, 2002). The theory is structured within a dialectical framework and addresses the tension between opening and closing boundaries in concealing or revealing private information (Petronio, 2002). Communication privacy management theory extends the psychological construct of self-disclosure to also address desires for privacy. Private information rather than disclosure became the focus of the theory over time because of the caveats inherent in private information that exceed the concept of disclosure, such as sharing a burden or sharing information about other people or coordinating sharing information about collectively owned information.

Communication privacy management theory uses the metaphor of boundaries to provide a framework for understanding how people regulate intentionally revealing personal information to others with also acknowledging ownership of private information and managing what is revealed about the private life (Petronio, 2002, 2004, 2007). The original development of the theory was called communication boundary management theory, but it has developed to underscore private disclosure as its cornerstone. The main elements of communication privacy management theory are privacy ownership, privacy control, and privacy turbulence. The boundary metaphor indicates how people enact rules to manage and regulate the sharing of private information (Petronio, 2002, 2010).

Theoretical assumptions. The first theoretical assumption of communication privacy management theory requires us to understand managing private information as a dialectical tension of needing both privacy and openness simultaneously (Petronio, 2002, 2010). Conceptualizing privacy management within a framework of contradictory impulses that at any given moment require weighing multiple viewpoints is important because it recognizes the interplay of different considerations for revealing or concealing information (Petronio, 2002, 2010). Securing protection for the self by concealing information or restricting access to information is considered alongside revealing information and establishing interconnected privacy boundaries and more open parameters for sharing information. The second theoretical assumption is that privacy management functions as a rule-based process, not an individual decision. People manage their privacy both personally and in their judgment about revealing or preserving and coordinating information about another person or information that exists within a collective boundary such as a family. The needs for privacy and granting access to information function to influence the choices people make about revealing or concealing information (Petronio, 2002, 2004). When people share private information, they expect to be able to negotiate privacy rules for sharing the information further.

Communication privacy management theory includes five core principles that follow from the theoretical assumptions. First, people believe they have a right to define and control their own private information. Second, people control their private information through privacy rules. Third, when people are given access to private information, they become co-owners of the information. Fourth, people believe they are able to negotiate mutual privacy rules with other people who become co-owners of private information. Fifth, the process of negotiating privacy boundaries is imperfect, and boundary turbulence results from ineffectively negotiated privacy rules or from situations where privacy rules are not mutually understood or where context shifts shared understanding (Petronio, 2002).

Privacy ownership. From the perspective of communication privacy management theory, privacy ownership refers to boundaries of private information, where people believe they are the sole owners of their private information and trust they have the right to protect their information or to grant access to the information (Petronio, 2002,

2007). Ownership of private information can be restricted or can be shared with other people. The original owner of the private information can grant other people access to private information, making them co-owners "authorized" by the original owner, and in that case the co-owners have fiduciary responsibility for further protecting the private information (Thompson, Petronio, & Braithwaite, 2012). Co-ownership boundaries maintain the original owner's private information and acknowledge the nature of privacy co-ownership in groups such as families and in online relationships. Co-ownership can include one additional person or multiple co-owners, and linkages between the original owner and co-owner(s) can be short-term or long-term (Petronio, 2002, 2010). Co-owners of private information can also be accidental, as in the case of discovering private information or overhearing private information. Conceptual developments for understanding communication privacy management theory and the notion of co-ownership assume a relational orientation to sharing private information because any assumption of fiduciary responsibilities moves from an individual to a relational orientation for responsibility of private information (Petronio, 2002, 2010).

Privacy control. Privacy control within communication privacy management theory is the engine that regulates conditions of granting or denying access to private information (Petronio, 2002, 2010). Because people believe they own the rights to their private information, they also believe they should be able to control their private information, and this assumption of privacy control remains even after giving authorized access to another person or people. People develop rules to control the boundaries and flow of private information (Petronio, 2002, 2010). Core criteria provide a consistent orientation to the way people manage their private information generally, but catalyst events such as a major illness diagnosis can shift the decision rules about access to private information (Petronio, 2002, 2010). People have different motivations for changes in their privacy rules and decisions about revealing and concealing, and the risk–benefit analysis changes in different situations (Child et al., 2011). For example, when people who wrote online blogs came to realize that what they posted could be hurtful to themselves or to other people, they were motivated to delete some of the messages they posted earlier because of the realized risks for revealing the information (Child et al., 2011). As situational changes continue to occur over time, privacy control rules then require ongoing coordination and negotiation of privacy rules with co-owners of private information who are granted legitimate access to the information (Petronio, 2002, 2004, 2010). Collective co-ownership and need to negotiate beyond the dyad exist in groups including families and could also exist in a health-care group.

Privacy turbulence. The third core component of communication privacy management theory is privacy turbulence. Because we do not live in a perfect world, privacy regulation can be unpredictable and can function differently from how people anticipate, even when they think they have carefully negotiated privacy control rules (Petronio, 2002, 2004, 2010). In situations where privacy control breaks down as a process, privacy turbulence erupts (Petronio, 2010; Petronio & Sargent, 2011). Turbulence can be prompted by mistakes such as accidentally overhearing private information. Turbulence can be prompted by intentionally sharing private information about another person. Turbulence can be prompted by lack of pre-existing rules for a situation or by violating those rules. Turbulence can range from minor disruption to major eruptions and violations (Petronio, 2002, 2010). When privacy turbulence occurs, privacy management systems might need to renegotiate systems regarding privacy rules and expectations for regulated boundaries that can be clearer in the future (Petronio, 2002, 2010).

Boundary coordination. Communication privacy management theory relies on the image of protecting private information through individual and collective boundaries (Petronio, 2002). Boundaries are coordinated based on understanding boundary permeability, boundary linkage, and boundary ownership (Petronio, 2002, 2004). The boundaries ideally serve as a sort of border for containing a piece of information. Although the boundaries for one individual might seem clear, boundary coordination also involves implications for how each owner of private information approaches and sets rule criteria for their own privacy boundaries.

Boundary permeability addresses thick or thin divisions for keeping private information from being shared with another person or another group (Petronio, 2002). Thick permeability means there is little possibility that information can be shared outside of the owner(s) of the information. Thin boundaries refer to information that is shared to another person or to a group. With these boundaries, the sphere of what is shared with another person or people expands and becomes more permeable.

Boundary linkage addresses connections among owners of private information. For example, spouses are linked to each other such that private information is consistently shared within the boundaries of the relationship (Petronio, 2002). In a health-care context, doctors and patients are linked such that private information about the patient is shared between doctors and patients and among other doctors in the group. These linkages might be strong or weak links depending on the context of how information is shared.

Boundary ownership addresses the rights and responsibilities people have about the information that belongs to them. Boundary ownership is closely connected to the person for whom the information is vulnerable. Thus, in the case of doctors and patients, the doctors might be the people who originally have access to the information, but the ownership of the information belongs primarily to the patient because the patient is connected to the health and illness information in a way that poses vulnerability.

Regulating confidentiality. Sometimes the concomitant needs to maintain privacy and reveal private information to another person or group are connected to the ability to meet a goal. In the health-care context, patients have to disclose private information without being able to explicitly negotiate how to keep this private information confidential. The nature of the health-care system involves sharing patients' private information with other health-care providers. Health-care providers see patients with an expectation that they keep patient information private, but the concept of privacy changes the dynamics of how information is viewed. Patients sharing private information with health-care providers cannot explicitly negotiate boundaries for who on the health-care team will have access to the information (Petronio & Reierson, 2009). The health-care provider with whom the patient originally shares private information becomes the co-owner, but then a team of health-care providers might have access to the information, particularly if it is relevant for next steps in treatment. However, the patient may not necessarily perceive that he or she has granted permission to share further or has given up control over the private information. Assumptions of privacy control in health-care contexts can become blurred. In sharing private information, the health-care provider becomes a confidant. Patients, however, do not necessarily know what information is shared further and how their information is shared within the health system.

Health and illness issues and communication privacy management theory. Research using communication privacy management to explore health privacy issues has been a growth area. Communication privacy management theory has developed alongside Health Insurance Portability and Accountability Act (HIPAA) regulations that provide organizational clarity about regulation and privacy of patient information. Communication privacy management theory addresses situations beyond the organizational reach of HIPAA. One study from the communication privacy management framework investigated physician disclosure of medical mistakes and provided evidence that physicians might disclose to their family as a means of relief, or they might keep the information hidden even from their families (Petronio, 2006). A subsequent study addressed the impact of medical mistakes for physicians and their families (Petronio et al.,

2013). Family members tend to be the safest and most trustworthy recipients of information. Family members can provide emotional support and responsiveness and can offer the many attributes identified as unique to close relationships (see chapter 2). However, drawing family members into institutional health-care predicaments blurs the boundaries between work life and family life (Petronio, 2006).

Communication privacy management theory provides a lens to understand issues of concern in physicians revealing medical mistakes to patients and physicians revealing a medical mistake to their own families. With regard to physicians disclosing medial mistakes to the patient and/or to the patient's family, understanding the dialectical tension for revealing or concealing and the image of boundaries sheds light on the ethical and legal implications for disclosing medical mistakes but the parallel concerns of physicians' own emotions and concerns about potential medical malpractice litigation (Petronio et al., 2013). A mistake disclosure management plan based on the theory suggests first considering physician preparation and addressing physician emotions and physician information seeking. The next step addresses mistake-disclosure strategies that protect the physician–patient relationship by considering timing, tone, content, sequencing, and apology (Petronio et al., 2013). Consistent with the theory, privacy boundaries and steps for renegotiating privacy dilemmas are considered in addition to the content of the mistake.

With regard to physicians revealing mistakes to their own families, boundary linkages between work and family require clarity in the amount and clarity of information revealed (Petronio, 2006). Boundary ownership issues address the responsibility others have once the mistake is revealed (Petronio, 2006). Physicians revealing information about their medical mistake to their family reverses the role of their serving as caregiver and positions them as recipient of support. Seeking support from family amidst potential emotional and professional upheaval might be volatile, because the information disclosed could potentially disrupt professional life and thus also disrupt family life in the case of litigation, organizational response, or peer evaluation of the mistake. Family members might feel vulnerable for knowing the information, might feel caught in the burden of knowing about the mistake of their family member physician, and might also feel distress about what happened with the patient and about whether the patient obtains full disclosure of information about his or her own body (Petronio, 2006). When physicians reveal private information about a medical mistake, they are sharing private patient information, and patients are not able to negotiate the boundary around their own information. Family members coping with the aftermath of medical mistakes face privacy dilemmas about loyalty, dissemination of information, personal struggles, and uncertainties.

Beyond the context of medical mistakes, the health-care context poses additional concerns for family and close friends in facing dilemmas of confidentiality and privacy (Petronio et al., 2004). Family and friends supporting a patient through illness serve as health-care advocates and can provide helpful comfort, social support, and beneficial aid. However, family and friends in this role are exposed to private information that can introduce complications. A person accompanying a close friend or family member to medical visits can be exposed to information outside normative boundaries of what is revealed or what is kept private. A treating nurse or physician does not have context to know the parameters of what might be disclosed to the family member or friend (Petronio et al., 2004). Family members might be unexpected or reluctant confidants, as they may not wish to know the information shared with them, or they might feel they need additional information in order to advocate for the patient (Petronio, 2004). The unofficial role blurs boundaries. Health-care providers are trained to ask about conversation in front of an accompanying family member or friend, but sometimes the information disclosed is beyond what the patient expects to be shared. We cannot assume that close friends and family members share the same information about vulnerable health-care situations that we would share. People might not fully share health information with a partner, even when it would be helpful in making choices about one's health (Checton et al., 2012). Some patients report sharing everything with their spouse or partner, but other patients report not sharing health issues or physical symptoms or ailments (Checton & Greene, 2014). Patients who avoid sharing information with their partner might be driven by personal boundaries (e.g., keeping fears and concerns to themselves) or by collective boundaries (e.g., sharing fears and concerns only with the partner, but clarifying that information would not be discussed with others) (Checton & Greene, 2014; Petronio, 2002).

A number of studies focus on ways that privacy issues influence patient care (e.g., Duggan & Petronio, 2009; Helft & Petronio, 2007; Petronio & Sargent, 2011), and influence confidentiality and control choices about disclosure, for instance with stigmatized illnesses such as HIV and AIDS (Ngula & Miller, 2010), and about e-health information (Jin, 2012). Physicians have two privacy boundaries they regulate with patients; first, they have their own personal privacy boundaries and judgments about situations where they share personal information with patients; second, they serve as guardians or co-owners of patients' private information and are included within the patient's privacy boundary surrounding health-care information and any information patients share during their time together (Petronio, DiCorcia, & Duggan, 2012). As physicians consider sharing their own information, they might share their own feelings about options for treatment or their own experiences with similar circumstances. Emotional objectivity and personal experiences shape their own boundaries about what is revealed to patients. As co-owners of patients' private information they make decisions about treatment plans with patients based on information they gather from tests and throughout the process they decide what to share with patients at each stage of treatment and who else to include in the process of sharing (Petronio et al., 2012).

Illness and patient care bring complications for disclosure. Patients are asked to reveal significant amounts of private information (Duggan & Petronio, 2009). Nurses and other people connected to patient care also receive personal disclosures. Hospitalized patients and patients receiving long-term treatment spend long hours in health-care contexts over time. In addition to the stakeholder role in protecting patient information, nurses and the support provided can create a haven for patients to talk, and family matters become an inseparable part of caring for the patient (Petronio & Sargent, 2011). Patient disclosure to nurses might feel like an infringement of the nurses' professional boundary, or they might welcome the opportunity to support patients beyond providing professional care (Petronio & Sargent, 2011). Patients' emotional needs to disclose feelings about their illness experience and to share private information in order to feel better understood as a person might drive patients' disclosure. The intersection of the nurses' privacy boundaries and the patients' sharing of private information requires privacy rules for how the information might be shared further, and these negotiations do not necessarily fall within the scripts of information specific to biomedical care (Petronio & Sargent, 2011).

Family privacy boundaries, parental privacy invasions, relational issues, and negotiations of potential turbulence at multiple stages of health care add additional complications to the process of revealing private information (Petronio, 2013). Authorized co-owners of private information may involve multiple people or groups and may require renegotiation at multiple turning points. The notion of co-ownership in health care requires seeing privacy and disclosure as relational in nature (Petronio, 2013). The relationships involve providers and patients as interconnected with family and close friends. Disclosure predicaments identified through the lens of communication privacy management theory shed light on the ethics of physician–patient confidentiality and the contradictions inherent in navigating the health-care provider–patient relationship while also considering implications for family relationships and patients' close relationships connected to receiving health care.

RELATIONAL TURBULENCE MODEL AND RELATIONAL TURBULENCE THEORY

The relational turbulence model poses a perspective on communication that highlights how relationship transitions in personal relationships polarize emotions and cognitive appraisals and disrupt the exchange of messages between people (Solomon, 2016). The relational turbulence model is an evidence-based model inductively derived from evidence of more frequent experiences of conflict, more frequent and intense negative emotions, and heightened relationship thinking during the transition from casual to serious involvement in dating relationships (Solomon, Weber, & Steuber, 2010). Since the original proposed model, the scope of the relational turbulence model has expanded beyond focusing on developing courtships to shed light on well-established relationships, such as transitions in marriage (Solomon, 2016). More recently, the model was transformed to focus on three key theoretical advances, moving from a model that depicts associations between phenomena to a theory. Relational turbulence theory identifies processes and mechanisms through which relational uncertainty and interference from a partner shape subjective experiences including emotions, cognitive processes, and subsequent behavioral sequences (Solomon et al., 2016). Because the theory developed from insights based on the model, and because the theory has only recently been published as a theory, I describe theoretical assumptions first for the relational turbulence model and then for the expanded logic of relational turbulence theory.

Theoretical assumptions. The relational turbulence model first assumes that relationship transitions create upheaval for romantic relationships, and that disruptions to the status quo require new patterns of interaction (Solomon et al., 2010). The relational turbulence model identifies relationship qualities that account for reactivity during times of transition in romantic relationships (Solomon & Knobloch, 2004; Solomon et al., 2010). The model proposes that transitions correspond to relational uncertainty including doubts and questions people have about their relationship and dyadic coordination where behavioral sequences correspond with more frequent experiences of interference from a partner (Solomon, 2016). *Relational uncertainty* includes self uncertainty, or the questions people have about their own relational commitment; partner uncertainty, or the doubts that emerge about a partner's relational goals and investment; and relationship uncertainty, or the doubts people have about the future of the relationship itself (Knobloch & Solomon, 1999). Path modeling suggests that multiple facets of relational uncertainty function as distinct phenomena but also are correlated (Knobloch, Miller, & Carpenter, 2007).

Changes in patterns of interaction include shifts in dyadic coordination. Consistent with interdependence theory, the relational turbulence model proposes that people in intimate relationships have enmeshed action sequences in that achieving goals or activities relies on the relational partner's behavior (Solomon, 2016). Relationship transitions challenge and disrupt the action sequences and dyadic coordination of action sequences.

Relationship transitions challenge the interdependence patterns in action sequences. According to the relational turbulence model, times of relational transitions include more frequent experiences of *interference* from a partner. As relationships adapt to the turbulence of transition, disruptive patterns of interference shift to coordinated actions that facilitate the achievement of goals and performance of routine or everyday activities (Solomon, 2016). Essential features of interdependence in the model stem from Berscheid's (1983) descriptions of interdependence features. According to the model, partner influence as engagement in everyday goals and activities functions differently from partner interference in accomplishing everyday goals and activities and differently from partner facilitation when a partner enhances involvement in everyday goals and activities (Knobloch & Solomon, 2004). Partners developing relationships increasingly involve each other in their activities such that involvement becomes less disruptive and more facilitative as relationships become more intimate (Knobloch & Solomon, 2004).

The relational turbulence model proposes that relational uncertainty and partner interference predict polarized emotional and cognitive appraisals and disrupt the exchange of messages between people in close relationships. Multiple studies address a myriad of negative outcomes that characterize the transition from casual to serious dating relationships. Previous studies document relationship challenges including negative emotions, bias cognitions, and difficult communication during relational transitions (Solomon & Theiss, 2011). Negative emotional experiences include feeling hurt, jealous, angry, and sad in response to partner behavior and in general (Solomon & Theiss, 2011). During relationship transition from casual dating to serious involvement, higher relational uncertainty and interference also correspond to romantic partners' evaluations of irritating circumstances within the relationship as more serious, the other person's hurtful behavior as more intentional, and assessed social networks as more disruptive to the relationship (Solomon & Theiss, 2011). The model predicts that people experience more relational uncertainty, more interference from a partner, more biased cognitive appraisals, stronger emotions, and distinctive communication at moderate levels of intimacy, and moderate levels of intimacy were assumed to correspond with the transition from casual to serious dating (Solomon & Knobloch, 2001; Solomon & Knobloch, 2004). Applications of the model indicated intimacy was less consistent in predicting outcomes than relational characteristics or characteristics of interdependence (Solomon & Theiss, 2008).

Over time, the relational turbulence model has moved beyond cross-sectional research designs and experiences of individuals to include longitudinal and dyadic studies that shed light on the process of developing interdependence over time and the role of relational uncertainty and goal interference across contexts. The model was initially developed and tested in the context of negative outcomes that characterize the transition from casual to serious romantic involvement. To that end, tests of the model contextualize and shed light on characteristics of relationships that contribute to romantic partners' influence, interference, and facilitation from a partner and how these processes yield specific outcomes (Knobloch & Solomon, 2004). The model offers explanations for turmoil during transitions from casual dating to serious involvement.

Theoretical developments since the inception of the relational turbulence model fall along two main lines. First, the context of the model has developed to pose implications for transitions in close relationships more broadly than during transition from casual dating to serious involvement. To that end, more recent descriptions and applications of the theory shed light on transitions that evoke relational uncertainty and disrupt interdependence over the life span of a close relationship. Second, initial applications and tests of the theory proposed that intimacy and relational development prompted relational uncertainty and experiences of interdependence (Knobloch & Solomon, 2004; Knobloch, 2007). More recent explications move the explanatory framework from a model that poses relationships among variables to a theory that addresses questions about the mechanisms that link relationship qualities to emotional, cognitive, and communicative responses to transitions that occur over the life span of romantic relationships (Solomon et al., 2016).

Expanded conceptualization: Relational turbulence theory. The expanded theoretical explanation of relational turbulence advances the earlier model by articulating processes that give rise to associations between identified phenomena. Relational turbulence theory specifies the distinctive processes through which relational uncertainty and interference from a partner shape cognitions and emotions (Solomon et al., 2016). The expanded theoretical explanation also elaborates on the causal relationships among cognitions, emotions, and communication. In addition, the expanded theoretical explanation sheds light on how specific experiences shape an overall perception of the relationship as chaotic, and how this characterization predicts outcomes. Attentiveness to theoretical mechanisms allows for guiding tests, rather than applications, of the framework (Solomon et al., 2016). Relational turbulence theory as expanded from the model provides insight into how relational turbulence constitutes a global quality of romantic associations that shape personal, relational, and social outcomes with implications for qualities of personal relationships, communication, and well-being (Solomon et al., 2016).

Relationship transitions. The expanded theory positions any romantic relationship transition as having the potential to promote relational uncertainty and complicate patterns of interdependence. A transition in a close relationship is defined as a period of discontinuity between times of relative stability, during which individuals adapt to changing roles (Solomon et al., 2016). Relationship transitions are positive or negative developments that encompass changes or create a mismatch between previously held relationship beliefs or routines and new relationship circumstances (Solomon & Theiss, 2011). Changes to the internal environment (e.g., pregnancy), or changes to the external environment (e.g., military deployment) can spark transition. Changes to the environment can be minor (e.g., starting a new hobby) to life altering (e.g., cancer diagnosis). Changes can develop gradually (e.g., declining health), or can surface suddenly and without notice (e.g., termination of employment) (Solomon et al., 2016). Relational turbulence theory considers a relational transition ending not when the emergent conditions subside but when partners adapt to the new circumstances and establish new patterns of relating (Solomon & Theiss, 2011). Relationship transitions are pivotal junctures that bring the potential for reorganization and renegotiation and growth or, on the contrary, for relationship decline. Although often prompted by relationship transition, relational uncertainty and interdependence processes can shift in salient ways without a specific transition as prompt (McLaren, Solomon, & Priem, 2011). Thus, the theory addresses changes to the relational environment but does not specify transition as a condition of testing the theory, because it considers relational uncertainty and interdependence to be relevant processes without a specific transition.

Relational uncertainty and interdependence during transitions. Beyond the application and explication of relational turbulence in the transition from casual dating to serious commitment, evidence for relational turbulence theory includes experiences of interdependence as married people grapple with life changes. Discourse posted in online discussion boards and blogs of women coping with breast cancer or the experience of infertility revealed that women experience uncertainty as a polarizing phenomenon in their relationships. In online discourse from women experiencing breast cancer, the women revealed experiences of uncertainty about telling other people about their cancer, questions about what life with their spouse would be like after cancer, worry about living with side effects of treatment, and worries about their future (Solomon et al., 2010). Challenges with interdependence included unmet expectations for support, challenges for physical constraints and activities of daily living, and disruptive reactions from relationship partners (Solomon et al., 2010).

Women experiencing infertility documented similar challenges to interdependence. Coming to terms with challenges in having a biological child prompted relationship transitions in which couples revised their plans for having a family, changed their conception of family, or came to terms with routes to creating their family (Steuber & Solomon, 2012). Relational uncertainty was connected in questions people asked about their partner's commitment to a relationship that could not produce a biological child. People coping with infertility reported goal interference including needing to change sexual behavior to coordinate with fertility and working around scheduled appointments with fertility clinics (Steuber & Solomon, 2012).

Similarly, people report relationship transitions and upheaval during the post-deployment transition for military service members. Military personnel who had recently returned home reported relational uncertainty and interference from partners. Higher uncertainty and interference predicted openness and aggression, which in turn predicted appraisals of affiliation and dominance in the relationship (Theiss & Knobloch, 2013). Military couples faced relational uncertainty challenges about sharing information, coordinating new routines, and managing emotions. Military personnel and partners experienced openness and aggressiveness as two features of relational communication predicted by the mechanisms of relational turbulence (Theiss & Knobloch, 2013). The military application provided evidence that features of relational communication are markers of relational turbulence that mediate the associations between the mechanisms of relational turbulence and appraisals of relational meaning.

Health and illness issues and relational turbulence theory. Relational turbulence theory and the constructs of the theory developed from an early explanatory framework of relational changes involved in moving from casual dating to more serious relationships. More recently the expanded conceptualization and theoretical development address turbulence in relationship transitions across the life span of stable relationships. Applications of the theory address issues that are more closely aligned with relational explanatory frameworks than health but that pose implications for better understanding the interconnections between close relationships and health-care contexts. In keeping with the theory, this chapter first addresses applications of relational turbulence theory that have direct health implications and then poses implications for considering health-care contexts more broadly than has yet been tested by the theory.

The two areas of research where components of relational turbulence theory have been applied to health contexts are breast cancer and infertility. Relational turbulence theory suggests that transitions in romantic relationships spark more extreme reactions to relationship events, and personal relationships and communication can function as sources of stress for people adjusting to diagnosis and treatment of breast cancer (Weber & Solomon, 2008). When moving from a known context to an unknown context such as hearing diagnosis of breast cancer or beginning or changing treatment, the relational contexts within which people live also experience change.

Breast cancer patients experience substantial distress during their diagnosis, treatment, and survivorship. Discussing their breast cancer with relationship partners or close friends at different points in treatment can facilitate psychological adjustment. The social support component of coping with illness is not necessarily a unique point of adjustment. However, the ways in which breast cancer creates distress by changing features of women's personal relationships and communication experiences is a dimension different from the constructs addressed in the social support literature (Weber & Solomon, 2008). Relational turbulence theory provides insight into the transformations that occur within relationships during times of transition, and breast cancer diagnosis, treatment, and survivorship serve as transitions. Transitions create change that involves the reorganization and reintegration of identities, roles, relationships, or behaviors, which may require one to alter one's current conduct or to modify how one defines oneself or one's relationship (Knobloch & Solomon, 1999).

Relational uncertainty focuses on people's confidence in their perceptions of relationship involvement (Knobloch & Solomon, 1999). The diagnosis of breast cancer connects to doubts and concerns and questions about personal relationships. Relational uncertainty is considered alongside illness uncertainty such that relational uncertainty connects to questions about a partner or close relationship, about a partner's desire for the relationship, and about ambiguity of relational norms or about the future (Knobloch & Solomon, 1999). Relational uncertainty was connected to each theme identified in online discourse about breast cancer (Weber & Solomon, 2008). Women struggled to reconcile their pre-diagnosis identity with relational identities that emerged throughout breast cancer treatment. Physical and mental fatigue, loss of hair, growth of facial hair, abnormal odors, nausea, burning sensations from radiation, and unfamiliar discomforts were connected to feelings of uncertainty about their relational identities (Weber & Solomon, 2008). The transition from feeling sturdy and healthy to feeling worn down mentally and physically caused women to question both casual and intimate relationships (Weber & Solomon, 2008). Coping with immediate and long-term side effects also required women and their relationship partners to adjust their routines, goals, and expectations (Weber & Solomon, 2008). Information needs sometimes prompted relational distress and taxed women and their families to manage a host of information needs with an eye toward how their choices affected other people in their lives. Partners and close friends who provided support also could be sources of relational and communicative tensions, including such issues as claiming to be grieving about the diagnosis of the partner or close friend. In addition, breast cancer patients described feeling misunderstood, isolated, or alone, at least indicating lack of shared meaning between their cancer experience and the experience close friends described in providing intended support (Weber & Solomon, 2008). Physical and emotional changes also shifted symbols of sexuality and how to address sexual identity following treatment. As women adapted new identities, managed information, coordinated ownership over the disease, felt misunderstood by others, and came to terms with their altered sexuality, they also worried about how their relationships would change their identity, relational life over time, and sexuality (Weber & Solomon, 2008).

Treatment decisions can be influenced by genetic understanding, environment, social factors, and personal behaviors on breast cancer, among other issues (Parrott, Silk, & Condit, 2003). In the context of breast cancer treatment decisions as connected to goal interference, research provides evidence for relationship-embedded decisions in addition to considering medical information, self-efficacy, and avoiding adverse experience (Weber, Solomon, & Meyer, 2013). In addition, people in the study who were other-focused tended to rely on the input of other people or the role that other people had in their life when making a difficult treatment decision (Weber et al., 2013). For women who engaged in a relationship-embedded decision style, their primary concern about breast cancer treatment was extending their life so they could spend more time with loved ones, including spouses, children, and grandchildren (Weber et al., 2013). For women engaged in a relationship-embedded decision style, the need to gather information appears to be overshadowed by a desire to be with their family; women in this study did not emphasize the steps they needed to take to make a treatment decision, but instead focused on being with their family and appeared to have low need for information (Weber et al., 2013).

Research about breast cancer treatment decisions did not directly test relational turbulence theory but offers insight into potential partner interference. In applying relational turbulence theory, interference from a partner occurs within relationships to the extent that one partner impedes the goals or activities of another partner (Solomon & Knobloch, 2004). Because transitions require partners to renegotiate roles, identities, relationships, and behaviors, they also increase opportunities for goal interference (Weber & Solomon, 2008). One part of breast cancer treatment decisions is considering medical information, potential new treatments such as clinical trials, self-efficacy, and information from a variety of sources. Considering relationship-embedded decisions in women's choices about breast cancer treatment through the lens of relational turbulence theory implies that women integrate information they think would be best for their close relationships. Considering relationship-embedded decisions poses implications that exceed previous tests of the theory to imply what people perceive in a relationship connected to illness treatment, which may be different from what relational partners or close friends perceive. Broader considerations for health and illness changes as a relational transition are proposed in the next chapters of this volume.

In the breast cancer context, information-sharing boundaries were identified as a source of distress discussed by breast cancer patients and by their close friends and family members (Weber & Solomon, 2008). When women faced changes in their sense of sexuality, they were concerned beyond the physical side of treatment. Women expressed concerns about sharing information with their spouses but not wanting to frighten them or put them off with their post-cancer appearance (Weber & Solomon, 2008). Both theories speak to issues of relationship transition as points of relational uncertainty, and the experience of shifting choices as connected to relationships goals and potential interference from partners or close friends in decision-making, in disclosure, or in next steps is coping.

Relational uncertainty surfaces within couples making sense of infertility. The difficulty inherent in balancing the treatment process with maintaining a marriage can contribute to doubts about the marital bond (Steuber & Solomon, 2008). The management of blame directed either toward the self or toward the partner can instigate sentiments of relational uncertainty. In addition to challenging decisions about treatment, couples make decisions about disclosure within a relational context characterized by doubts and ambiguities (Steuber & Solomon, 2008). Couples might experience difficulties engaging in negotiation about what can be shared because they are coping with their own relational uncertainty. Partner interference also surfaces within infertile couples, as people coping with infertility highlighted tensions arising when their partner wanted to respond to infertility differently from how they did (Steuber & Solomon, 2008). Partner interference also included frustrations when the partner prioritized infertility over the normalcy of the relationship or, conversely, failed to appreciate the perceived gravity of the condition (Steuber & Solomon, 2008).

Disclosure and privacy can be interconnected with relational uncertainty and partner interference. Examples from the infertility context suggest that relational uncertainty increases when partners negotiate treatment for, and disclosure about, infertility (Steuber & Solomon, 2012). Disclosure discrepancies emerged when spouses differed in their perceptions or behaviors related to sharing infertility-related information with people outside the marriage. From examining spouses' accounts of their own disclosures about infertility to third parties, their feelings about those disclosures, and their perceptions of each other, researchers provide evidence for the complexity of co-owning information about disclosure sometimes resulting in disrupted coordination or boundary turbulence (Steuber & Solomon, 2012). Disclosure prompted privacy dilemmas about who has the right to know the information, unclear boundaries, mistaken violation of rules, and sometimes intentional leaks of information (Steuber & Solomon, 2012). As Petronio (2002) emphasized in communication privacy management theory, manifestations of boundary turbulence and disclosure discrepancies required renegotiations of privacy rules.

Disclosure discrepancies also were connected to discomfort with spousal disclosures consistent with the theoretical constructs of partner interference in relational turbulence theory (Steuber & Solomon, 2012). Couples who experienced interferences with their everyday routines as connected to infertility might be more likely to discuss discrepancies in disclosure about their infertility, thereby limiting boundary turbulence (Steuber & Solomon, 2012). Couples with facilitative patterns of interdependence might assume coordination in their disclosure boundaries without engaging in conversations that would clarify the expected disclosures to others (Steuber & Solomon, 2012). Experiences of interference might be disruptive in the short term but might prompt communication behaviors that promote coordinated behavior and limit future privacy boundary violations (Steuber & Solomon, 2012). Couples participating in research about infertility disclosure also reported relatively low levels of relational uncertainty in that they self-selected to take part in a research study implying marital stability (Steuber & Solomon, 2012). In considering how disclosure about infertility to third parties connects to both theories, future considerations would continue to uncover relational characteristics of the transition at each stage and attempt at infertility treatment, as co-navigating expectations for infertility assume relational stability but also can challenge assumptions for relational progression and relational goals. When we consider the interconnection between privacy boundaries and relational turbulence, we also are inherently talking about how relationships are entangled, or how the interdependent sequences are manifest in partners' behavior.

Applications of the theories in the context of stressors associated with breast cancer, and applications of infertility disclosures addressing markers of boundary turbulence in sharing private information, integrate both relational turbulence theory and communication privacy management theory. Diagnosis and changes in illness treatment choices can serve as a relationship transition and also can obscure the boundaries that define who owns and controls private information. As patients and their relational partners and close friends receive new information about illness choices and trajectories, poorly coordinated boundaries for information sharing can lead to violated expectations and privacy rules (Duggan & Petronio, 2009; Petronio, 2002). Health-care treatment transitions necessitate the reorganization and reiteration of information sharing in close relationships. Sharing private information fosters intimacy and makes individuals vulnerable, and people in close relationships supporting someone through treatment develop norms for disclosing and withholding information (Duggan & Petronio, 2009; Petronio, 2002). The health-care system poses multiple challenges and complexities for sharing information otherwise negotiated within a close relationship (Duggan & Petronio, 2009; Petronio, 2002). Changes in the circumstances for individuals receiving health care and their close friends and family who are with them during the illness transitions can lead to problems coordinating information sharing and privacy (Duggan & Petronio, 2009; Petronio, 2002). When individuals have different standards for information sharing, or when the health-care context shifts expectations for information, they might experience boundary turbulence in information disclosure (Duggan & Petronio, 2009; Petronio, 2002). Furthermore, patients and partners or close friends might experience changes in illness treatment functioning as a relationship transition connected to relational uncertainty and partner interference (Solomon & Knobloch, 2004; Steuber & Solomon, 2011). Disclosure or new information can function as a marker of relationship turbulence. In addressing infertility, a number of contextual variables may affect whether couples effectively coordinate boundaries around shared infertility-related information (Steuber & Solomon, 2012).

PART III Integrated Theory of Health and Illness Trajectories and Relational Processes

7 Theorizing Close Relationships and Health and Illness Trajectories
Co-created, Co-generative, and Systematic Processes

> *I don't think literature would be possible in a determined world. We might go through the motions but the heart would be out of it ... I think the more you write, the less inclined you will be to rely on theories like determinism. Mystery isn't something that is gradually evaporating. It grows along with knowledge.*

– Flannery O'Connor

> *I write because I don't know what I think until I read what I say.*

–Flannery O'Connor

> *When it comes to the past, everyone writes fiction.*

–Stephen King

ENGAGED THEORIZING

> When Frances turned thirty-three, she started to become someone she did not know. She had always relied on her body to serve her well. Ted, who Frances met on the ski lift, was equally reliant on his body. Doing pleasurably strenuous activities together was a fundamental cornerstone of their relationship. At the age of thirty-three, Frances began to get signals from her body that all was not well. She felt tired as soon as she woke up in the morning, even though she had had eight hours of sleep. Most disturbing to her was that her body hurt. She felt aches and pains similar to those she experienced after a ten-mile hike. At times, when Ted caressed her hair or massaged her shoulders, she yelped in pain. Frances tried to ignore her symptoms, but over the next six months they got worse. She was tired all the time, which made it difficult for her to concentrate at work as a lawyer. She was regularly abrupt with Ted or avoided him altogether. Ted showed his concern by inviting her to participate in the activities they enjoyed, which had often worked in the

> past. Now, however, Frances was too tired or in too much pain to engage,
> and too confused and worried to explain. Their world had changed, and
> they didn't know why.

> – Kivowitz & Weisman, 2013. *In Sickness as in Health: Helping Couples
> Cope with the Complexities of Illness.*

> Engaged theorizing, like good conversation, puts us and our knowl-
> edge at risk. If we are open to the other, we do not know where the
> conversation is going; we do not know how they and we will change.
> In productive engagement with the world, a world of possibilities that
> was not seen before can open, and can place demands to grow and
> change. If we enter one-sided and protected we may do a good thing
> for the other, but engagement allows a different risk, mutual learning,
> concept formation.

> – S. Deetz, 2008. "Engagement as Co-generative Theorizing."

I chose the brief references to Flannery O'Connor and Stephen King
alongside each other because they are known for such different writing. O'Connor's writing wrestles with morally flawed characters
engaged in questions of morality or ethics. Her characters face transformation through opportunities to be more fully human, and her
Catholic sense of unfolding mystery is evident in her attentiveness
consistent with a divine sense of grace and humor. Stephen King spent
half a century writing horror stories, and the horror of his writing is in
the portrayal of characters who engage as terrifyingly real villains or
inner monsters. Their quotes give a hint into their engagement with
the subject matter as they write, with an unfolding that occurs during
the process.

   The story of Frances comes from a book on helping couples cope
with the complexities of illness and provides a glimpse into the process of listening to the body and making new sense of the self and of
the relationship as the body changes with illness. This story indicates
how the physical body redirects attention during illness, a theme that
connects to the ideas of embodiment described in this volume.
The body shifts from being engaged in pleasurably strenuous activities
to carrying aches and pains. Individual and relational identity and
connection are shifted.

The image of engaged theorizing as good conversation is especially salient for relationship researchers. We remain in the research not because we have more to say, but because we have more to understand. In this chapter, I build on the idea of writing and theory as engagement, with hopes that we can grow and change as researchers and practitioners, that we develop the attentiveness to unfolding new concepts.

THEORY AS CO-CREATED

Co-created theory engages what we understand with what we do not yet know. Rather than applying relationship theories to health contexts (or rather than applying health behavior theories to relationship contexts), co-created theory engages the complexities of the subject matter. In health and illness, and in close relationships, the subject matter itself is complex. Co-created theory engages the complexities of the parts of the subject matter we know and the parts of the subject matter for which we have language. *But it goes beyond that.* Co-created theory also engages the mystery, the unfolding, the parts of the subject matter we do not yet know, the part of the self we do not know. Sometimes the emergence is manifest in the body, and other times the emergence is manifest in new understanding in relationships. Sometimes emergence is manifest in multiple ways. Sometimes we notice it. Other times we come back to it again and again before we can find meaning. Like a new relationship or a newly recognized illness, we cannot fully understand without continuing to engage.

In this chapter, I map out an integrated, co-created theory of relationship processes and health and illness trajectories. In order to understand co-created theory we first address strengths and limitations in interconnections of individual factors, dyadic factors, turning points in diagnosis, management and treatment of illness, turning points in relationships, and the societal, economic, and cultural factors within which relationships are embedded. Beyond the complexities of those interconnections, co-created, co-generative, and systematic theorizing allows for emergence, for recognizing moments of something that can be new. Mapping out the integrated theoretical framework shows processes and pathways through which relationship processes and health and illness trajectories are co-created, co-generative, systematic processes. The integrated theory explains how dual and interdependent lenses of relationship processes and health and illness trajectories are communicatively coproduced at particular turning points and over time.

SYSTEMATIC UNDERSTANDING

Systematic understanding of close relationships and health and illness trajectories first requires an ability to see social scientific theories and humanistic understanding not as dichotomous *either/or* explanations but as mutually appropriate *both/and* options, as mutually compatible and offering different lenses. The chapters so far present multiple lenses for understanding the foundations of health and illness and close relationships. To that end, researchers can recognize the strengths and challenges in social scientific theories of relationships as also recognizing the complexities of the health and illness context. A systematic understanding of close relationships and health and illness trajectories recognizes tensions, contradictions, and synergies as opportunities for emerging understanding. Emerging understanding moves beyond additional application of a theory we already know to instead playing with the tension, contradictions, and synergies that emerge by engaging with the subject matter. In outlining systematic understanding, my intention is to recognize and illustrate co-created theoretical *process as generative* rather than to elaborate two connected hypothetico-deductive models. The communication, behavior, understanding, and choices emerge from the interaction between the health and illness systems and the close relationships systems such that emergence and generativity are the foundation of mapping out theory. In describing emergence or generativity of interconnected systems, the end goal is not to take into account all of the contributing variables, but to recognize competing tensions and stakeholders and how interactions are communicatively produced.

IMAGES OF THEORETICAL GENERATIVITY

Image of creating ongoing possibilities: Mirror-in-mirror. If I could choose a theme song for my understanding of theory, it would be Arvo Pärt's 1978 composition of "Spiegel im Spiegel (Mirror in Mirror)." The piece was originally written for a single piano and violin and refers to an infinity mirror which infinitely reflects back ongoing parallel images. I am not a musician, and as an "outsider" to music, I lack the language for attempting to capture the particular pathways through which the music speaks to me. I know that when I listen to it, the interconnection between two performers captures something of the other and allows for me to sense both structure and alteration, to experience variation of ascending and descending, to know of nuance for which I do not have language, and about which language feels limiting rather than expanding. Complexities emerge in the image of reflecting on the mirror, of moving away from the mirror, and of returning over and over to the reflection. The mirror-in-mirror image is both the tangible mirror that reflects back and the process of image within the reflection.

The mirror-in-mirror image provides a metaphor for *way of being* as reflected in *asking questions* that allow for engaged emergence, for co-generativity, and for seeing differently. We notice differently when we are drawn into questions instead of applying what we already know to a new situation. We pay attention differently when we are drawn into human conversation for what might unfold rather than for repeating what we already know. Asking good questions sustains and allows for people to be drawn in and to keep noticing questions differently.

In coproduced theory as mirror-in-mirror, we allow for emerging questions.

What draws attention? What else exists that does not draw attention? How do we make meaning of what we see? How do we respond to the questions? Like the mirror-in-mirror image, our response might evoke further attentiveness, shifting meaning, and ongoing variation in how we respond to the questions. Co-generative theory sheds light, makes meaning, and engages with emergent questions and new ways of seeing.

Image of embodied generativity: Walking a labyrinth. I have a long fascination with walking labyrinths, an image of process and embodiment as generative. By labyrinth, I do not mean a maze where there are potential false turnings and blind endings where one can get lost and never escape. Instead, I mean a labyrinth as a single unicursal path where the only choice is whether to go in. The labyrinth does not engage the thinking mind, but invites a physicality of the intuitive, pattern-seeking, symbolic senses to come forth. Walking a labyrinth immerses the physical self in a process world where the walking becomes the process of seeing between lines of linear thought to the potential for more creative imagination and intuition. The labyrinth calls to "stay awhile," to be distant from the hope of the known self, to let emergence be silent, like spring flowers just about to open. Walking a labyrinth brings me questions and curiosity. Sometimes the labyrinth path is a wide open space, or so narrow it requires focus to keep one foot in front of the other; sometimes the labyrinth path is marked by rocks or bricks with a smooth pathway, or grassy, or elevated slightly above the rocks. Although a single path, the labyrinth includes twists and turns that require the walker to turn and to change direction in order to move forward, to see new optics when the straight path is not possible.

The labyrinth exists within context of other spaces. In downtown Boston, I walk a labyrinth dedicated to the victims of the Armenian Genocide located in a quiet corner; across one busy street corner the walk looks into Faneuil Hall, across another corner to the bustle of children taking a spin on a carousel of animals native to Boston (lobster, cod, fox, squirrel, falcon, harbor seal), and across another corner to the ferries to the harbor islands. The immersive experience of quiet reflection amidst these wildly disparate images offers an image of context as emergence. An intentional stepping into the path, to step back from the possibilities in every direction, to allow the possibility of seeing differently. At another favorite labyrinth, there is a small sign reading "it is solved by walking." Walking the labyrinth is an image of engaging without needing an outcome, of engaging to allow for emergence, of engaging the physical body with imagination.

Engaged scholarship as co-created research. The theme of engaged scholarship is articulated in organizational communication scholarship as being immersed in the lives of real-world groups and organizations (Barge, Simpson, & Shockley-Zalabak, 2008). I begin with a description of engaged scholarship as manifest in organizational communication research and then move to the broader idea of engagement as offering multiple lenses of coproduced theory of health and illness in close relationships. The conversation in organizational communication was articulated in 2002 to include organizational practitioners and scholars to mutually shape understanding and interests; this "engaged communication scholarship" explores the theory, praxis, and pedagogy of organizational engagement with the goal of engaging meaningfully with practitioners (Simpson & Seibold, 2008). Engagement moves beyond translating scholarship into practice and instead considers theoretical perspectives with practical questions and concerns (Simpson & Seibold, 2008).

Engaged scholarship can be generative, but that requires a commitment to embracing aspiration and expectation without predetermined constraint, of seeing new possibilities for action, of trusting in the possibility of new insights, new possibilities, new realities (Barge et al., 2008). Engaged scholarship utilizes a range of theoretical tools in studying a particular context as opposed to studying a particular theory or construct (Simpson & Seibold, 2008). Engaged scholarship is developed and executed in partnership with practitioners by developing relationships (Simpson & Seibold, 2008). The reflexive and recursive practices can enrich theory and can ensure a more complex ethical foundation by engaging what we become in producing knowledge rather than what we do with the knowledge. Engaged scholarship allows the possibility of emergent theory rather than focusing on expanding our audience and making scholarship more relevant or accessible to practitioner audiences (Simpson & Seibold, 2008).

One way that engaged scholarship can allow for emergence is by recognizing the constitutive nature of language as reflecting a way of attending to the world and recognizing how language relates to knowledge (Deetz, 2008). Language and knowledge-producing practices can become impoverished when they no longer help us attend to differences. Impoverished ways of talking about the world reproduce and protect what we already know instead of organically growing in relation to changing human need and life circumstances (Deetz, 2008). To that end, approaches to understanding focus on the interplay between the ways that scholars theorize the subject and the practices they inspire within the contextual life of what is addressed. Constitutive engagement considers communication as generative such that theoretical resources can intervene in the productive process. Communicative practices can challenge understanding or, on the contrary, can reproduce what is already known. Engaged scholarship embraces multiple perspectives but also requires attentiveness and reflection about how values and theories inform action. Reflection allows for stepping back to consider essential practices that might be done differently so as to engage in a process of continuous learning and of seeing differently.

The necessity of multiple lenses. The lived experience of health and illness and the nature of people in close relationships require an ongoing commitment to exploring emerging complexities. Instead of making sense of the world through processes of simplification that deny the complexity and details of experience, allowing for complexities means creating context and listening in ways that evoke details of individual experience and recognizing a multiplicity of lenses. Stories about health and illness illustrate the details such that the complexities and authentic experiential nature of each person resist simplification.

One manifestation of multiple lenses is the nonverbal context alongside verbal language. Nonverbal behaviors in the face, the voice, and the body indicate tone, affect, emotion, and experience beyond what words capture. Communication about health and illness addresses both biomedical components about patients' symptoms and the structure and functions of organs and experiential components about beliefs, emotions, family connections, and beliefs about illness (Duggan & Parrott, 2001). Traditional medical training in the United States has focused on prompting verbal patient disclosure about relevant biomedical symptoms. As broader understanding of health and illness includes information better measured in affective tone and rapport, we then look to the importance of nonverbal communication behaviors and of patient disclosure of information that sheds light on their illness experience (Duggan & Parrott, 2001). Applications of social scientific understanding of theory provide evidence for physicians and patients' interaction adaptation (Duggan & Bradshaw, 2008). Physicians and patients shifted during different interactions: as interactions evolved, physicians and patients became more similar to each other in smiling and head nodding; they became more different from each other in negative behaviors, increasing divergence in their negative eye behaviors, sentence disfluencies, and talk about barriers to wellness (Duggan & Bradshaw, 2008). This analysis of physician–patient communication illustrates social-scientific evidence for within-interaction change as an indication of relationship-centered health care, and poses that divergence may indicate a power-imbalanced interaction (Duggan & Bradshaw, 2008).

Establishing a context that promotes disclosure about the illness experience gives a different and broader lens for communication about health and illness than just asking biomedical questions. Studying relationships in health and illness contexts illustrates the necessity of multiple lenses. In integrating lenses of biopsychosocial understanding with systematic processes and generativity, we recognize illness as a point of vulnerability in the bodily experience and in close relationships. The unanticipated, nonlinear experience of a frightening diagnosis or injury requires finding new ways to navigate, a shifting appreciation for the relative predictability of close relationships, attentiveness to different cues. It requires finding new ways to navigate that integrate the subtle expressions and allow for emergence that moves beyond just promoting disclosure through particular communication behaviors.

Multiple lenses as noticing complexities. Multiple lenses can allow for better noticing of subtleties, complexities, and nuances. In the *Handbook of Systems and Complexity in Health*, the editors Joachim Sturmberg and Carmel Martin (2013) begin the introduction with Albert Einstein's quote that "the world will not evolve past its current state of crisis by using the same thinking that created the situation." The way we theorize and talk about the world is the way we think about the world. The behavior of system components varies with context and can be co-generative with context (Sturmberg & Martin, 2013). Multiple lenses can allow for generativity in noticing and addressing complexities instead of reproducing the part of the world we know.

Complexity study and theory aims to understand how things are connected with each other and how these interactions work together. Complexity science and complexity theories represent a convergence of different types of ideas and theories to address the nonlinearity and dynamics of real-world systems (Sturmberg & Martin, 2013). Complexities in medicine do not follow the linear mantra of history, examination, diagnosis, and treatment of a single diagnosis to suggest appropriate treatment; complexities in medicine instead recognize that a single patient comes with multiple biological, psychosocial, relational, historical, and experiential components. Seeing the health-care interaction as a complex adaptive system moves past the biomedical mantra such that sensitivity, intuition, commitment, and pragmatic preparedness become as important as a sound grasp of medical knowl-edge (Heath, 2013). Heath (2013) delineates two distinct groups of health-care professionals interested in complexity theory. The first group comes with understanding and talent in mathematics to offer possibilities of mathematical modeling of chaos and complexity; the second group is motivated by understanding chaos and complexity as a metaphor to make sense of the experience of caring for patients and to reunite the apparent polarities described as the art and science of medicine. To that end, complexity can be understood in the uncertainty and necessarily messy links between science and the humanities in health care (Heath, 2013). Our lenses to interact with the world determine the direction of our thoughts. Multiple lenses allow for uncertainties and recognize the (sometimes painful) limitations of a model and the potential capacities for different metaphors, different angles, and different lenses.

There is a socioeconomic gradient in almost all major disease categories, meaning that people and families who are socioeconomi-cally disadvantaged are at risk of a compounding multiplicity of health and social problems (Heath, 2013). Multiple morbidity is a major component of health inequalities and can be understood in part as a consequence of the wider societal determinants of ill-health (Heath, 2013). Health care that is driven and evaluated increasingly by proto-cols derived from studies of single-disease conditions seems likely to disadvantage systematically those with complex and overlapping health and illness experiences (Heath, 2013). Multiple lenses require patient narratives that allow for illustrating the context of the broader life story, and communication processes and responses that manage multiple health and illness issues and address the full diversity of the experiences. Biomedical science based on generalizations of symp-toms recognized as disease allows for progress in clinical medicine, but the process of being asked biomedical questions can leave individuals feeling unrecognized and misunderstood, and the reality of their symptoms unheard (Heath, 2013).

The necessity of understanding multiple lenses also extends to multiple explanatory frameworks of complexities of a global and socioeconomic spectrum. The illness experience is further confounded when people have more than one diagnosis. When we give examples of illness, we talk about management of a single disease, which is useful to the extent that it allows for guidelines for managing symptoms. However, the limitations of this approach become clear when we consider that few people have only one diagnosis, and people who are poor, old, or lower on the socioeconomic gradient often have multiple and compounding issues.

The urge to simplify misses the opportunity for multiple lenses. The complexities addressed in the *Handbook of Systems and Complexity in Health* include almost a thousand pages of well-considered, well-researched sense-making to expand the understanding of health-care processes and outcomes. To that end, the handbook includes areas of understanding on the complex notions of health, health care, health-care reform, and the interconnected, multidimensional aspects of sense-making around health. Additional complexities are to be considered when we also integrate systems and complexities of close relationships.

COMMUNICATION AS CONSTITUTIVE

Understanding theory as seeing multiple lenses also suggests that seeing is theory-laden. What people see is framed through the lenses of attentiveness such that observations themselves are theory-laden. The treatment of observation as if it preceded and could be compared to theoretical accounts hides the theoretical choices implicit in conceptualization and instrumentation of the observation (Deetz, 1992). If we understand theory as process of being in the world, then we also recognize observations, questions, and attentiveness as manifestations of the theoretical lens through which we see the world. Theory as process involves recognizing interests and values. As illustrated in the complexities of definitions, and theories presented so far in this book, definitions and theories are inherently connected to interaction, and our process of being in the world serves as a lens through which we understand health and illness, as well as how we understand and experience close relationships.

Recognizing the possibilities of multiple lenses allows for meaning to continue to emerge. Choosing words to express experience is challenging, and the fears and uncertainties amidst emergent symptoms and ongoing choices cannot be adequately captured by words. The specialist vocabulary of medicine may hinder flexibility and may limit capacity for crucial conversation. Throughout the ongoing experience with illness, multiple lenses may allow for multiple innovative ideas and new understanding. Language and knowledge have informing reciprocities in interactions over time and in broader society. Communication as an emergent property is manifest in a patient's presentation of symptoms in choosing words and using words differently and giving different nonverbal context and expression to the lived experience of symptoms. Communication as an emergent property is manifest in a close relationship when someone tries to articulate the aches and pains, and in feeling too tired to engage, and in the close friend or relationship partner's words and nonverbal context and expression of empathy, understanding, or of resistance, confusion, or of commitment to "conquer" the symptoms "together."

A constitutive view of communication sees experiences of reality as a product of communicative activity (Deetz, 1992). A constitutive view of communication addresses process of explanation, of language and nonverbal behavior as the pathway through which people *construct and create* social reality (Deetz, 1992). Understanding communication as constitutive questions people, disease, and health and illness and instead positions communication as the discursive process of producing and understanding experience. Experiences are understood as constituted through communication such that a communicative situation is not a moment of information or type of message exchanged but a situation in which communicative activities constitute participants and the situation they believe themselves to be situated within (Mokros & Deetz, 1996). Communication and knowledge inform reciprocities in that the capacity to communicate is contingent on definitional qualities that continuously work their way through us; definitional qualities become naturalized and enable us to engage with others (Mokros & Deetz, 1996). Constitutive explanations as a meta-theoretical framework make possible the critical appraisal of communication practices with plausible alternative modes of communication practices.

To that end, understanding communication as constitutive allows for the reflective appraisal of practices and processes through which we make sense of the world and communicatively enact our beliefs and positions. Understanding communication as constitutive allows for reflective appraisal and for seeing below the surface to recognize multiple lenses. The end goal is not to develop a model with more interconnected variables for how communication occurs, but to engage aspects of theories and address how communication process creates and manifests reality. Understanding communication as constitutive translates into unpacking and disentangling emergent processes.

Communication as constitutive of health and illness. Examples from health-care interactions illustrate how communication is not a mere tool for expressing social reality but also a means of creating social reality and potentially also creating disenfranchisement and making claims about others' experiences. In one example transcript, a child psychiatrist interviews a thirteen-year-old girl following her suicide attempt, and first asks her to offer her understanding of her difficulties, in her own words (Mokros & Deetz, 1996). The girl says she feels alone and like she is not needed and no one cares for her. Her language indicates an understanding of her relational world. The language of asking her to describe her experience "in her own words" indicates listening to a narrative of potentially emergent value. Her words indicate a sense of social isolation, and the depth with which she describes her feeling of alienation seems to surprise even her, as indicated in a parenthetical aside in a softened and speeded voice asking herself aloud "why do I keep saying that?" The psychiatrist asks if she knew of a potential precipitant for her "sadness," substituting the term sadness as consistent with a clinical diagnosis of depression, thus shifting the lens of understanding and meaningfulness. Sadness is an intrapersonal experience that is different from the girl's relational or interpersonal description of social isolation (Mokros & Deetz, 1996). The definition and communicative reconstruction then is consistent with treatment through medication rather than addressing her potential productive agency in building a more connected relational life (Mokros & Deetz, 1996). The professionalized medical dialogue in this case likely produced the identity of the psychiatrist and the value of the professional as well as disqualified the validity of the experience of the girl as desiring or needing better relational connection with her family. This interpretation is not to suggest lack of caring, lack of goodwill, intentionality, or even awareness on the part of the psychiatrist, but instead to illustrate the communicative process of disenfranchisement and the communicative production of reality of the health and illness experience.

Communication as co-constructing interactions about disability. A second illustration examines interpersonal communication processes in the ways medical students approach standardized patient educators with visually apparent disabilities during medical interviews and indicate emotionally toned predispositions of values and beliefs by what is said or avoided in health-care conversation. Disability as a particular aspect of health communication provides an opportunity to examine the "elephant in the room," indicating a powerful, but not always explicit, experience that drives and dominates discourse in both overt and subtle ways. Language may serve as a dialectical tension that restricts discourse and allows the dominant group to keep

278 INTEGRATED THEORY OF HEALTH AND ILLNESS TRAJECTORIES

disabled "others" in place (Duggan, Bradshaw, & Altman, 2010). Language can shape the self-concept of the patient, the allocation of resources away from the patient, and the beliefs of other physicians. Language can indicate underlying attitudes toward individuals with disabilities include social discomfort, exaggerated empathy, and fear of contracting or being contaminated by the disability, attitudes that may be related to misunderstandings or lack of knowledge about physical disability. In contrast, language about disability can promote empowering exchanges by emphasizing "person first" language and discourse about the person as a whole. Language about disability can promote self-differentiation, or, in contrast, invasive questions can challenge privacy. From videotaped interactions between family medicine students, the researchers examined the communication process of asking about the physical disability (Duggan et al., 2010).

Using the word "disability" and integrating disability implications with the presenting issue of shoulder pain allows for interconnections with multiple identities of a patient and to absorb and accept what the patient says (Iezzoni, 2006). Asking about a disability and then integrating disability disclosure indicates the provider has absorbed, and is acting upon, what the patient said. Time delays before asking about the disability may indicate cultivation of patient communication cues, but waiting too long to ask about a disability within the interaction may indicate provider non-responsiveness (Duggan et al., 2011). Clinicians who ask and integrate disability with new pain complaints seem to inherently recognize that the patient's life exceeds the initial visit explanation; nevertheless, they may be usefully cautioned against premature conclusions about integrating biomedical and psychosocial concerns, while encouraging reflective practice and insights into ways communication shapes medical outcomes.

Asking indirectly about disability involves naming implications of the disability rather than using the word "disability." Late timing in such cases may indicate uncertainty and lack of clarity in the progression of the interaction. Medical students who ask about injury or illness might be cautioned regarding language choices and the possibility for escalating disability assumptions (Duggan et al., 2009; Duggan et al., 2010). Failing to integrate disability disclosure may indicate discomfort, negativity, or avoidance. Redirecting the conversation, switching topics, or reverting to biomedical questions following disability disclosure may be interpreted as communicatively treating disability information as irrelevant and missing the patient's sense of self and relationships. Once the disability is named, patients may perceive greater obstacles for socially acceptable ways to return to the topic than if the disability was never addressed. We also observed that over-accommodation through overly positive or affirming language, or third-person language, may have the most potential for restricting communication. The danger in over-accommodation is that these behaviors themselves can be interpreted as rapport building; patients with disabilities may perceive this language as inferring what otherwise is normative behavior as exceeding expectations. Students responding to standardized patient-led disclosure instead of initiating questions about disability confirm the utility of the case's deliberate educational construction, which allows medical students to hear the person refer to disability and provide an abundance of clues highlighting language preferences from the disability community. Interpreted through a lens of politeness, this group of medical students may have been hesitant to offend by asking about disability but, instead, they noticed and responded to disability disclosure. Asking about previous medical history provides a general way of potentially addressing disability, but the question may be too broad and may indicate uncertainty in framing disability questions. Reflection about communicatively constitutive language sometimes prompted medical students to consider ways individuals with disability live in adapted but normal circumstances and may prefer to consider their disability as not "problematic," but as a dimension of self-identity (Duggan et al., 2009; Duggan et al., 2010).

Qualitative analysis of videotaped feedback sessions following medical interviews provides evidence of learning to connect disability with pain, everyday life, and treatment. Medical students learned to recognize patients' expertise in their own condition and in health-care navigation; medical students also examined how their language implies attitude and communicatively shapes interactions (Duggan et al., 2009). Qualitative analysis provided evidence of the ways examining disability can serve as a cornerstone for reflectively enacting relationship-centered patient care and encouraging reflective practice overall (Duggan et al., 2009).

Identified learning occurrences allow for identifying evidence-based theoretical processes as emergent, refining teaching and curriculum to better encourage reflective medical practice, and potentially modifying physician perspectives on disability (Duggan et al., 2009; Duggan et al., 2011). Building on knowledge, skills, and attitudes necessary to thoughtfully and deliberately provide care and serve as patient advocates for individuals with disabilities (Saketkoo et al., 2004), their study identified learning areas that provide evidence of medical students' reflection about parameters of treating patients with disabilities and about promoting patient empowerment. One of these ways of empowering patients is to recognize patients with disabilities as experts in their own condition and in navigating the health-care system, a theme that operates in the current study as an undercurrent across all of the identified learning areas. Specifically, this series of studies suggests that innovations in medical education can provide opportunities to learn how to work toward relationship-centered communication, which inherently involves freedom from negative assumptions or attitudes about disability (Duggan et al., 2009).

Medical students expressed learning how to ask about disability, how to consider disability implications for patients' everyday lives, and how treatment includes disability-particular services. Analysis suggested medical students' awareness of disability conditions, yet they lacked the vocabulary to effectively articulate disability implications (Duggan et al., 2009). Reflections indicated that medical students who had not adequately addressed disability during the interview articulated lessons learned about ignoring disability disclosure. Students' reflections in feedback suggested increased breadth and depth in understanding patients with disabilities as multi-competent and as individuals whose relational roles include workers, caretakers, and support providers. Medical students' reflections indicating attitudes about disability suggested that they learned to recognize the ways they interpreted disability disclosure. Particularly poignant examples include describing themselves feeling tense and awkward in facing disability, difficulties asking about disability, and challenges about communication. Students with previous disability experience also were better able to anticipate patients' needs (although all of these students had limited patient experience overall). Medical students who commented on the ways "disability did not interfere" considered assumptions of "normal" communication. Reflection about disability attitudes prompted students to recognize when they asked but did not integrate disability disclosure into treatment, and the potential negative attitudes portrayed in naming the disability, but then switching topics or reverting to biomedical conversation following disability disclosure (Duggan et al., 2009). Feedback experience seemed to prompt medical students to particularly examine the life world of the patient and to uncover multiple layers of a patient's life, allowing for a holistic sense of self, relationships, and sexuality for individuals with disabilities. Medical students expressed appreciation for the nonevaluative feedback as an opportunity to dispel inaccurate assumptions, to understand their own attitudes and aversions about disability, and to recognize the gap between their performance and what they would have liked to accomplish (Duggan et al., 2009).

Instances of learning from conversations with patients with disabilities provided evidence of increased knowledge about medicine overall. For example, learning about standardized patient educators (people who role-play the patient but live with physical disabilities in everyday life) in medical education and strategies for improved medical interviews emerged as learning constructs. Medical students commented on their interview organization and time management and the ways the experience informed relationship-centered care. Finally, students described that improved understanding about patients' needs and opinions are balanced with doctors' professional advice (Duggan et al., 2009).

A CONSTITUTIVE COMMUNICATION APPROACH TO CLOSE RELATIONSHIPS

Research and theory indicates that communication is not only a tool for expressing social reality but also a means for creating relationships, identities, and tasks. A constitutive approach focuses on the communication as the relational process rather than focusing on communication as contained within relationships between people. A constitutive communication approach to close relationships considers how different theories and explanatory frameworks, how different contexts and research traditions, as disparate as they might seem, can productively work together to allow larger understanding about communication than one theoretical tradition alone (Manning, 2014). A constitute approach engages plurality in understanding and theorizing.

For example, picking up "threads" of interpersonal communication research across multiple theoretical traditions and lenses and weaving them into a tapestry of understanding may allow for more nuanced theorizing, richer practical findings, and more opportunities to engage inter-contextual research within a discipline as well as interdisciplinary understanding (Manning, 2014; Manning & Kunkel, 2014). A constitutive approach potentially disrupts the common fallacy that a theory is locked in a singular paradigm or tradition. A constitutive approach instead asks how a theory (or multiple theories) can be translated or enacted across contexts or research traditions or disciplines.

Qualitative research includes interpretive theoretical approaches that offer revelations and meaning that can be missed when "reality" is measured and articulated by quantitative measures and statistics. Increasingly sophisticated statistical tools provide increasingly accurate measurement models. However, measurement models also face ongoing limitations in that knowledge generated is a product of the theory and methods appropriated. Qualitative relationship studies offer revelations for the process of how people interact in the construction of meaning-making. Interpretive approaches provide a starting place for meaning-making of what cannot be captured by statistical measurement models.

Interpretative qualitative research focuses on the meaning-making process as a reflective, complex, and continuous process. Several key aspects of qualitative relationship studies offer a view of meaning-making in action, allowing for marginalized voices to emerge, evoking senses of experiences in actions and articulations, and a constitutive form of sense-making (Manning & Kunkel, 2014). Qualitative relationship studies offer a view of meaning-making in action by shedding light on the paradoxical and contradictory elements at play and on how different ideas or actions come to the forefront depending on situation and context and how elements change across time (Manning & Kunkel, 2014). The emergent process of meaning-making can allow rich insights into processes, practices, or rituals in close relationships (Manning & Kunkel, 2014). Qualitative relationship studies allow for marginalized voices to emerge in describing the complex and nuanced accounts of realities and experiences that may emerge differently from dominant voices (Manning & Kunkel, 2014). Qualitative relationship studies evoke understanding of experiences in feeling, emotion, and latitude of understanding actions and articulations of people (Manning & Kunkel, 2014). Qualitative relationship studies serve as a constitutive form of sense-making in ongoing assumption and analysis of how the relationship is constructed through interaction process (Manning & Kunkel, 2014). In some qualitative studies, theory is generated from the data in an iterative process. Inductively analyzing the data might also be compared to existing theory as a heuristic for better understanding meaning-making (Manning & Kunkel, 2014). Qualitative relationship studies allow for flexibility in sense-making that sheds light on both data and theory.

RECOGNIZING PRODUCTIVE TENSIONS IN THEORY

In addition to qualitative approaches, theorizing that reaches across traditions allows for constitutive insights for readers. Disentangling concepts allows for recognizing productive tensions that allow for more fully realized theoretical frameworks. Positioning theories within the time and place that influenced the intellectual history helps inform how the ideas came together and can be pulled apart. The creation of theory itself is a productive process. Continued tests of a theory help us see the complexities, strengths, and limitations of the theory. A constitutive view recognizes that any theory is by definition incomplete. Instead, a constitutive view allows for considering breadth and complexity as allowing for emergent patterns. Certainly the complexities of close relationships during illness trajectories require attentiveness to emergent processes in responding and relating. Because no experience of illness is exactly like any other, there cannot be a prescriptive way to assure that a patient engages in a healing relationship with a health-care provider. Because no two experiences of relationship are exactly the same, there cannot be a prescriptive way to assure that people will engage in supportive, validating interactions during the ongoing illness trajectories. However, understanding theoretical explanations for how communication is manifest in supportive interactions allows for awareness and increasing attentiveness and reflectivity about the emergence of healing and supportive interactions. Understanding communication as constitutive allows attentiveness and reflectivity about the process of meaning-making in interactions.

SYSTEMATIC UNDERSTANDING OF THEORIZING: COMMUNICATION IN CO-GENERATIVE PROCESSES

Systematic understanding of close relationships and health and illness as co-generative process engages a willingness to take a holistic view of the interconnected complexities. Communication processes in close relationships and in health and illness trajectories co-constitute an ongoing, dynamic process of emergence. In clinical encounters, we do not focus on patient or clinician but on the communicative process of interactions over time as opportunities for emergence. The processes that continue to shift over time integrate responsiveness and adaptation. Openness to emergence requires capacity for patterns that cannot be predicted or cannot be known. The vulnerability of illness might be seen as experience that continues to emerge over time. In close relationships, we do not focus on patient or friend or relationship partner but again on the communicative process of interactions over time and on the potential for creativity.

Emergence over time. Emergence and responsiveness are manifest over time rather than at one given point. In health-care interactions, as the popular surgeon, writer, and public health advocate Atul Gawande describes, emergence and responsiveness are processes of incremental care (Gawande, 2017). Incremental care involves physicians coming to know their patients over the course of years. Physicians learn and take into account not just their patients' medical records, but also their living situation, their family history, their stress levels, their nutrition, and how all these factors interrelate over time (Gawande, 2017). Incremental care is hands-on and relational; it is patient and takes the long view. It is marked less by tests and results and more by listening and conversation; it depends on medical skill, to be sure, but more importantly on trust and the physician's ability to communicate (Gawande, 2017). Unless a person is dangerously ill, incremental care is not about episodic, heroic interventions, but about consistent and sustained paying attention over time. Incremental care is practiced by those who are willing to admit, "I'm not sure what's going on," who can resist the allure of the quick-fix prescription or sophisticated medical test, and who have a tolerance for the anxiety that comes with watching and monitoring (Gawande, 2017).

Similarly, emergence and responsiveness are manifest over time in close relationships. In illness experience, short-term interests can be reconsidered to instead address the long-term commitments of close friends or relational partners. Actions and attitudes of compassion in close relationships address the longer-term commitment in supporting the person with the illness through the ups and downs of symptoms. In long-term, close relationships, a caring attitude can be expressed through facial expression, through language, or through words built in the ecosystem of the close relationship over time. The subtle manifestation of caring in a long-term relationship may be understood even when the actions and expressions are quite subtle or are particular to the relationship. In the story of Sherry at the beginning of Chapter 1 of this book, the group of women regularly enjoyed Sherry's cakes. Sherry is a great cook, and expert pastry chef, creating eight-layer cakes that could be featured in a baking magazine. When she was ill and uncertain of her diagnosis, the most compassionate and caring shared language was our description of the "Sherry worthy" cake, language built over time and across shared celebrations.

Nonlinearity. A key property of the systematic processes in health-care interactions and in close relationships is nonlinearity such that process allows for co-emergence within the interaction as well as over the course of continued wrestling with, understanding, and decision-making in connected illness trajectories and close relationships. This understanding of systematic co-emergence requires multiple, broad lenses of understanding. The communicative behavior in health-care interactions can change over time, and the communicative behavior in close relationships can change over time. The process of interest is not in patterns of language already spoken but in the potential for additional unfolding, differently nuanced utterances, subtleties in nonverbal cues, and differences between words and nonverbal cues.

Emergence in internal and embodied understanding. Systematic understanding allows emergence in internal states. Emergence in the internal state means meaning-making may not yet have words for the person having a shift in experience. The person may not feel ready to describe the emotional experiences connected to illness in words. Body responsiveness to an experience or to a turning point in treatment or to a set of physical symptoms may not feel like they fit the previous words. Silence is not necessarily to be interpreted as agreement with a previous conversation or with the perceived orientation of the other people involved in the connected systems (health-care providers and/or people in close relationships). In allowing emergence of the internal state, the experience and the expression might differ in time or in noticing shifts. Feeling states can include a different way of experiencing the body, of experiencing affect and emotion, of experiencing bodily rhythms, of constituting meaning. In attending to emergence, the internal world of the other is not assumed to fit previous scripts. Knowing or noticing an experience with the body during illness trajectories might not yet (and might not ever) have language.

EMERGENCE IN CLOSE RELATIONSHIPS AND IN INTERPERSONAL PROCESSES

Attending to generative processes requires attentiveness to the process of relating and the potential dynamic new ways of being in close relationships. Illness interrupts earlier relationship scripts. The process of relating requires new ways of relating, the rules of which are not yet clear. Trajectories of illness connect to an immersion that can make visible the relationship challenges as experienced so far in the relationship and can pose a fragmented uncertainty for hopes of the future. Choices emerge where assumptions about the relationship no longer hold consistent. Complex processes of relating during illness can be described as chaotic in that people experience a presence of stability simultaneously with potential for radical change (Scott, 2013). In relationships, the experience of relational stability indicated in support through physical presence during procedures might feel paradoxical to the amplification of feeling misunderstood and feeling the body exists outside of individual or relational identity. The coherence of relational identity is interrupted by illness.

Expectations for collaboration in shared activities or in decisions that benefit the relationship over the individual can be challenged by logistics of illness. Assumptions about the relationship may not hold consistent. For example, a spouse or closest friend might not feel right about being physically present during treatment, as illness can feel different from other life changes. Relational interactions can face different views in choices. The ongoing communicative construction of the relationship and in sense-making and decisions during illness trajectories exist within a context fraught with intensity.

Logistical and clinical variables define the boundaries of a fully co-generative sense of potential. The demands of illness treatment can take precedence in the time and scheduling of appointments and in the related (im)balance of responsibilities and upheaval in routines and normative enactment of relational roles. Power dynamics are inescapable in clinical consultation, where biomedical language and the health provider's expertise are not possible to translate into a reciprocal interaction. That said, the inescapable power differential between provider and patient and the task-oriented process of health care, although a challenging boundary for creative generativity, do not necessitate the possibility of shifting beyond authoritative communicative or decision-making models to generative processes.

Emergence and co-creative or co-generative processes in close relationships require stepping back from assumptions to enable the possibility of interactions of greater value. Emergence and co-generative processes require and offer possibility of transcending ideas, rules, and patterns. Interactions have potential to imaginatively envision something new. As with the internal world, we are likely not to have language or context to articulate a "goal" or to fully explain relational processes during the trajectories of new experiences or new relational sensations.

Opportunities for emergence require theoretical breadth as well as multiple tools that allow for disentangling complexities and recognizing where tensions and paradoxes can be noticed with a different lens. The end goal is not to reach an unquestionable state or to achieve increasing accuracy. Instead, opportunities for emergence means engaging in process. Theory of systematic co-generativity means recognizing the interconnected conversation in the world where the complexities of illness trajectories meet the complexities of close relationship processes. Interpretation of qualitative data alongside continued development and sophisticated tests of underlying factors still falls short of the constitutive, co-generative, systematic process of emergence necessary to map out close relationships in health and illness contexts. Systematic understanding and recognizing generative processes is not necessarily met through more sophisticated methods and expertise, but by recognizing constitutive processes where tensions and paradoxes exist. Instead of producing evidence through which our claims are supported, we identify how considering some aspect differently can be compelling.

In mapping out an integrated theoretical understanding of close relationships in health and illness contexts, I consider how engaged research promotes curious inquisition between people who make sense of the world differently. Pathways predicting emergence might be seen as organized around recognizing contradictions and points of difference and what is not explained by a theoretical lens.

DESIGNING INTERACTIONS THAT ALLOW FOR EMERGENCE

The experience of a serious or life-threatening illness can make everyday experiences appear odd and distant. The experience of a serious or life-threatening illness can be a highly self-reflexive moment with mismatch between ongoing continuous experience and a new perception of experience. Before moving to processes of co-generative opportunities, it is necessary to first recognize how the concepts and communication processes become highly scripted and how the scripts can become limitations rather than vehicles for creativity and generativity.

LANGUAGE LIMITATIONS AND CONSTRUCTION OF MEANING

The inherent difficulties in defining health and illness and in defining close relationships highlight a need to first recognize the nature and source of human experience, knowledge, and meaning as a process. Processes that allow for emergence allow for people to become what they can envision. Outlining the theoretical foundations is intended to allow for ongoing conversation that allows for generative process and creative choices to emerge. Generative processes and creative choices require attentiveness, listening, and reflectivity in recognizing contrasting points of experience and explanatory frameworks. Difference is the presence of a contrasting understanding, contrasting construction, counter-claim, or challenge to our own construction of meaning (Deetz, 1992). As people encounter new patterns and structures in their interactions, they also have the potential to encounter new consequences and new ways of engaging. This is a process question that is a different conception from obtaining full breadth of information and making medical decisions based on best predictability of information. Encountering new patterns and structures is also a different question from making relationship decisions that touch on the topics of medical treatments and how to adapt relationship roles to allow for physical recovery from medical treatment. Emergent engagement instead re-conceptualizes the process through which we attend to, talk about, make sense of, and respond to ongoing changes in both the illness trajectory and relationships. Emergent engagement shifts past repetitive patterns in scripts in health care and in close relationships. Emergent engagement considers instead how the core problems and issues might be conceptualized and then reconsiders over time how the core problems and issues continue to shift. The interconnected worlds of illness trajectories and close relationships require disrupting the scripts that are learned in one set of circumstances and do not hold consistent when we consider the interconnectivity.

Language and nonverbal symbols as currently used in health care do invite the possibility for emergence. When we add the layers and complexities of language and nonverbal symbols in close relationships we can further disconnect, limit, and narrow creativity. Paradoxically, our very attempts to address relationship-centered health care or to talk through close relationship processes are limited by language. Patient-centered practitioners (relationship-centered health care, as described in Chapter 1) focus on improving different aspects of the patient-physician interaction by employing measurable skills and behaviors. However, the questions included in patient-centered care focus on communication as information rather than on the possibility for emergence of anything that is new. As with sophisticated methods and statistical tools, the topics and questions provide a helpful start, but the language confirms experiences consistent with the lens of the observations and measures. Patient-centered care replaces the physician-centered system with one that revolves around the patient, at least as measured by information obtained. Opportunities for engaging patients more broadly than traditional medicine are defined by or in consultation with patients rather than by physician-dependent tools or standards. Questions for patient-centered care understand that patients must be asked to rate or judge their health care; this is in contrast to health-care providers' belief that they understand patients and patients' care. Questions for patient-centered care begin to address what is important to people, how well the team delivers health care, and what improves patient outcomes. Questions for patient-centered care shift from conceptualizing "what is the matter" with patients or in relationships to "what matters" to patients and in relationships. This shift addresses a broader topic and priority structure and allows for better responsiveness for patient priorities. This "patient centered" process of interviewing addresses some of the structural limitations in physician-driven interviewing. However, the questions do not address constitutive process. The questions do not address opportunities for emergence. Integrating the possibility for relationship emergence introduces additional need for co-creating interactions.

SCRIPTS CAN LIMIT EMERGING UNDERSTANDING

Questions and measures of patient-centered care focusing on the information-sharing process or on the information-sharing script address biopsychosocial topics but miss the potential for emergence or generativity. Questions and measures of patient-centered care include a range of topics and variables that are helpful and necessary in shifting the lens of understanding from a biomedical model to a psychosocial model. Similarly, the questions and measures are helpful in shifting the process of communication as controlled by the health-care provider to a process of more reciprocal questions and answers between patients, providers, and health-care organizations. To that end, one of the leading non-profit advocacy and membership organizations, Planetree International, works with a growing network of health-care provider organizations across the continuum to implement comprehensive person-centered models of care (https://planetree.org). Among other resources, they offer a person-centered care certification program. Their "questions to ask your hospital about patient-centered care" include questions about eight topics (http://planetree.org/wp-content/uploads/2015/08/PCC AM-Hospital.pdf). The topic *access to information* includes questions such as "How will I access my medical records while I am in the hospital? Will it be real time information that someone will explain to me? Do I have the option of adding my own perspective for the healthcare team to read and review?" The topic *involvement of family and friends* includes questions such as "Are there limitations on when I may have family/friends with me? How will my family and friends be trained to help care for me, both while I am in the hospital and when I am discharged?" The topic *personalized care* includes questions such as "How do you document my personal health and treatment goals to share them with my care team? How will you adjust mealtimes and routine checks around my schedule [preferences for schedule]?" The topic *care coordination* includes questions such as "How will you communicate with my primary care physician and other specialists about my care and treatment in the hospital? While I am in the hospital, how will you assist me in scheduling follow-up appointments, filling prescriptions and learning basic skills to manage my care once I'm discharged?" The topic *patient preferences and comfort* includes questions such as "Will I be able to see outside from my room and adjust my lighting and room temperature? What types of complementary and integrative therapies such as massage are available to me and how would I access them?" The topic *responsiveness to patient or family concerns* includes questions such as "What process should I (or my family member/friend) use to raise a concern while in the hospital? Do you have a process for a team to rapidly assess a patient who is deteriorating? Can a patient or family member initiate the team?" The topics *patient input in hospital operations* and *patient feedback* give the question "Do you have a patient and family advisory council, other committees or patient focus groups that I (or my family) can participate in to provide my input about my experience?"

These questions do not give us a new way to think about health or illness or to talk about health and illness. These questions allow for mapping out interdependence in topics and for listening to topics and concerns from patients, but the questions are grounded in communication about information. Breadth is observed in topics, but not in the constitutive process. This health-care illustration marks progress in that the measurement of core competencies of medicine has shifted in the last 20 years from a biomedical model to also include humanistic components, including communication. The questions illustrate limitations in recognizing generative processes. Outlining how the constitutive and emergent possibilities are manifest in language and nonverbal processes allows a different angle, a different but complementary way of seeing. Emerging systematic approaches can allow for better articulating the problems and issues in the health-care interaction and in how the health-care interaction connects to issues in close relationships. Connected systems of close relationship processes and health and illness will require addressing generative processes.

CO-GENERATIVITY AND EMERGENCE THROUGH REFLECTION

My use of co-generativity and emergence are intended as openings for recognizing something as different. In health-care interactions and in close relationships, this means drawing out qualities that cannot yet be determined. This conceptualization allows for new ways of seeing. Instead of coming to health-care interactions or to interactions in relationships with the theoretical accounts of what is already conceptualized, we come to understand what current conceptualizations and variables are included, but also we uncover implicit opportunities that cannot be seen on the surface. If we understand theory as process of being in the world, then we also recognize observations, questions, and attentiveness as manifestations of the theoretical lens through which we see the world. Reflection offers the potential for deeper understanding. Reflection offers potential for mirror-in-mirror, for a lens that first acknowledges how the understanding is a product of current knowledge of variables and socially constructed and sometimes distorted representations.

Reflection counters a current understanding. Traditionally, reflection involves conscious and deliberate mental energy to explore one's *understanding* of a problem rather simply solving the problem (Eva & Regehr, 2008). Reflection involves developing self-knowledge and improving self-awareness beyond just thinking about an event. Thus, reflective practice involves evaluating an experience such that new knowledge gained from the experience can be integrated into an existing knowledge structure (Sandars, 2009). These definitions implicitly or explicitly describe a conscious attention paid to one's intention. According to these definitions, reflection requires learners to appreciate and develop their metacognitive ability, assessing cognitive performance to identify specific strategies to control their learning or thinking.

Sometimes the subtleties of everyday interactions allow new light, bring shades of color, and we are able to look beyond a certain narrow or predictable way of seeing. In the vulnerabilities of illness trajectories and close relationships, seeing beyond the predictable involves discovering how to see through a different lens. Seemingly straightforward statements about illness and about choices for treatment, or about roles and relationships, integrate with subtle clues that contextualize the broader illness experience and can shape the color of the prism. When we see the mirror-in-mirror, how the lens reflects an ongoing manifestation of image, we also can see emergence.

Reflection can shift the lens of seeing through internally examining a trigger experience or exploring an issue of concern, creating or clarifying meaning, and changing conceptual perspective (Boyd & Fales, 1983). Conceptually, reflection is described as encouraging a deeper approach to learning. However, research documents the process of reflection and distinguishes types of reflective portfolios, but research does not provide evidence to link competence, self-assessment, or self-understanding with formal reflective exercises (Buckley et al., 2009; Mann, Gordon, & MacLeod, 2009). For developing physicians, reflections often focus on scientific reasoning and research evidence about providing appropriate patient care, maintaining professional relationships, and self-care (Mann et al., 2009). Reflection can also be used for exploration, appraisal, and meaning-making of experiences. Reflection can potentially benefit balanced functioning, learning, and professional and personal development (Wear et al., 2012). Attentiveness to communication behaviors offers a lens to understanding the process of navigating interconnected encounters.

Through a communication-as-constitutive lens, we investigate the systematic properties and how language and nonverbal behavior produce the conditions for reflection and then for co-creating interactions. We investigate conceptions and terms to see the communicative processes of enacted sense-making (Shaughnessy, Allen, & Duggan, 2017). Reflection provides intentionality aimed at the nature of thoughts, feelings, and actions. Through reflection, we seek to understand and challenge assumptions, meaning, and action. We can consider possible alternatives to the current practices. We can imagine and explore options that have the possibility of providing creative new answers (Shaughnessy et al., 2017). Generating new answers can challenge routines, scripts, or established orders. The generative processes have potential to bring new ways of communicating and new vocabularies for moving forward differently. We might find ourselves saying "this is not quite the right word but ... ?" or "I may not fully understand but do I hear ... ?" Counterintuitive options can emerge from reflection about potentially emergent options. The interplay of lenses amidst moving variables allows for complexities to be identified and for new knowledge and understanding to emerge.

REFLECTION ON COMMUNICATION IN HEALTH-CARE INTERACTIONS

In the complicated worlds of health care, reflection is one tool through which people can examine different and emergent pathways forward and different language for interactions (Vicini, Shaughnessy, & Duggan, 2017a). Reflection can promote professional self-awareness that is crucial to responding empathetically to patients and to recognizing patients' lives connected to illness (Duggan et al., 2009). We asked family medicine residents to write reflective entries across an entire academic year (Shaughnessy & Duggan, 2013). Our work indicates how written reflection can promote critical self-reflection and show where communication questions or challenges previous knowledge.

Reflection offers the experiential material to integrate analysis of communication processes by examining explicit and tacit points of reflection and by explicating the explicit and the intuitive and unconscious aspects of reflective exercises (Shaughnessy et al., 2017).

Reflection allows for unpacking the multifaceted aspects of compli-cated experiences, and bridges learning experiences with communica-tion foundations (Shaughnessy & Duggan, 2013). Experiences identified as material for reflection allow for medical educators, com-munication scholars, and practitioners to recognize the concept and the value of reflection and to develop competency to use it purposely in theory development and in professional life (Shaughnessy et al., 2017). To that end, projects in reflective practice in medicine build on understanding of interpersonal communication processes and addresses challenges of interdisciplinary research and translational work (Duggan, 2006). Reflection in health-care contexts applies a practice-derived educational tool that helps learners visualize reflec-tion and thereby more readily grasp its concepts (Vicini et al., 2017a). Examples illustrate the multiple facets of the image and pose ques-tions for how theory built on the images can more comprehensively explain how and why replaying situations or events in our minds can better trigger people to inquire and find new information to resolve tensions observed in reflections about communication behavior. Identified examples illustrate the development of attitudes coincident with those defined by medicine, including physicians' developing abilities to critically assess themselves and their actions in order to learn from their experiences and improve patient care (Duggan et al., 2015; Vicini, Shaughnessy, & Duggan, 2017b). A vital part of assem-bling illness scripts and integrating biomedical information with recognition of the life world of the patient is the construction of meaning, based on experience through the process of reflection (Duggan et al., 2015).

The parsimony in distinguishing between content or report functions and meta-communicative verbal and nonverbal expressions of relational regard can be duly narrow and may mask depth of rela-tional meaning (Burgoon & Hale, 1987). Observable and conscious communication behavior can be intentional, manifest, and clearly observable. Other components such as clinical and scientific reason-ing support the observable behavior. Deeper below the surface are personal reflection and unconscious thoughts not yet manifest in communication. These aspects of personal reflection can be accessed through reflective writing and perhaps dialogue where an individual explores and appraises experiences, clarifying and creating meaning for the benefit of balanced functioning, learning, and development (Aukes et al., 2007). In medicine, this type of "sense making" reflection serves as the ballast to keep the physician upright in learning and working effectively (Aukes et al., 2007). Both the manifest and implicit components play a role in maintaining balance in learning and working.

In considering reflection about communication in medicine, we suggest that explicitly stated, surface-level behavior is the manifestation of experience, and also symbolizes broader organizational and institutional context (Duggan et al., 2015). Recognizing and navigating the subtleties of implicit communication involves interpreting cues in context, and seeing and appreciating the reality and the boundaries of patients' concerns and comforts. Communication behaviors may provide a glimpse into deeper meaning than appears on the surface. For example, communication behaviors indicative of rapport, such as smiling, friendly tone of voice, forward leaning, and direct eye contact, may cross boundaries and instead may be interpreted as patronizing, particularly toward patients with physical disabilities (Duggan et al., 2011).

Physicians' reflection about communication might consider explicit messages where patients express frustration with feeling misunderstood, and subtle, implicit message cues that patients feel misunderstood. Physicians' reflection about communication offers insight into explicit messages and mindful awareness of attending to deeper experience. Explicit, surface messages are connected to research evidence about providing appropriate patient care, maintaining professional relationships, and self-care (Aukes et al., 2007). Personal reflection involves more careful exploration and appraisal of experience that clarifies meaning and benefits balanced functioning, learning, and development as well as what exists within the person (Duggan et al., 2015). Thus, physicians' reflections about below-surface communication can clarify and confirm subtle meanings of messages within context cues that offer delicate balance but depth of understanding. Patient experiences, concerns, and responses to illness be expressed through implied "clues" instead of direct statements. Clues might include subtle expressions of concern or worry, attempts to explain symptoms, speech clues (e.g., repeating an illness statement), personal narratives, or suggesting unresolved concerns (e.g., seeking a second opinion) (Lang, Floyd, & Beine, 2000). Communication behavior involves not only explicit statements but also recognizing what lies below the surface.

For medical residents, the training is a time of rapid learning, mistakes, and new experiences. With the challenges coming so fast, allotting time for reflection on the learning process can benefit them in the long run. Reflection can help residents understand patient behavior, communicate better, comprehend the learning process, and recognize their growth as a doctor and potential for future improvement (Duggan et al., 2015; Shaughnessy et al., 2017).

REFLECTION AS EMERGENCE

Most authors who write about reflection emphasize the conscious and deliberate aspects of reflection, such that written reflections can be used to assess the learner's metacognitive ability. Writing reflective exercises for oneself (i.e., not submitted for assessment) may allow learners to avoid the tacit or explicit expectations present when writing for others to assess and may allow them to explore their experiences in ways not necessarily available to their consciousness (Shaughnessy et al., 2017). In a recent analysis of family medicine physicians' reflections written across an academic year, we identified themes based on written reflections that were not written for subsequent assessment. We developed a theory of reflection such that identified instances in which writings not typically characterized as "reflective" may signal a degree of tacit self-discovery without conscious intention (Shaughnessy et al., 2017). We expanded the definition of reflective theory to include unconscious descriptions of events and goal setting. Our expanded understanding of reflection provides evidence-based theoretical explanation to suggest that understanding medicine includes both consciously integrated aspects of understanding of the self as doctor and processing medical learning more generally (Shaughnessy et al., 2017).

The goal of reflection, as used in medical education, is to create learners with an explicit (deliberate) approach to practice. However, a broader perspective on learning and reflection might be required; one that does not require explicit reflection but that still allows growth and self-understanding to occur (Shaughnessy et al., 2017). Explicit reflection identifies a narrative outlook in which one places a unifying or form-finding construction on the events of one's life, or at least on parts of one's life (Shaughnessy et al., 2017). Our research provides evidence for a broader perspective on reflection, and we provide evidence that noticing and writing indicates an unconscious process that is still important as a process of sense-making.

Failing to see a unity in one's life – to see one's life as a story – does not necessarily mean that self-development is not possible. Further, self-understanding may not require a tendency toward narrativity. People may develop and grow without realizing the changes. People may develop self-understanding and expertise without an explicit narrative reflection but sometimes in a process not staged in consciousness (Duggan et al., 2015; Shaughnessy et al., 2017). The ability to be explicitly reflective as a cognitive process is traditionally described as necessary (Wear et al., 2012). However, deliberate practice does not fully explain the difference between expert and non-expert performance. Musicians, as an illustration, develop their ability through practice without ongoing, intentional reflection. From religious traditions to the descriptions of medical practice as an "art," self-development often is described as a tacit, unconscious process that does not involve reflection or imagining one's life as a story. The concepts of "flow" and "wu-wei" describe conscious processing of events in the moment as a *hindrance* to performance rather than a benefit.

We provide similar evidence of emergence in examples of family medicine residents' writing indicating unsolicited attentiveness to their inner lives – the emotions, perceptions, reflections, experiences, competence, beliefs, and practices – that forms the core of who we are as individuals (Vicini et al., 2017b). The inner life is not directly seen by others, but shapes our personal humanity and how our values and virtues are reflected in our actions (Vicini et al., 2017b). Cultivating, nurturing and developing one's inner life is just as important as developing one's technical prowess or ability to make complex clinical decisions (Vicini et al., 2017b). This development involves beliefs and emotions, ethics and spirituality, all topics that often are considered to be outside of the normative realm of training (and even the practice of medicine). In a protected opportunity for development, people can express the multiple dimensions of their humanity noticed in movement of the inner life (Vicini et al., 2017a). Developing physicians can question troubling human experiences. They can face the ethical issues that surface. This claim of reflection as emergent, and the evidence for noticing longings, doubts, joys, struggles, and ongoing "wrestling with sense-making" is consistent with noticing what the body holds but that might not be manifest yet in words, or in "wondering why we keep saying that" as described in illustrating communication as constitutive.

In close relationships, people face similar complexities in circumstances where reflection can examine different pathways forward. For example, consider psychotherapy as addressing both the manifest and the emergent in close relationships. Evidence-based approaches to interventions come from tested theories as also connected, and emerging from, years of working with people addressing dilemmas in close relationships.

EMERGENCE IN DILEMMAS OF INTIMACY

Dilemmas of intimacy in couples provide a conceptualization for examining competing tensions and in the processes of therapy to allow for new emergence. Therapy that allows for emergence moves past the places of "being stuck" in what is not working in a close relationship. Understanding dilemmas of intimacy may allow for moving past the dilemmas. As identified by Karen Prager from three decades of research on intimacy, dilemmas of joy versus protection from hurt, I versus we, and the past lives in the present, can be understood as outgrowth of the rewards and risks of intimate relating (Prager, 2014). Some couple partners withdraw and avoid intimacy, whereas others sabotage it; some people minimize their own aims to get along with their partners, whereas others attempt to mold their partner to fulfill their own needs; still others break up one relationship after another to seek the partner who will fulfill unmet dreams (Prager, 2014). In her three dilemma model, we can identify complexities in the coexisting joys and emotional risks involved in intimate relating.

Intimacy promises that people's needs can be known, accepted, and fulfilled; intimate partners reward us when they allow us to know them and when they participate with us in the give and take of support, love, affirmation, and joy (Prager, 2014). The promise of intimacy brings risk in that more shared intimacy also means taking risks of feeling hurt or deeply wounded in our most vulnerable aspects of ourselves (Prager, 2014). Patterns and scripts come together to form a couple such that both people seek to maximize the rewards of intimacy and minimize its risks, but a couple's pattern of intimate relating combines inviting, approach behaviors with defensive behaviors that protect against hurt (Prager, 2014). Conceptually, intimacy has been difficult to define because the word describes several different but related concepts (Prager, 2014), but it includes dimensions of self-disclosure and validation, caring, and understanding in the receiving of the other's disclosure (Reis & Shaver, 1988). In an intimate interaction, both partners gain access to or learn more about the other's inner experience, from private thoughts, feelings, and beliefs, to characteristic rhythms, habits, or routines, to private sexual fantasies and preferences (Prager, 2014). This knowledge endures beyond a particular interaction and informs and deepens the intimate relationship. Four interrelated needs are identified: need to share the self, need to be accurately understood, need to be valued and accepted, and need to know another person inside and out, which together compose the need for intimacy (Prager, 1995, 2014). Most people will continue to yearn for or seek out intimate relationships despite disappointments, hurts, and losses from previous relationships (Prager, 2014).

Intimacy dilemmas are conflicts between two intimacy-related values or motives. Intimacy dilemmas can be internalized to the individual or can be manifest in conflicts between partners; intimacy dilemmas can be best understood when we recognize intimacy as a simultaneously rewarding and anxiety-provoking aspect of couple relationships (Prager, 2014). People can respond to intimacy dilemmas in ways that disrupt the relationship, and people may avoid intimate relationships altogether because they are overwhelmed by the risks of intimacy (Prager, 2014). The *joy versus protection from hurt* dilemma involves seeking intimate contact and the deep and abiding need for closeness, but people sometimes respond insensitively or cruelly to vulnerabilities or do not share joys we experience (rejoice with us), and people may reject, abandon, or withdraw from expressions of love or yearning (Prager, 2014). The *I versus we* dilemma involves forging common life goals and aims on one hand and our desire to pursue individual dreams, interests, and friends on the other; some people give too much of themselves whereas other people attempt to change partner to harmonize with their individual desires (Prager, 2014). The *past lives in the present* dilemma recognizes developmental histories. In psychological conceptualization, this dilemma rests in confrontation of risk or rejection that taps into a vulnerable aspect of the self (feeling unattractive or holding a conviction that some part of the self is unlovable), or in seeking love and intimacy unfulfilled as a child or in seeking relationships but re-experiencing pain, disappointment, unmet needs, or insecurity manifest in earlier development or childhood (Prager, 2014). From a broader social construction perspective, experiences exist within a broader conception of core issues in the interaction systems where they are constituted.

Reflection attends to the process of difference and counter-claims of understanding. Attending to process difference can include behavioral, cognitive, and affective aspects of couples' handling intimacy and its dilemmas, as consistent with a psychological lens (Prager, 2014). Therapeutic intervention involves attitudes, beliefs, expectations, and problematic emotion regulation strategies in one or both people in the couple (Prager, 2014). Therapy to address intimacy dilemmas addresses the defenses that have been carefully (sometimes deliberately) developed to protect people from feeling hurt (Prager, 2014). Addressing the complications of intimacy dilemmas cannot be done by "forcing intimacy" on people who are reluctant and want to stay in protective but safe corners (Prager, 2014). Addressing the complications of intimacy dilemmas requires recognizing competing tensions with "opposing" needs; addressing intimacy dilemmas creates experiences of oneness and togetherness, paradoxically, with awareness of difference in the honest and self-revealing emergence that indicates differences as well as similarities with intimate partners (Prager, 2014). People may respond by distancing themselves from one another to avoid feeling too much emotion, or they may become more enmeshed in submerging their own needs or wants or in pushing the other to change (Prager, 2014). Interventions are ongoing and can allow for people to recover, sustain, and more thoroughly enjoy the close connection that brought them together (Prager, 2014). The process of addressing intimacy dilemmas requires creating and designing interactions that address manifest communication and that also allow for emergence. Attentiveness and reflection can allow for seeing differently. Communication processes and co-created communication can allow for responding differently.

CONCLUSION

Human interaction can unfold in predictable ways and familiar patterns, or human interaction can be designed to allow for generativity and emergence, for difference. The ideas in this chapter assume a reciprocal process of noticing, reflecting, sharing, and making decisions, and the reciprocal process continues to unfold as new knowing continues to emerge. The ideas of co-created, co-generative, and systematic processes can become part of human interaction, but that will require particular interaction processes with health-care providers and between people in close relationships. Human interactions first need to be approached with fully present *attentiveness and reflection*. Being fully present means using words and actions that indicate curiosity and that take seriously the current and emergent concerns and an explicit interest in the response of the people involved in decisions and in support. Such interactions require patience and care and often require requests for further understanding at the moment and as illness trajectories continue to unfold. Shared decision-making around the complexities of health and illness and the complexities of close relationships also requires *concrete* details as they emerge. Concrete details address particular descriptive information on which people can base their own evaluations and responses. Concrete details describe the issue itself rather than abstractions of what someone else has experienced.

In the emotionally charged complexities of health and illness in close relationships, human interaction is more productive when people can take *ownership* of their own feelings and actions. Conversely, statements that shift ownership can muddy the potential for co-created and co-generative interactions. For example, a statement like "your choice made me so angry" or "your decision to forgo the surgery makes the family disappointed" inappropriately shifts responsibility for feelings to the other person. Anger or disappointment require not just the action of another person, but also some unmet hopes, desires, expectations, or anticipations that reside within the individual who "feels" angry or disappointed. Claims and facts in health-care decisions can quickly become distorted and misappropriated when they are presented as unowned "should" or "ought" statements. Responsibility and decisions can be misappropriated to some invisible realm of "medicine." Values and assumptions are often embedded in unowned or misappropriated ownership. Reciprocal, co-created interactions require reflection to know what a person is really feeling, thinking, or doing, and how that knowing connects to current and emerging information. Reciprocal, co-created interactions also are more productive when they include *acknowledgment* in (accurately) indicating understanding rather than trying to influence. The vulnerability of interconnected health and illness trajectories and close relationships brings up all sorts of messages that can be misaligned in emergent knowing and in interpretations. Acknowledgment in understanding (and clarifying meaning when needed) allows for affirming and valuing each participant. New information in health care can otherwise be overlooked, denied, or partially understood. New emotional and embodied information and changes in choices over time necessitate ongoing listening and acknowledgment.

Theoretical co-generativity may be akin to knitting a more complex narrative of life events and relationships. Theoretical co-generativity allows for describing events from different perspectives, include multiple explanations, and exploring complex and even contradictory emotions. In many ways, theoretical co-generativity and creativity is the opposite of the need for absolute truth; instead of searching for simple, generalizable facts, self-aware people appreciate the complicated nature of their life stories.

Considering options for new, creative, inventions requires an ability to reflect or to skeptically encounter how the system properties could distort issues or could distort the potential to uncover a different path forward. The potential for a newly emerging way forward engages possibility and the potential for new alternatives. The process of new understanding is not just shifting cognitions, but a way of considering concept formation rather than applying what is already known. The possibility for new language and new conceptualization engages beyond applying what we already know. Increasing   self-awareness,   for   example,   allows   for   more possibilities than the current conceptualizations. Current theories and conceptualizations certainly can be helpful explanatory frameworks, but generative processes move to engage how repetitive failures in solving core problems might illustrate a need to consider differently rather than applying a response.

8 Integrated Co-generative, Systematic Processes and Considerations for Interdisciplinary Understanding

I realize I left you hanging in sharing part of Sherry's story. Welcome to the life of the patient, to the world of illness and close relationships where so much happens, but at the same time where little glimpses never provide the full picture, and where the story never really ends. Illness changes the way we engage, and we do not necessarily bring others up to speed. Similarly, we cannot fully tell the story of another person. We offer a perspective. From the perspective of co-generative, systematic processes, I offer glimpses into the further unfolding of Sherry's story in the applications in this chapter.

The theoretical propositions in this book are intended as a framework through which we gain a broader and more cohesive understanding as we continue to engage. The foundations in this book provide an initial framework from which we can participate in the co-construction of new knowledge and new ways of interacting.

In this chapter, I apply the theoretical propositions to relational trajectories and delineate how the integrated theoretical processes pose considerations for relational and health and illness changes over time. I consider illustrations of health and illness trajectories where close relationships help people successfully find meaning and purpose despite enormous medical challenges and illness-related vulnerabilities. To that end, I show how integrated pathways can promote resilience and relational thriving in the face of adversity. I show how integrated pathways similarly explain other relationships where illness serves as a catalyst for relational decline, for shattered assumptions, or for decreased ability to navigate the relationship instability, disorientation, and disillusionment of the ongoing illness trajectory.

RECOGNIZING COMPLEXITIES IN DEFINITIONS AS EMERGENT

Definitions of health and illness far exceed the biomedical explanation for malady. Language and experience bring new contradictions in understanding the self, the body, and our changing relationships. Sherry's story of initial sharing gives some sense of the language of diagnosis and unfolding complexities.

> *One of the first people Sherry called was Anne. Anne had her ringer turned off but noticed mid-morning that Sherry called.*
> *No message. She had missed a call from Sherry at home, but again, no message. At 10 pm, a few minutes into mindless television, the phone rang.*
> *"Hey, Sherry!" Anne answered the call, "I saw you called a couple of times today, but no message. What's going on?" Her friend of over two decades had a mass in her brain. She did not want to leave a message. Sherry explained that the mystery of the language struggle had been solved. The mass was located in the speech center of her brain. She was in the hospital and had been there for a few days. "Where?" "What?" "How?" Anne tried to make sense of what Sherry was saying.*
> *"I can't think of what to say," Anne responded, "I need to process this."*
> *"I know it's a lot to take in," Sherry said patiently, "you don't have to say anything now."*
> *"A lot to take in?" Anne thought, "A LOT TO TAKE IN? You've got a brain tumor, but you're worried about me?" But she didn't say it aloud. The cruel irony of a professor –*
> *a Communication professor – with a tumor in that part of her brain that controlled speech was not lost on Anne, even at that point.*
> *"Will you call everyone for me?" Sherry asked. By everyone, Anne knew she meant the circle of friends. The women with whom*

*we had just spent three days on Martha's Vineyard a few short
weeks ago for our annual end of the school year retreat. Women
who had gathered with spouses and partners to celebrate Sherry's
tenure in March. Women who had gathered for the Breast Cancer
Walk when Rita was diagnosed. Women who had celebrated
a son's Bar Mitzvah and a daughter's first child. Women who were
there on opening night for Roberta's play and drank toasts at
Bonnie's retirement party. Women who sometimes also
disappointed each other, missed the event, said the wrong thing,
kept pushing on the wrong thing we say, and sometimes deeply
hurt each other's feelings.*

*"I have bad news, Sherry is in the hospital and the emergency
room doctor has given her the diagnosis of a brain tumor,
inoperable, and she needs to have a biopsy." Anne's voice told
a serious story. The information seemed too much to grasp at one
time, but it sunk in fast, at least this part of the understanding.
We all waited for more information. Room number and visiting
hours; doctors were saying be prepared for the tumor to be
malignant.*

*When one or more of us went to visit Sherry, we found ourselves
staying for hours. Doctors came and went. We wondered whether
we were invading Sherry's privacy and kept offering to step out
when another doctor came in for another check or to let Sherry
know about the next set of tests. Each time we began to leave,
Sherry told us to stay. It seemed to strengthen Sherry to have people
around her, even during private times.*

Each chapter in this book addresses definitions and theoretical
cornerstones in understanding the interconnections between health
and illness and close relationships. Those interconnections are manifest in struggling with initial diagnosis and then throughout the
process of decisions and experiences with illness. Each chapter provides multiple lenses of understanding, beginning with definitions of
health and illness, defining characteristics of close relationships, and

theoretical attributes in connecting health and illness with close relationship processes. What we see in each chapter of this volume is that recognizing complexities is necessary in order to fully explain processes. Recognizing complexities as emergent allows for approaching an open system that adapts within an environment that also includes emergent qualities. When we consider health and illness and close relationship processes both as complex but open systems, we allow for expanding what we already know. For example, we allow for understanding how Sherry's initial story of diagnosis and sharing about the tumor allows for getting our heads around how we can be supportive and what we might expect during treatment. Focusing on emergence for Sherry allows her to co-participate across multiple systems of her own understanding and sense-making. An open system bridges this initial understanding with what develops over time, which might include one of us going through surgery with her, absorbing the impact of decisions that don't rest well with her extended family, and listening to newfound understanding over the years. Changes in the relationship may become part of explicit conversation, or changes might allow for a different sense of presence or for unfolding sense-making that does not have a particular end.

The process of modeling human behavior from a traditional social-scientific framework sometimes requires that we reduce the complexities of the systems in order to explain one part of the system at a time. For example, addressing privacy implications allows for recalibrating rules for sharing information; we reconsider what information is disclosed with whom during which part of treatment. The privacy implications are an important part of the system, but the theory proposes how ongoing emergence exceeds privacy. This process of modeling human behavior does not imply that the process of theoretical testing is inadequate, as something to be improved upon. Instead, recognizing interconnected systems as potentially co-generative allows for wrestling with the necessary tension in imposing a limited but testable framework for part of the system with the ongoing generative potential of unpacking and disentangling complexities. Note that wrestling with the necessary tension does not imply a need to resolve the tension. Perhaps, instead, finding language for the tensions allows for recognizing new contradictions. Similarly, wrestling with the tension between the testable frameworks for parts of the system does not mean that we need to constrain the potential for emergence in definitions or interconnections of attributes within the system or of attributes about the broader contexts. Defining complex problems requires multiple lenses, each of which provides a helpful explanatory framework, but where multiple lenses allows for new understanding to emerge.

In defining health and illness in terms of both disease (the disorder of structure) and illness (the broader experience of malady), we begin to recognize complexities as emergent in defining what we think we know and in recognizing complexities beyond what current language can label or explain. A definition of health and illness might often be reduced to a set of disease symptoms, and that is helpful when the goal is to recognize clusters of symptoms, to provide an accurate diagnosis, and to renegotiate relationships in such a way that allows for rest and recovery as symptoms are treated. A more complex understanding of health and illness positions the breadth of potential health as emergent in addressing physical health, mental health, and ongoing well-being as interconnected to a broader environment. The broader environment allows for dynamic emergence in promoting better human functioning and strengthening capacities for people, for communities, and for societies to more fully flourish through resilience and ongoing fulfillment. Strengthening capacities of communities and societies in understanding and addressing health, then, requires acknowledging the social production of health and disease, the living and working circumstances of people's lives, and the disparities in communities in the distribution of resources and services. Strengthening capacities necessarily shifts understanding by positioning health and illness definitions within cultural contexts, where emergence of evidence moves beyond what is objectively measured to address what else might emerge that is not yet measured.

Narratives and relationships allow potential for co-constructing experience and understanding. Co-construction allows for emergent definitions in health-care interactions and in close relationships through listening as a joint action. Emergent understanding of health and illness is not wholly determined by what is already understood or measured but by responsivity and engagement with information and experience around health and illness.

On some level, we wondered how Sherry could go through what seemed unexplainable. On another level, we had enough experiences that we could relate to life unfolding differently from how we thought it would. It brought one of us back to a night in the hospital more than forty years ago, where she sat alone in a strange hospital bed, feeling terrified. Sometimes illness shifts future plans to wondering how long the future will be.

The loneliness of living differently from what we know can be manifest in feeling like our own thoughts are our best company. For some people, visitors arriving in the morning is a welcome sense of normalcy. As friends, we might be determined to fill the daylight space, both in the hospital and at home. However, we also know that we all handle these situations in different ways and that we have different desires. We might find that our desires are not what we thought we would desire; our current hopes have changed from what we negotiated earlier with a close friend or relational partner. We know that Sherry is hesitant to accept support, and we teased her about whether she had queried the hospital staff about sharing the kitchen so she could bake cakes for visitors.

Considering close relationship processes as emergent addresses a relational co-construction of cognition, behavior, and understanding. Considering close relationship processes as emergent, generative, and relationally co-constructed is different from looking at individuals as they influence, and are influenced by, their relationship with another person. Instead, considering close relationship processes as emergent requires cognition, behavior, and understanding at the dyadic level. Interdependence in behaviors, cognition, emotion, and meaning require considering close relationships as transactions. Close relationship processes involve mutual interdependence such that the qualities of the people involved and the unique dynamics of the relationship mutually influence each other. The scientific study of relationship processes begins with the assumption that relationship processes involve complexities that extend beyond any particular process. This means that understanding relationships begins with explicating cornerstone concepts such as love, commitment, jealousy, respect, willingness to sacrifice, loneliness, disclosure, and positivity. But those concepts are not enough without considering the interconnection and the particular aspects of the people in close relationships.

Reciprocal relationships. Reciprocal relationships function differently from role relationships in that reciprocal relationships involve an assumption of mutual influence as the process of validating and enacting the relationship. Role relationships, on the contrary, involve tasks to be met as the primary process of engaging. Role relationships such as the doctor–patient relationship, the therapist–client relationship, or the parent–child relationship may involve some degree of reciprocity, but not in the same ways that patterns are revealed over time and across situations. Close relationship processes connect to human development and to the stability (or instability) of lives as negotiated and enacted. Relationship integration can involve shared goals including the goals of health promotion. Close relationships prompt strong emotional responses, both positive and negative. Communication processes allow for the co-creation of close relationships that integrate individual attributes with the manifestations of structure and function in a particular close relationship. Close relationships can perpetuate or, on the contrary, can help resolve challenges and vulnerabilities at the deepest levels, including health and illness behaviors.

Beyond the emergence in defining health and illness or in understanding close relationship processes, attributes that integrate the health and illness context with relationship processes shed light on emergent vulnerabilities and on shifted expectations. Attributes of the health and illness context begin to offer a glimpse of the potential for co-generative emergence. People do not commit to close relationships with the expectation they will face ongoing trauma or that a serious diagnosis will challenge the core assumptions of their roles and relationships. The diagnosis of illness brings an unanticipated vulnerability that requires changing expectations. A chronic illness or an ongoing health problem changes relational identity and can shift identity, confidence, and the way relationships are negotiated. Fragmented ambiguities can emerge with heightened uncertainty. Physical and emotional needs and desires change and may require different connections and behaviors in close relationships. The experience of illness can shift self-concept and individual and relational identity. The emotional experience may be heightened, or people in close relationships may reach a threshold of what they can address in emotional processing.

The illness experience can be prolonged, complicated, and lonely. Relationships can take on new qualities with illness diagnosis and during the trajectories of treatment, and the illness experience can exacerbate relational challenges. People have to find new ways to cope and to deal with the stress and challenges of illness, all of which can pose challenges that strain close relationships. Some illnesses bring the additional burden of stigma and can leave people wanting to hide details of the illness or treatment. Physical manifestations of illness, as well as the ongoing necessity to schedule life around treatments, can shift perception and use of time. Some aspects of relationships can facilitate better health, but other aspects of relationships can interact with illness challenges to exacerbate the worst in close relationships. In some relationships, people successfully find meaning and purpose despite enormous medical challenges and illness-related vulnerabilities. For example, people find new meaning in the experience and expression of compassionate love, of trust and forgiveness, or of coming to new understanding of resilience.

Returning to the story. The early gatherings at the hospital almost felt like ordinary Martha's Vineyard Community Association (MVCA) luncheons, but with the challenges of getting to the hospital and parking. We bring food. We share lunch and treats and chocolate ganache cake. One mantra of the MVCA is that cake is always a good idea. The table is where we gather and solve the problems of the world, as well as some of our own. That day was no exception, from all outward appearances, as were the days that followed. But there was a quietness, a tautness that was unusual. We spent the first hour avoiding the conversation that we knew had to happen, so we had extended commentaries about the ringtones on Rita's cell phone (a separate tone for each MVCA member), navigating in the city, the lack of hospital gown styles. One question broke the ice, and then a barrage followed. We are all professors and we thrive on information – but we are friends, and we want to respect Sherry's boundaries and this story is first hers, not ours.

Sometimes teaching communication interferes with spontaneity – you tend to overthink a situation. To everyone's relief, Sherry shared a chronological explanation of how she came to be in the hospital with a brain tumor, less than the two weeks after we had all been together on the Vineyard. Then there were questions related to treatment. Radiation is a one-time process, so Sherry needs to decide whether to do it now or wait until the situation worsens. Surely this is not the life she expected. Rita shares what she learned about her own cancer treatment and suggests things Sherry may want to discuss with the doctors: whether she could fly after the biopsy, or the side effects of the steroids.

Doctors and nurses drifted in and out, with medical orders, pills, blood pressure gauges, as well as explanations – details about the biopsy process and what to expect the next day. Colleagues from Sherry's university stopped by, adding to the array of bakery products. Underlying the lighter conversations, there were hints of deep-seated fears: would we all grow old together; will this be as painful as my neighbor's biopsy; do the doctors agree on the course of treatment?

Sherry remained remarkably calm, somewhat relieved to know the "something" that was wrong. We all played our part, sharing stories, joking, asking questions, and, of course, passing around the desserts. There is an acceptance that comes with this group of women; we love and support each other amidst our quirks, weaknesses, strengths, and gifts. Today it's Sherry's turn to be the center of our attention, something she never seeks, but with grace and good humor, she accepts our love and support. In turn, we are humbled to be invited to share this journey with her, a journey of newfound vulnerability and new understanding.

Ten days after the biopsy Sherry received definitive results. On Monday morning, Sherry had an appointment with the neurosurgeon. We kept our cell phones nearby. On Monday afternoon, Anne was the bearer of the news: Sherry had a stage 2 cancerous tumor, but a "frisky" stage 2. It felt strange to be happy about the news because a stage 2 cancer is still cancer with serious ramifications for treatment and health issues. However, all were scared that the tumor would be worse, and Sherry also seemed to be prepared for worse news. The best news of the day was that the doctor spoke about the ramifications of the treatment five, ten or fifteen years down the road, which gave us all hope.

The doctor said they are going at it with everything they've got: chemo, radiation – all the weapons in their arsenal – five days a week for six weeks starting immediately. The last bit of information concerned possible side effects during her treatment. If we are doing "treatment with Sherry" then we need to know what to expect. The doctors listed some significant positive and negative side effects. A positive effect is that Sherry's word retrieval, speech, and writing difficulties should improve significantly, particularly with steroid treatments. To facilitate a more rapid recovery, the once-a-day steroid dosage was doubled to twice a day. Possible negative steroid side effects to monitor included soreness in her mouth and "'roid rage." Additional side effects from the radiation included fatigue and hair loss, while the side effects from the chemotherapy would be mild.

Radiation treatment poses potential additional long-term side effects including the worsening of speech after treatment, and memory loss.

The medical team encouraged Sherry to focus on living as normally as possible. Sherry should expect to regain lost language skills, and to plan on eventually being able to return to work. These early days in the journey are helpful but also just initial indicators of the longer trajectory. Changes in the person do not end when the treatment ends. Relationships are shifted in unanticipated and nonlinear ways.

RELATIONSHIP PROCESSES AND THEORIES AND HEALTH AND ILLNESS OUTCOMES AS EMBEDDED WITHIN SOCIAL STRUCTURES

Sherry's story is one of resources and access to excellent medical care. Sherry has health insurance, a stable marriage, friends who have the flexibility to be with her for long periods of time, the aptitude to figure out anything, and a strong sense of herself. She has a work environment where she can be flexible with her time. She has good humor over the "bad haircut" when she gets the first glimpse of herself after the biopsy when she touched her head where her hair had been shaved. Iodine used to prep her scalp before the procedure now left stains the color of red clay along the roots of the hair that remained. A dark-blue line marked the center of the shaved area where a bit of blood still dripped from the incision line. "ARGGHHH! I don't think my stylist can fix this haircut." The breadth and depth of what emerges is sometimes painful and disorienting. For others, the social structures limit instead of offer potential.

Once we have established the complexities in definitions of health and illness and in relationship processes, we consider the interconnections in pathways connecting multiple processes to outcomes. Those pathways cannot be disentangled from the disparities in healthcare access or from support systems. Illness can serve as a catalyst for relational decline and for shattered assumptions. Illness can decrease the ability to navigate relationship goals, and can bring instability, disorientation, and disillusionment. Conversely, relationships can buffer against the negative challenges of illness. Interconnections of pathways between relationship processes and health and illness trajectories then require considering the broader social networks and societal-level attributions and biases in which they co-occur.

Social-scientific empirical work and theoretical work provides evidence that high-quality relationships and strong social networks connect with better physical and mental health. The robust correlational evidence connecting relationship processes and health requires considering the broader psychosocial, environmental, and biological factors that can account for the correlation. Macro-analytic sociological research provides evidence that social integration and cohesion connect to morbidity and mortality. Social networks and social integration are considered critical components of conceptual models and theoretical explanations linking individual behavior and attitudes through processes of shaping the flow of resources. Social networks are embedded within macro-social environments and broad social forces such that networks and psychobiological processes connect. Social and economic conditions coexist with social networks and social integration. Within those conditions, physiological biomarkers connect to markers of disease outcomes including physical and mental illness. Social support can be considered a behavioral pathway linking social processes and health. We can only disentangle the biobehavioral pathways linking close relationships and health when we also consider broader disparities in health and illness and in health care and then the psychological processes as occurring within social structures.

THE PHYSICAL BODY IN HEALTH AND ILLNESS IN CLOSE RELATIONSHIPS

The literature addressing physical health does not directly connect to literature about how "knowing" is manifest in the body. Research about mind–body connections addresses theoretical propositions and biomarkers but leaves much to be explored and explained. What I have known for years in my own way of being in the world is that the particulars of my knowing are closely connected to the physical body. I can relate to the stories of people who describe taking on the pain or fatigue of others and whose bodies feel porous and who feel the experiences of others. I have learned to listen to my body and to be attentive to my breath. I have learned to step back when my "tightly wound" body is overwhelmed with sound or scent or tension held in the back. I was not entirely surprised following surgery one year by my body rejecting a series of what should have been permanent stitches. What I know of sharing my experiences with close friends is that mostly people do not understand, but they know that much about the set of experiences is important to me. They have learned to give space around the parts they do not understand. When I hear other stories of wisdom in the body, I know we still have much to explore and integrate in research on mind and body health connections and close relationships. The physical experience involves mind, body, and spirit. Close relationships can sometimes foster a sense of well-being and coherence with the experience of the physical body. Physical spaces can similarly foster a sense of healing and calm as manifest in a person's posture and demeanor as the face lightens, the breath relaxes, and muscles release.

Serious illness challenges assumptions and understandings of the role of the body. We might learn to know in the body what we cannot yet describe in language of the mind. Serious illness manifest in the body challenges the already complex interplay of how people feel in their body and how thoughts, emotions, and relationship processes connect to the physical body. Reconsidering the physical body as inherently connected to the illness experience and to close relationships sheds light on an aspect of illness experience not usually addressed in the social science literature on relationships. Although biomarkers of illness are included in empirical and theoretical research on close relationships, an inherent *way of being* as manifest in the physical body is underdeveloped and underexplored. When we consider the body as a site of identity, as knowing how to be in the world, then we understand illness as a lived experience. Considering the body as perceiving and interacting with the world means the physical body "holds" and manifests information. This is a broader understanding of lived experience such that meaning-making can occur in the body. Considering an embodied way of living shifts from the body to be "treated" in addressing symptoms of disease and considers illness as a disruption or a point of fragmentation in more holistic knowing. Time and space considerations change with illness. The body can feel foreign, and language to "conquer" or "kick" symptoms treats the symptoms as distinct from an embodied and holistic experience of being in the world. The body in illness can be reduced to a contrasting duality in opposition to the lived experience in measuring reductions in symptoms as success in treating disease. Limited language for the embodied experience in illness reveals the challenges in disconnecting the experience of the body from the relational experiences or the illness experiences. Trauma literature provides initial evidence for psychological experiences where people disengage and treat information that may be known in the body as foreign, and that foreign part of the body becomes fragmented from the other parts of self or of relationships.

RELATIONSHIP THEORIES AS EXPLAINING PART OF THE SYSTEM

Theories serve as explanatory frameworks through which we come to richer and deeper understanding. Theories of close relationships address part of the systems in understanding close relationship process in health and illness contexts. Relationship theories address interconnection and interdependence among people as dyadic (or as more than two people, but the dyad is an illustration of interconnection). To that end, relationship theories reduce the complexities of the systems in order to explain one part of the system at a time, but those parts of the system are helpful and important. For example, interdependence theory in psychology addresses how people in close relationships affect each other and how behavior in specific interactions shapes the general course of a relationship. Relational turbulence theory in communication identifies specific relationship qualities that exacerbate the experience of negative emotions, promote negative cognitions, and complicate communication between partners at points that prompt strain in a relationship. Communication privacy management theory in communication addresses how people form rules around shared boundaries of disclosing private information and the distressing sense that can occur when people do not adhere to the privacy rules. As illustrations of relationship theories, each of these theories provides helpful and testable predictions applicable to health and illness.

In the context of health and illness, each relationship theory offers helpful insight. Interdependence theory provides a framework for better understanding how people are interconnected during the process of understanding and making decisions together about health and illness and how interconnected processes can translate into potentially better adaptive coping. Communication privacy management theory provides a framework for understanding how people form and communicate rules about how their health and illness information might be shared, and poses the assumption that co-ownership of private health and illness information assumes fiduciary responsibilities. Relational turbulence theory provides a framework for understanding how an illness diagnosis or a next step in treatment can function as a point of particular uncertainty that is necessary to navigate in moving forward in a close relationship. Each of these cornerstone theories provides potentially rich application and explanation for relationships with health providers and for close relationship processes during the process of coming to terms with illness. The limitations in these theories, and the limitation in applying relationship theories to a particular context, lies in the limitation of not being able to consider the broader systems and the potentially emergent opportunities for doing something different from the framework addressed by the theory.

We might notice emergence in our engagement with a particular theory. When we work with a theory we continue to learn and develop new ways of engaging and applying the theory. The authors of particular theories described in this book can all describe stories of reshaping, refining, changing, and growth in concepts and application. The authors and researchers who develop theories also can describe the practical tasks of articulating parameters and domains in their explanatory frameworks.

EMERGENCE AND CO-GENERATIVITY IN THEORY

Emergence might be manifest within the self, within a close relationship, within an interaction, or over time in the synergies among multiple component parts. Allowing for emergence in close relationships and in health and illness can be hard. The feeling of being discovered, wanting to hide, or avoiding exposing vulnerability can be strong, and the noises around quieter wisdom can be loud. Considering emergence and co-generativity in theory gives a lens for changing purposes, changing connections with other people and with health providers, and the changing environments of our everyday lives in illness and in our experiences navigating next steps in health care.

As I keep returning to brief glimpses of Sherry's story, I am well aware of the very narrow parameters of what I share of her story. At best, you get a sense of the emergence and co-generativity of initial diagnosis as connected to a friendship network. Five years past that initial story, Sherry is doing very well. She continues to see her oncologist, and we are all grateful for ongoing MRI reports that "look good." The details so important in those few months now give shadow and shade and another lens for ongoing seeing in the context of what changes over time. Her story continues to be important, but exists among additional areas of growth and change, experiences of life and time, of joys and disappointments, some of which we share with the friendship group and some of which we experience in the sweet confinement of being alone. Some of us listen better than others to different aspects of emergence and co-generativity in everyday life and in the research languages that allows us to shed light on what becomes manifest.

A theoretical lens of systematic processes as co-created and co-generative provides opportunity to consider what we do not yet know from current theories. Co-generative theoretical understanding engages in the potential for creativity in moving forward differently by recognizing tensions, contradictions, and synergies as opportunities. Emergence and co-generativity between health and illness trajectories and close relationship processes shift from application to engagement with the multiple subjects that offer competing tensions. The physical body then becomes one source of understanding health and illness, as it adapts and responds to next steps in treatment. Instead of struggling against the symptoms or the bodily implications of (invasive) treatments, the physical embodiment is recognized as a source of emergent information and acknowledged as such. Co-created experiences of illness and of close relationships each become "conversational partners" as also connected to the body in the engagement of sense-making, reflecting about vulnerability, acknowledging differences and new symptoms and sensations, and recognizing that the conversation cannot yet fully be described because it remains ongoing. The multiple lenses offer opportunity to continue to expand understanding and to question what we think we already know. More complexity might be manifest, as in poetic inquiry, as something to be noticed instead of as a new variable to integrate into a tighter model. The constituent experiences may be experienced in explicit language or may be more implicit and emergent in attentiveness to new questions and new points of being. The vulnerability of illness then becomes one of the lenses through which we are attentive and notice what emerges.

Ongoing emergence in the illness trajectory interconnects, although not in a linear sense, with ongoing emergence in close relationships during the course of treatment. The understanding lies then in recognizing process instead of necessarily reaching for particular outcomes. Communication, language, and nonverbal behavior then are tools for expressing reality but also for creating reality and for noticing when language and nonverbal behavior constrain as opposed to when communication opens new potential. Emergence is considered as something that can occur over time within the relationship, within the illness trajectory, or within the physical body. The goal becomes understanding and offering a lens to see a different angle. Interactions with health-care professionals, with the physical body, and with others in close relationships then are considered as designing process for better understanding. This understanding and emergence is in contrast with tighter and more refined theoretical explanations. Emergence then requires noticing where scripts might limit instead of open possibility for better understanding. Reflection and finding language and noticing the body then become emergent processes in themselves. This co-generative and systematic approach to theory attends to the process of difference and poses implications for noticing where understanding seems not to be met. Considering options for new, creative, and inventive ways of engaging and co-generating requires a skeptical encountering of how system properties could potentially distort process. Generative theorizing engages how we might keep moving forward differently instead of repeating and testing frameworks that explain only part of the system.

INTERDISCIPLINARY AND LIFE-SPAN IMPLICATIONS

Theorizing close relationships and health and illness trajectories as co-created, co-generative, systematic processes offers implications for interdisciplinary and life-span understanding. Interdisciplinary implications include considerations across disciplines and interplay and collaboration in theory and methods that can allow for the ongoing mirror of next reflections. Different disciplines offer implications for cross-level linkages between relational theories and macro-level theories of social and economic context within which close relationships are embedded. Considerations for generative processes enlarge the scope of how the theoretical integration provides implications for renegotiating relationships across the life span, including age-related disabilities, for dementia and mental illness, and for connections with end-of-life care. Interdisciplinary and life-span perspectives offer new questions about how theoretical arguments are positioned and what can be better understood as co-developing. A life-span approach highlights the need to better understand the stage of illness as well as the ongoing trajectory of illness, often as interconnected and co-experienced with additional illnesses. A life-span approach highlights the need to also consider how relationships change and might be renegotiated over time to address what emerges and develops.

Interdisciplinary lenses offer the potential to recognize difference that can co-inform, which moves us beyond combining multiple theoretical perspectives to instead integrate how we might consider the questions from a different lens. For example, if the goal of family medicine is to provide relationship-centered health care, then we consider and design interactions that allow for emergence between doctors and patients, between patients and their families, between family members and close friends, among health-care provider peers. We don't try to adapt the questions we already know but to consider how current knowing can instead translate into doing the process differently. Interdisciplinary lenses give us a sense of the occasions when we wish to do things that require another way of understanding. Recognizing the co-created, co-generative, systematic processes keeps us engaged such that we can increase the complexity of our own thinking and to listen to difference in others' thinking, across disciplines, and as the purposes and environments continue to change. To that end, on with the journey, with a horizon more than we can see.

References

Ackerson, L. K. & Viswanath, K. (2009). The social context of interpersonal communication and health. *Journal of Health Communication*, *14* (Suppl. 1), 5–17. https://doi.org/10.1080/10810730902806836

Adler, N. E. & Rehkopf, D. H. (2008). U.S. disparities in health: Descriptions, causes, and mechanisms. *Annual Review of Public Health*, *29*, 235–252. https://doi.org/10.1146/annurev.publhealth.29.020907.090852

Afifi, T. D., Hutchinson, S., & Krouse, S. (2006). Toward a theoretical model of communal coping in postdivorce families and other naturally occurring groups. *Communication Theory*, *16*, 378–409. https://doi.org/10.1111/j.1468-2885.2006.00275.x

Afifi, T. D., Merrill, A. F., & Davis, S. (2016). The theory of resilience and relational load. *Personal Relationships*, *23*, 663–683. https://doi.org/10.1111/pere.12159

Afifi, W. A. & Morse, C. R. (2009). Expanding the role of emotion in the theory of motivated information management. In T. D. Afifi & W. A. Afifi (Eds.), *Uncertainty, information management, and disclosure decisions: Theories and applications* (pp. 87–105). New York, NY: Routledge.

Afifi, W. A. & Weiner, J. L. (2004). Toward a theory of motivated information management. *Communication Theory*, *14*, 167–190. https://doi.org/10.1111/j.1468-2885.2004.tb00310.x

Agnew, C. R., Arriaga, X. B., & Wilson, J. E. (2008). Committed to what? Using the bases of relational commitment model to understand continuity and change in social relationships. In J. P. Forgas & J. Fitness (Eds.), *Social relationships: Cognitive, affective, and motivational processes* (pp. 147–164). New York, NY: Psychology Press.

Agnew, C. R., Van Lange, P. A., Rusbult, C. E., & Langston, C. A. (1998). Cognitive interdependence: Commitment and the mental representation of close relationships. *Journal of Personality and Social Psychology*, *74*, 939–954. https://doi.org/10.1037/0022-3514.74.4.939

Antelius, E. (2009). Whose body is it anyway? Verbalization, embodiment, and the creation of narratives. *Health: An Interdisciplinary Journal for the Social Study of Health, Illness and Medicine*, *13*, 361–379. https://doi.org/10.1177/1363459308101808

Aron, A., Aron, E. N., & Smollan, D. (1992). Inclusion of other in the self scale and the structure of interpersonal closeness. *Journal of Personality and Social Psychology, 63*, 596–612. https://doi.org/10.1037/0022-3514.63.4.596

Aron, A., Aron, E. N., Tudor, M., & Nelson, G. (1991). Close relationships as including other in the self. *Journal of Personality and Social Psychology, 60*, 241–253. https://doi.org/10.1037//0022-3514.60.2.241

Aron, A., Fisher, H. E., & Strong, G. (2006). Romantic love. In A. L. Vangelisti & D. Perlman (Eds.), *The Cambridge handbook of personal relationships* (pp. 595–614). New York, NY: Cambridge University Press. https://doi.org/10.1017/CBO9780511606632.033

Aron, E. N. & Aron, A. (1996). Love and the expansion of the self: The state of the model. *Personal Relationships, 3*, 45–58. https://doi.org/10.1111/j.1475-6811.1996.tb00103.x

Arriaga, X. B. (2013). An interdependence theory analysis of close relationships. In J. A. Simpson & L. Campbell (Eds.), *The Oxford handbook of close relationships* (pp. 39–65). Oxford, England: Oxford University Press.

Arriaga, X. B. & Agnew, C. R. (2001). Being committed: Affective, cognitive, and conative components of relationship commitment. *Personality and Social Psychology Bulletin, 27*, 1190–1203. https://doi.org/10.1177/0146167201279011

Arriaga, X. B., Slaughterbeck, E. S., Capezza, N. M., & Hmurovic, J. L. (2007). From bad to worse: Relationship commitment and vulnerability to partner imperfections. *Personal Relationships, 14*, 389–409. https://doi.org/10.1111/j.1475-6811.2007.00162.x

Attridge, M., Berscheid, E., & Simpson, J. A. (1995). Predicting relationship stability from both partners versus one. *Journal of Personality and Social Psychology, 69*, 254–268. https://doi.org/10.1037/0022-3514.69.2.254

Aukes, L. C., Geertsma, J., Cohen-Schotanus, J., Zwierstra, R. P., & Slaets, J. P. J. (2007). The development of a scale to measure personal reflection in medical practice and education. *Medical Teacher, 29*, 177–182. https://doi.org/10.1080/01421590701299272

Badr, H. (2004). Coping in marital dyads: A contextual perspective on the role of gender and health. *Personal Relationships, 11*, 197–211. https://doi.org/10.1111/j.1475-6811.2004.00078.x

Balint, E. (1969). The possibilities of patient-centered medicine. Journal of the Royal College of General Practitioners, 17, 269–276.

Ballin, L. & Balandin, S. (2007). An exploration of loneliness: Communication and the social networks of older people with cerebral palsy. *Journal of Intellectual and Developmental Disability, 32,* 315–327. https://doi.org/10.1080/13668250701689256

Barge, J. K., Simpson, J. L., & Shockley-Zalabak, P. (2008). Introduction: Toward purposeful and practical models of engaged scholarship. *Journal of Applied Communication Research, 36,* 243–244. https://doi.org/10.1080/00909880802190113

Beach, M. C., Inui, T., & The Relationship-Centered Care Research Network (Frankel, R., Hall, J., Haidet, P., Roter, D., Beckman, H., Cooper, L. A., Miller, W., Mossbarger, D., Safran, D., Sluyter, D., Stein, H., & Williamson, P.) (2006). Relationship-centered care: A constructive reframing. *Journal of General Internal Medicine, 21,* S3–S8. https://doi.org/10.1111/j.1525-1497.2006.00302.x

Bengston, V., Rosenthal, C., & Burton, L. (1995). Paradoxes of families and aging. In R. H. Binstock, L. K. George, V. W. Marshall, G. C. Myers, & J. H. Schulz (Eds.), *Handbook of aging and the social sciences* (4th ed., pp. 253–282). San Diego, CA: Academic Press.

Berkman, L. F. (2000). Social support, social networks, social cohesion and health. *Social Work in Health Care, 31*(2), 3–14. https://doi.org/10.1300/J010v31n02_02

(2004). Social integration, social networks, and health. In N. B. Anderson (Ed.), *Encyclopedia of health and behavior* (pp. 670–674). Thousand Oaks, CA: SAGE Publications, Inc. https://dx.doi.org/10.4135/9781412952576.n192

Berkman, L. F., Glass, T., Brissette, I., & Seeman, T. E. (2000). From social integration to health: Durkheim in the new millennium. *Social Science & Medicine, 51,* 843–857. https://doi.org/10.1016/S0277-9536(00)00065-4

Berkman, L. F. & Syme, S. L. (1979). Social networks, host resistance, and mortality: A nine-year follow-up study of alameda county residents. *American Journal of Epidemiology, 109,* 186–204. https://doi.org/10.1093/oxfordjournals.aje.a112674

Berscheid, E. (1983). Emotion. In H. H. Kelley, E. Berscheid, A. Christensen, J. H. Harvey, T. L. Huston, G. Levinger et al. (Eds.), *Close relationships* (pp. 110–168). New York, NY: W. H. Freeman.

Berscheid, E. (1996). The "paradigm of family transcendence": Not a paradigm, questionably transcendent, but valuable, nonetheless. *Journal of Marriage and the Family, 58,* 556–564. https://doi.org/10.2307/353716

Berscheid, E. (1998). In Bradbury T. N. (Ed.), *A social psychological view of marital dysfunction and stability.* New York, NY: Cambridge University Press. https://doi.org/10.1017/CBO9780511527814.019

Berscheid, E. & Ammazzalorso, H. (2001). Emotional experience in close relationships. In G. J. O. Fletcher & M. Clark (Eds.), *Blackwell handbook of social psychology: Interpersonal processes* (pp. 308–330). Oxford, England: Blackwell.

Berscheid, E. & Regan, P. (2005). *The psychology of interpersonal relationships.* New York, NY: Prentice-Hall.

Bertera, E. M. (2005). Mental health in U.S. adults: The role of positive social support and social negativity in personal relationships. *Journal of Social and Personal Relationships, 22,* 33–48. https://doi.org/10.1177/0265407505049320

Bodenmann, G. & Randall, A. K. (2013). Close relationships in psychiatric disorders. *Current Opinion in Psychiatry, 26,* 464–467. https://doi.org/10.1097/YCO.0b013e3283642de7

Boomsma, D. I., Cacioppo, J. T., Muthén, B., Asparouhov, T., & Clark, S. (2007). Longitudinal genetic analysis for loneliness in Dutch twins. *Twin Research and Human Genetics, 10,* 267–273. https://doi.org/10.1375/twin.10.2.267

Borrell-Carrió, F., Suchman, A. L., & Epstein, R. M. (2004). The biopsychosocial model 25 years later: Principles, practice, and scientific inquiry. *Annals of Family Medicine, 2,* 576–582. https://doi.org/10.1370/afm.245

Borstelmann, N. A., Rosenberg, S. M., Ruddy, K. J., Tamimi, R. M., Gelber, S., Schapira, L., ... Partridge, A. H. (2015). Partner support and anxiety in young women with breast cancer. *Psycho-Oncology, 24,* 1679–1685. https://doi.org/10.1002/pon.3780

Bowen, K. S., Uchino, B. N., Birmingham, W., Carlisle, M., Smith, T. W., & Light, K. C. (2013). The stress-buffering effects of functional social support on ambulatory blood pressure. *Health Psychology, 33,* 1440–1443. https://doi.org/10.1037/hea0000005

Bowlby, J. (1982). Attachment and loss: Retrospect and prospect. *American Journal of Orthopsychiatry, 52,* 664–678. https://doi.org/10.1111/j.1939-0025.1982.tb01456.x

Bowler, K. (2018). *Everything happens for a reason, and other lies I've loved.* New York, NY: Random House.

Bowman, G. S. (2001). Emotions and illness. *Journal of Advanced Nursing, 34,* 256–263. https://doi.org/10.1046/j.1365-2648.2001.01752.x

Boyd, E. M. & Fales, A. W. (1983). Reflective learning: Key to learning from experience. *Journal of Humanistic Psychology, 23,* 99–117. https://doi.org/10.1177/0022167883232011

Bradbury, T. N. & Fincham, F. D. (1991). Clinical and social perspectives on close relationships. In C. R. Snyder & D. R. Forsyth (Eds.), *Handbook of social and clinical psychology: The health perspective* (pp. 309–326). Elmsford, NY: Pergamon Press.

Braithwaite, D. O. & Eckstein, N. J. (2003). How people with disabilities communicatively manage assistance: Helping as instrumental social support. *Journal of Applied Communication Research, 31*, 1–26. https://doi.org/10.1080/00909880305374

Brashers, D. E. (2001). Communication and uncertainty management. *Journal of Communication, 51*, 477–497. https://doi.org/10.1111/j.1460-2466.2001.tb02892.x

Brashers, D. E., Haas, S. M., Neidig, J. L., & Rintamaki, L. S. (2002). Social activism, self-advocacy, and coping with HIV illness. *Journal of Social and Personal Relationships, 19*, 113–133. https://doi.org/10.1177/0265407502191006

Brown, E., Orbuch, T. L., Bauermeister, J. A., & McKinley, B. (2013). Marital well-being over time among black and white Americans: The first seven years. *Journal of African American Studies, 17*, 290–307. https://doi.org/10.1007/s12111-012-9234-1

Buckley, S., Coleman, J., Davison, I., Khan, K. S., Zamora, J., Malick, S., ... Sayers, J. (2009). The educational effects of portfolios on undergraduate student learning: A best evidence medical education (BEME) systematic review. BEME guide no. 11. *Medical Teacher, 31*, 282–298. https://doi.org/10.1080/01421590902889897

Bugental, D. B. (2000). Acquisition of the algorithms of social life: A domain-based approach. *Psychological Bulletin, 126*, 187–219. https://doi.org/10.1037//0033-2909.126.2.187

Burgoon, J. K. & Hale, J. L. (1987). Validation and measurement of the fundamental themes of relational communication. *Communication Monographs, 54*, 19–41. https://doi.org/10.1080/03637758709390214

Burke, T. J., Randall, A. K., Corkery, S. A., Young, V. J., & Butler, E. A. (2012). "You're going to eat that?" relationship processes and conflict among mixed-weight couples. *Journal of Social and Personal Relationships, 29*, 1109–1130. https://doi.org/10.1177/0265407512451199

Burleson, B. R., Metts, S., & Kirch, M. W. (2000). Communication in close relationships. In C. Hendrick & S. S. Hendrick (Eds.), *Close relationships: A sourcebook* (pp. 245–258). Thousand Oaks, CA: Sage Publications. https://doi.org/10.4135/9781452220437.n18

Burt, R. S. (1982). *Toward a structural theory of action*. New York, NY: Academic Press.

Butler, E. A., Lee, T. L., & Gross, J. J. (2007). Emotion regulation and culture: Are the social consequences of emotion suppression culture-specific? *Emotion, 7,* 30–48. https://doi.org/10.1037/1528-3542.7.1.30

Butler, E. A. & Sbarra, D. A. (2013). Health, emotion, and relationships. *Journal of Social and Personal Relationships, 30,* 151–154. https://doi.org/10.1177/0265407512453425

Bylund, C. L. & Duck, S. (2004). The everyday interplay between family relationships and family members' health. *Journal of Social and Personal Relationships, 21,* 5–7. https://doi.org/10.1177/0265407504039837

Byrd, W. M. & Clayton, L. A. (2002). *An American health dilemma: A medical history of African Americans and the problem of race.* New York, NY: Routledge.

Cacioppo, J. T., Fowler, J. H., & Christakis, N. A. (2009). Alone in the crowd: The structure and spread of loneliness in a large social network. *Journal of Personality and Social Psychology, 97,* 977–991. https://doi.org/10.1037/a0016076

Cacioppo, J. T., Hawkley, L. C., & Thisted, R. A. (2010). Perceived social isolation makes me sad: 5-year cross-lagged analyses of loneliness and depressive symptomatology in the Chicago health, aging, and social relations study. *Psychology and Aging, 25,* 453–463. https://doi.org/10.1037/a0017216

Call, V., Sprecher, S., & Schwartz, P. (1995). The incidence and frequency of marital sex in a national sample. *Journal of Marriage and Family, 57,* 639–652. https://doi.org/10.2307/353919

Campo, R. A., Uchino, B. N., Vaughn, A., Reblin, M., Smith, T. W., & Holt-Lunstad, J. (2009). The assessment of positivity and negativity in social networks: The reliability and validity of the social relationships index. *Journal of Community Psychology, 37,* 471–486. https://doi.org/10.1002/jcop.20308

Canary, H. E. (2008). Negotiating dis/ability in families: Constructions and contradictions. *Journal of Applied Communication Research, 36,* 437–458. https://doi.org/10.1080/00909880802101771

Carel, H. (2009). "I am well, apart from the fact that I have cancer": Explaining wellbeing within illness. In L. Bortolotti (Ed.), *Philosophy and happiness* (pp. 82–99). Basingstoke, England: Palgrave Macmillan.

(2013). Bodily doubt. *Journal of Consciousness Studies, 20*(7–8), 178–197.

(2014). The philosophical role of illness. *Metaphilosophy, 45,* 20–40. https://doi.org/10.1111/meta.12065

(2015). With bated breath: Diagnosis of respiratory illness. *Perspectives in Biology and Medicine, 58,* 53–65. https://doi.org/10.1353/pbm.2015.0013

(2016). *Phenomenology of illness.* New York, NY: Oxford University Press.

Carel, H. & Kidd, I. J. (2014). Epistemic injustice in healthcare: A philosophical analysis. *Medicine, Healthcare and Philosophy, 17*, 529–540.

Carleton, R. N., Peluso, D. L., Collimore, K. C., & Asmundson, G. J. G. (2011). Social anxiety and posttraumatic stress symptoms: The impact of distressing social events. *Journal of Anxiety Disorders, 25*, 49–57. https://doi.org/10.1016/j.janxdis.2010.08.002

Carlisle, M., Uchino, B. N., Sanbonmatsu, D. M., Smith, T. W., Cribbet, M. R., Birmingham, W., & Vaughn, A. A. (2012). Subliminal activation of social ties moderates cardiovascular reactivity during acute stress. *Health Psychology, 31*, 217–225. https://doi.org/10.1037/a0025187

Cassel, J. (1976). The contribution of the social environment to host resistance. *American Journal of Epidemiology, 104*, 107–123. https://doi.org/10.1093/oxfordjournals.aje.a112281

Caughlin, J. P. & Huston, T. L. (2002). A contextual analysis of the association between demand/withdraw and marital satisfaction. *Personal Relationships, 9*, 95–119. https://doi.org/10.1111/1475-6811.00007

Chan, W. C. H. (2011). Being aware of the prognosis: How does it relate to palliative care patients' anxiety and communication difficulty with family members in the Hong Kong Chinese context? *Journal of Palliative Medicine, 14*, 997–1003. https://doi.org/10.1089/jpm.2011.0099

Checton, M. G. & Greene, K. (2012). Beyond initial disclosure: The role of prognosis and symptom uncertainty in patterns of disclosure in relationships. *Health Communication, 27*, 145–157. https://doi.org/10.1080/10410236.2011.571755
(2014). "I tell my partner everything ... (or not)": Patients' perceptions of sharing heart-related information with their partner. *Journal of Family Nursing, 20*, 164–184. https://doi.org/10.1177/1074840714521320

Checton, M. G., Greene, K., Magsamen-Conrad, K., & Venetis, M. K. (2012). Patients' and partners' perspectives of chronic illness and its management. *Families, Systems, & Health, 30*(2), 114–129. https://doi.org/10.1037/a0028598

Chen, Y. & Feeley, T. H. (2014). Social support, social strain, loneliness, and well-being among older adults: An analysis of the health and retirement study. *Journal of Social and Personal Relationships, 31*, 141–161. https://doi.org/10.1177/0265407513488728

Child, J. T., Petronio, S., Agyeman-Budu, E. A., & Westermann, D. A. (2011). Blog scrubbing: Exploring triggers that change privacy rules. *Computers in Human Behavior, 27*, 2017–2027. https://doi.org/10.1016/j.chb.2011.05.009

Cohen, S., Doyle, W. J., & Baum, A. (2006). Socioeconomic status is associated with stress hormones. *Psychosomatic Medicine, 68,* 414–420. https://doi.org/10.1097/01.psy.0000221236.37158.b9

Cohen, S. & Janicki-Deverts, D. (2009). Can we improve our physical health by altering our social networks? *Perspectives on Psychological Science, 4,* 375–378. https://doi.org/10.1111/j.1745-6924.2009.01141.x

Collins, N. L. & Feeney, B. C. (2000). A safe haven: An attachment theory perspective on support seeking and caregiving in intimate relationships. *Journal of Personality and Social Psychology, 78,* 1053–1073. https://doi.org/10.1037/0022-3514.78.6.1053

Collins, N. L. & Read, S. J. (1990). Adult attachment, working models, and relationship quality in dating couples. *Journal of Personality and Social Psychology, 58,* 644–663. https://doi.org/10.1037//0022-3514.58.4.644

Conrad, P. & Barker, K. K. (2010). The social construction of illness: Key insights and policy implications. *Journal of Health and Social Behavior, 51,* S67–S79. https://doi.org/10.1177/0022146510383495

Cooper, L. A., Hill, M. N., & Powe, N. R. (2002). Designing and evaluating interventions to eliminate racial and ethnic disparities in health care. *Journal of General Internal Medicine, 17,* 477–486. https://doi.org/10.1046/j.1525-1497.2002.10633.x

Cooper, L. A., Roter, D. L., Carson, K. A., Beach, M. C., Sabin, J. A., Greenwald, A. G., & Inui, T. S. (2012). The associations of clinicians' implicit attitudes about race with medical visit communication and patient ratings of interpersonal care. *American Journal of Public Health, 102*(5), 979–987. http://dx.doi.org.proxy.bc.edu/10.2105/AJPH.2011.300558

Corbin, J. M. (2003). The body in health and illness. *Qualitative Health Research, 13,* 256–267. https://doi.org/10.1177/1049732302239603

Cornwell, E. Y. & Waite, L. J. (2009). Social disconnectedness, perceived isolation, and health among older adults. *Journal of Health and Social Behavior, 50,* 31–48. https://doi.org/10.1177/002214650905000103

Corrigan, F. M. (2014). Threat and safety: The neurobiology of active and passive defense responses. In U. F. Lanius, S. L. Paulsen, & F. M. Corrigan (Eds.), *Neurobiology and treatment of traumatic dissociation: Toward an embodied self* (pp. 29–50). New York, NY: Springer Publishing Company.

Corrigan, F. M., Wilson, A., & Fay, D. (2014). The compassionate self. In U. F. Lanius, S. L. Paulsen, & F. M. Corrigan (Eds.), *Neurobiology and treatment of traumatic dissociation: Toward an embodied self* (pp. 269–287). New York, NY: Springer Publishing Co.

Cross, S. E. & Morris, M. L. (2003). Getting to know you: The relational self-construal, relational cognition, and well-being. *Personality and Social Psychology Bulletin, 29,* 512–523. https://doi.org/10.1177/0146167202250920

Croteau, C. & Le Dorze, G. (2006). Overprotection, "speaking for," and conversational participation: A study of couples with aphasia. *Aphasiology, 20,* 327–336. https://doi.org/10.1080/02687030500475051

Cumella, S. & Martin, D. (2004). Secondary healthcare and learning disability: Results of consensus development conferences. *Journal of Learning Disabilities, 8,* 30–40. https://doi.org/10.1177/1469004704041703

Curtis, K., Tzannes, A., & Rudge, T. (2011). How to talk to doctors – A guide for effective communication. *International Nursing Review, 58,* 13–20. https://doi.org/10.1111/j.1466–7657.2010.00847.x

Dailey, R. M., McCracken, A. A., & Romo, L. K. (2011). Confirmation and weight management: Predicting effective levels of acceptance and challenge in weight management messages. *Communication Monographs, 78,* 185–211. https://doi.org/10.1080/03637751.2011.564638

Dailey, R. M., Richards, A. A., & Romo, L. K. (2010). Communication with significant others about weight management: The role of confirmation in weight management attitudes and behaviors. *Communication Research, 37,* 644–673. https://doi.org/10.1177/0093650210362688

Dailey, R. M., Romo, L. K., & Thompson, C. M. (2011). Confirmation in couples' communication about weight management: An analysis of how both partners contribute to individuals' health behaviors and conversational outcomes. *Human Communication Research, 37,* 553–582. https://doi.org/10.1111/j.1468–2958.2011.01414.x

de Bie, R. P., Massuger, L. F., Lenselink, C. H., Derksen, Y. H., Prins, J. B., & Bekkers, R. L. (2011). The role of individually targeted information to reduce anxiety before colposcopy: A randomised controlled trial. *British Journal of Obstetrics and Gynaecology: International Journal of Obstetrics and Gynaecology, 118,* 945–950. https://doi.org/10.1111/j.1471–0528.2011.02996.x

Deetz, S. A. (1992). *Democracy in an age of corporate colonization: Developments in communication and the politics of everyday life.* Albany, NY: State University of New York Press.

Deetz, S. (2008). Engagement as co-generative theorizing. *Journal of Applied Communication Research, 36,* 289–297. https://doi.org/10.1080/00909880802172301

Diderichsen, F. (2010). *A conceptual framework for action on the social determinants of health: Social determinants of health discussion paper 2.* Geneva, Switzerland: World Health Organization.

DiGiacomo, S. M. (1992). Metaphor as illness: Postmodern dilemmas in the representation of body, mind and disorder. *Medical Anthropology*, *14*(1), 109–137. https://doi.org/10.1080/01459740.1992.9966068

Dillow, M. R. & LaBelle, S. (2014). Discussions of sexual health testing: Applying the theory of motivated information management. *Personal Relationships*, *21*, 676–691. https://doi.org/10.1111/pere.12057

Dorling, D., Mitchell, R., & Pearce, J. (2007). The global impact of income inequality on health by age: An observational study. *British Medical Journal*, *335*, 833–834. https://doi.org/10.1136/bmj.39349.507315.DE

Drigotas, S. M., Rusbult, C. E., Wieselquist, J., & Whitton, S. W. (1999). Close partner as sculptor of the ideal self: Behavioral affirmation and the Michelangelo phenomenon. *Journal of Personality and Social Psychology*, *77*, 293–323. https://doi.org/10.1037/0022-3514.77.2.293

Duggan, A. P. (2006). Understanding interpersonal communication processes across health contexts: Advances in the last decade and challenges for the next decade. *Journal of Health Communication*, *11*, 93–108. https://doi.org/10.1080/10810730500461125

(2007). Sex differences in communicative attempts to curtail depression: An inconsistent nurturing as control perspective. *Western Journal of Communication*, *71*, 114–135. https://doi.org/10.1080/10570310701354492

Duggan, A. P. & Bradshaw, Y. S. (2008). Mutual influence processes in physician-patient interaction: An interaction adaptation theory perspective. *Communication Research Reports*, *25*(3), 211–226. https://doi.org/10.1080/08824090802237618

Duggan, A., Bradshaw, Y. S., & Altman, W. (2010). How do I ask about your disability? an examination of interpersonal communication processes between medical students and patients with disabilities. *Journal of Health Communication*, *15*(3), 334–350. https://doi.org/10.1080/10810731003686630

Duggan, A. P., Bradshaw, Y. S., Carroll, S. E., Rattigan, S. H., & Altman, W. (2009). What can I learn from this interaction? A qualitative analysis of medical student self reflection and learning in a standardized patient exercise about disability. *Journal of Health Communication*, *14*, 797–811. https://doi.org/10.1080/10810730903295526

Duggan, A. P., Bradshaw, Y. S., Swergold, N., & Altman, W. (2011). When rapport building extends beyond affiliation: Communication overaccommodation toward patients with disabilities. *The Permanente Journal, 15*(2), 23–30. https://doi.org/10.7812/tpp/11–018

Duggan, A. P., Dailey, R. M., & Le Poire, B. A. (2008). Reinforcement and punishment of substance abuse during ongoing interactions: A conversational test of inconsistent nurturing as control theory. *Journal of Health Communication, 13*, 417–433. https://doi.org/10.1080/10810730802198722

Duggan, A. P. & Kilmartin, B. (2016). Parental and sibling behaviors that encourage daughters' continued eating disorders: An inconsistent nurturing as control perspective. In L. Olson & M. Fine (Eds.), *The darker side of family communication: The harmful, the morally suspect, and the socially inappropriate* (pp. 49–68). Bern, Switzerland: Peter Lang Publishing, Inc.

Duggan, A. P. & Le Poire, B. A. (2006). One down, two involved: An application and extension of inconsistent nurturing as control theory to couples including one depressed individual. *Communication Monographs, 73*, 379–405. https://doi.org/10.1080/03637750601024149

Duggan, A. P. & Le Poire Molineux, B. A. (2013). The reciprocal influence of drug and alcohol abuse and family members' communication. In A. L. Vangelisti (Ed.), *The Routledge handbook of family communication* (2nd ed., pp. 463–478). New York, NY: Routledge.

Duggan, A. P., Le Poire, B. A., & Addis, K. (2006). A qualitative analysis of communicative strategies used by partners of substance abusers and depressed individuals during recovery: Implications for inconsistent nurturing as control theory. In R. M. Dailey & B. A. Le Poire (Eds.), *Applied interpersonal communication matters: Family, health, and community relations* (pp. 150–174). New York, NY: Peter Lang.

Duggan, A. P., Le Poire, B. A., Prescott, M., & Baham, C. S. (2009). Understanding the helper: The role of codependency in health care and health care outcomes. In D. E. Brashers & D. Goldsmith (Eds.), *Communicating to manage health and illness* (pp. 271–300). New York, NY: Routledge.

Duggan, A. P. & Parrott, R. L. (2001). Physicians' nonverbal rapport building and patients' talk about the subjective component of illness. *Human Communication Research, 27*, 299–311. https://doi.org/10.1093/hcr/27.2.299

Duggan, A. & Petronio, S. (2009). When your child is in crisis: Navigating medical needs with issues of privacy management. In T. J. Socha & G. H. Stamp (Eds.), *Parents and children communicating with society: Managing relationships outside of home* (pp. 117–132). New York, NY: Routledge.

Duggan, A., Robinson, J., & Thompson, T. L. (2012). Understanding disability as an intergroup encounter. In H. Giles (Ed.), *The handbook of intergroup communication* (pp. 250–263). New York, NY: Routledge.

Duggan, A. P. & Thompson, T. L. (2011). Provider-patient communication and health outcomes. In T. L. Thompson, R. L. Parrott, & J. Nussbaum (Eds.), *The Routledge handbook of health communication* (2nd ed., pp. 414–427). New York, NY: Routledge.

(2014). Social interaction processes in healthcare contexts. In C. Berger (Ed.), *Interpersonal communication: Handbook of communication science* (pp. 493–516). Berlin, Germany: De Gruyter Mouton.

Duggan, A. P., Vicini, A., Allen, L., & Shaughnessy, A. F. (2015). Learning to see beneath the surface: A qualitative analysis of family medicine residents' reflections about communication. *Journal of Health Communication, 20*(12), 1441–1448. https://doi.org/10.1080/10810730.2015.1018647

Dykstra, P. A. & Hagestad, G. O. (2016). How demographic patterns and social policies shape interdependence among lives in the family realm. *Population Horizons, 13*(2), 54–62. https://doi.org/10.1515/pophzn–2016–0004

Earnshaw, V. A., Bogart, L. M., Dovidio, J. F., & Williams, D. R. (2013). Stigma and racial/ethnic HIV disparities: Moving toward resilience. *American Psychologist, 68*, 225–236. https://doi.org/10.1037/a0032705

Eastwick, P. W. & Hunt, L. L. (2014). Relational mate value: Consensus and uniqueness in romantic evaluations. *Journal of Personality and Social Psychology, 106*, 728–751. https://doi.org/10.1037/a0035884

Eggly, S., Barton, E., Winckles, A., Penner, L., & Albrecht, T. (2015). A disparity of words: A comparison of offers to participate in cancer clinical trials by patient race. *Health Expectations, 18*, 1316–1326. https://doi.org/10.1158/1055–9965.DISP12–A11

Eggly, S., Harper, F. W. K., Penner, L. A., Gleason, M. J., Foster, T., & Albrecht, T. L. (2011). Variation in question asking during cancer clinical interactions: A potential source of disparities in access to information. *Patient Education and Counseling, 82*, 63–68. https://doi.org/10.1016/j.pec.2010.04.008

Eggly, S., Tkatch, R., Penner, L. A., Mabunda, L., Hudson, J., Chapman, R., Griggs, J. J., Brown, R., & Albrecht, T. (2013). Development of a question prompt list as a communication intervention to reduce racial disparities in cancer treatment. *Journal of Cancer Education, 28*, 282–289. https://doi.org/10.1007/s13187-013-0456-2

Engel, G. L. (1977). The need for a new medical model: A challenge for biomedicine. *Science, 196* (4286), 129–136. https://doi.org/10.1126/science.847460

Ertel, K. A., Glymour, M. M., & Berkman, L. F. (2009). Social networks and health: A life course perspective integrating observational and experimental evidence. *Journal of Social and Personal Relationships, 26*, 73–92. https://doi.org/10.1177/0265407509105523

Eva, K. W. & Regehr, G. (2008). "I'll never play professional football" and other fallacies of self-assessment. *Journal of Continuing Education in the Health Professions, 28*, 14–19. https://doi.org/10.1002/chp.150

Farber, S. K. (2013). The mind-body connection: Why we all need to be touched. Retrieved April 1, 2018 from www.psychologytoday.com/blog/the-mind-body-connection/201312/the-mind-body-connection

Fehr, B. & Sprecher, S. (2009). Prototype analysis of the concept of compassionate love. *Personal Relationships, 16*, 343–364. https://doi.org/10.1111/j.1475–6811.2009.01227.x

Fehr B. A., Sprecher, S., & Underwood, L. G. (Eds.). (2009). *The science of compassionate love: Theory, research, and applications.* Oxford, England: Wiley-Blackwell.

Fekete, E. M., Deichert, N. T., & Williams, S. L. (2014). HIV-specific unsupportive social interactions, health, and ethnicity in men living with HIV. *Journal of Social and Personal Relationships, 31*, 830–846. https://doi.org/10.1177/0265407513506796

Felmlee, D. & Sprecher, S. (2006). Love: Psychological and sociological perspective. In J. E. Stets & J. H. Turner (Eds.), *Handbook of sociology of emotions* (pp.389–409). New York, NY: Springer.

Ferris, J. (2009). Why should communication scholars pay attention to disability? *Spectrum, 45*(1), 9–10.

Fife, B. L., Weaver, M. T., Cook, W. L., & Stump, T. T. (2013). Partner interdependence and coping with life-threatening illness: The impact on dyadic adjustment. *Journal of Family Psychology, 27*, 702–711. https://doi.org/10.1037/a0033871

Fincham, F. & Beach, S. R. H. (2007). Forgiveness and marital quality: Precursor or consequence in well-established relationships? *The Journal of Positive Psychology, 2*, 260–268. https://doi.org/10.1080/17439760701552360

Fingerman, K. L., Hay, E. L., & Birditt, K. S. (2004). The best of ties, the worst of ties: Close, problematic, and ambivalent social relationships. *Journal of Marriage and Family, 66*, 792–808. https://doi.org/10.1111/j.0022–2445.2004.00053.x

Finkel, E. J. & Campbell, W. K. (2001). Self-control and accommodation in close relationships: An interdependence analysis. *Journal of Personality and Social Psychology, 81*, 263–277. https://doi.org/10.1037/0022–3514.81.2.263

Finkel, E. J., Simpson, J. A., & Eastwick, P. W. (2017). The psychology of close relationships: Fourteen core principles. *Annual Review of Psychology, 68,* 383–411. https://doi.org/10.1146/annurev-psych–010416–044038

Fitness, J. (2009). Anger in relationships. In H. Reis & S. Sprecher (Eds.), *Encyclopedia of human relationships* (pp. 94–97). Thousand Oaks, CA: Sage.

(2015). Emotions in relationships. In M. Mikulincer, P. R. Shaver, J. A. Simpson, & J. F. Dovidio (Eds.), *APA handbook of personality and social psychology: Vol. 3. Interpersonal relations* (pp. 297–318). Washington, DC: American Psychological Association. https://dx.doi.org/10.1037/14344–011

Fitness, J. & Fletcher, G. J. O. (1993). Love, hate, anger, and jealousy in close relationships: A prototype and cognitive appraisal analysis. *Journal of Personality and Social Psychology, 65,* 942–958. https://doi.org/10.1037/0022–3514.65.5.942

Fitzsimons, G. M., Finkel, E. J., & vanDellen, M. R. (2015). Transactive goal dynamics. *Psychological Review, 122,* 648–673. https://doi.org/10.1037/a0039654

Fortenbury, J. (December 30, 2013). Love in the time of chronic illness: When should you disclose medical conditions to a date? When is illness too much for a relationship to survive? The Atlantic, Retrieved April 1, 2018 from www.theatlantic.com/health/archive/2013/12/love-in-the-time-of-chronic-illness/282477/

Fox, S. A. & Giles, H. (1997). Let the wheelchair through: An intergroup approach to interability communication. In W. P. Robinson (Ed.), *Social groups and identity: The developing legacy of Henri Tajfel* (pp. 215–248). Oxford, UK: Heinemann.

Frank, A. W. (1995). *The wounded storyteller: Body, illness, and ethics.* Chicago, IL: University of Chicago Press.

(2002). *At the will of the body: Reflections on illness* (2nd ed.). Boston, MA: Houghton Mifflin.

Frank, G. (2000). *Venus on wheels: Two decades of dialogue on disability, biography, and being female in America.* Berkley, CA: University of California Press.

Frankel, R. M., Eddins-Folensbee, F., & Inui, T. S. (2011). Crossing the patient-centered divide: Transforming health care quality through enhanced faculty development. *Academic Medicine, 86,* 445–452. https://doi.org/10.1097/ACM.0b013e31820e7e6e

Franks, M. M., Wendorf, C. A., Gonzalez, R., & Ketterer, M. (2004). Aid and influence: Health-promoting exchanges of older married partners. *Journal of*

Social and Personal Relationships, 21, 431–445. https://doi.org/10.1177/0265407504044839

Friedli, L. (2009). *Mental health, resilience, and inequalities.* Copenhagen, Denmark: World Health Organization Regional Office for Europe. Retrieved from World Health Organization.

Frost, D. M. (2013). The narrative construction of intimacy and affect in relationship stories: Implications for relationship quality, stability, and mental health. *Journal of Social and Personal Relationships, 30,* 247–269. https://doi.org/10.1177/0265407512454463

Gaines, S. O., Jr. (2016). *Personality and close relationship processes.* New York, NY: Cambridge University Press. https://doi.org/10.1017/CBO9781316271926

Gangestad, S. W., Garver-Apgar, C. E., Simpson, J. A., & Cousins, A. J. (2007). Changes in women's mate preferences across the ovulatory cycle. *Journal of Personality and Social Psychology, 92,* 151–163. https://doi.org/10.1037/0022-3514.92.1.151

Garcia, R. L., Kenny, D. A., & Ledermann, T. (2015). Moderation in the actor–partner interdependence model. *Personal Relationships, 22,* 8–29. https://doi.org/10.1111/pere.12060

Garnett, B. R., Masyn, K. E., Austin, S. B., Miller, M., Williams, D. R., & Viswanath, K. (2014). The intersectionality of discrimination attributes and bullying among youth: An applied latent class analysis. *Journal of Youth and Adolescence, 43,* 1225–1239. https://doi.org/10.1007/s10964-013-0073-8

Gawande, A. (2014). *Being mortal: Medicine and what matters in the end.* New York, NY: Metropolitan Books, Henry Holt and Company.

(January 23, 2017). The heroism of incremental care. *The New Yorker.*

Geist-Martin, P., Ray, E. B., & Sharf, B. F. (2003). *Communicating health: Personal, cultural and political complexities.* Belmont, CA: Wadsworth Publishing Co.

Giles, H., Coupland, N., & Coupland, J. (Eds.). (1991). *Context of accommodation: Development of applied linguistics.* Cambridge, England: Cambridge University Press.

Giles, H., Reid, S. A., & Harwood, J. (Eds.). (2010). *The dynamics of intergroup communication.* New York, NY: Peter Lang.

Glymour, M. M., Weuve, J., Fay, M. E., Glass, T., & Berkman, L. F. (2008). Social ties and cognitive recovery after stroke: Does social integration promote cognitive resilience? *Neuroepidemiology, 31,* 10–20. https://doi.org/10.1159/000136646

Goldsmith, D. J. (2004). *Communicating social support.* New York, NY: Cambridge University Press. https://doi.org/10.1017/CBO9780511606984

Gorman, B. K. & Sivaganesan, A. (2007). The role of social support and integration for understanding socioeconomic disparities in self-rated health and hypertension. *Social Science & Medicine, 65,* 958–975. https://doi.org/10.1016/j.socscimed.2007.04.017

Gouin, J., Carter, S., Pournajafi-Nazarloo, H., Glaser, R., Malarkey, W., Loving, T., . . . Kiecolt-Glaser, J. (2010). Marital behavior, oxytocin, and wound healing. *Brain Behavior and Immunity, 24,* S8–S8. https://doi.org/10.1016/j.bbi.2010.07.026

Granger, D. A., Kivlighan, K. T., Blair, C., El-Sheikh, M., Mize, J., Lisonbee, J. A., . . . Schwartz, E. B. (2006). Integrating the measurement of salivary α-amylase into studies of child health, development, and social relationships. *Journal of Social and Personal Relationships, 23,* 267–290. https://doi.org/10.1177/0265407506062479

Green, L. R., Richardson, D. S., Lago, T., & Schatten-Jones, E. C. (2001). Network correlates of social and emotional loneliness in young and older adults. *Personality and Social Psychology Bulletin, 27*(3), 281–288. https://doi.org/10.1177/0146167201273002

Greene, K. (2009). An integrated model of health disclosure decision-making. In T. D. Afifi & W. A. Afifi (Eds.), *Uncertainty, information management, and disclosure decisions: Theories and applications* (pp. 226–253). New York, NY: Routledge.

Greenhalgh, T. (2016). *Cultural contexts of health: The use of narrative research in the health sector.* (No. 49). Copenhagen, Denmark: World Health Organization Regional Office for Europe.

Guerrero, L. K. & Andersen, P. A. (1994). Patterns of matching and initiation: Touch behavior and touch avoidance across romantic relationship stages. *Journal of Nonverbal Behavior, 18,* 137–153. https://doi.org/10.1007/bf02170075

Guiaux, M., van Tilburg, T., & van Groenou, M. B. (2007). Changes in contact and support exchange in personal networks after widowhood. *Personal Relationships, 14,* 457–473. https://doi.org/10.1111/j.1475–6811.2007.00165.x

Ha, J. (2008). Changes in support from confidants, children, and friends following widowhood. *Journal of Marriage and Family, 70,* 306–318. https://doi.org/10.1111/j.1741-3737.2008.00483.x

Haider, A. H., Sriram, N., & Cooper, L. (2011). Unconscious race and social class bias in medical students – reply. *Journal of the American Medical Association, 306,* 2454–2455. https://doi.org/10.1001/jama.2011.1771

Harvey, J. H. (1995). *Odyssey of the heart: The search for closeness, intimacy, and love.* New York, NY: Freeman.

Harvey, J. H. & Pauwels, B. G. (1999). Recent development in close-relationships theory. *Current Directions in Psychological Science, 8,* 93–95. https://doi.org/10.1111/1467–8721.00022

Hawkley, L. C. & Cacioppo, J. T. (2010). Loneliness matters: A theoretical and empirical review of consequences and mechanisms. *Annals of Behavioral Medicine, 40,* 218–227. https://doi.org/10.1007/s12160-010-9210-8

Hawkley, L. C., Thisted, R. A., Masi, C. M., & Cacioppo, J. T. (2010). Loneliness predicts increased blood pressure: 5-year cross-lagged analyses in middle-aged and older adults. *Psychology and Aging, 25,* 132–141. https://doi.org/10.1037/a0017805

Hazan, C. & Shaver, P. (1987). Romantic love conceptualized as an attachment process. *Journal of Personality and Social Psychology, 52,* 511–524. https://doi.org/10.1037/0022–3514.52.3.511

Heath, I. (2013). Complexity, uncertainty, and mess as the links between science and the humanities in health care. In J. P. Sturmberg & C. M. Martin (Eds.), *Handbook of systems and complexity in health* (pp. 19–24).

Helft, P. R. & Petronio, S. (2007). Communication pitfalls with cancer patients: "Hit-and-run" deliveries of bad news. *Journal of the American College of Surgeons, 205,* 807–811. https://doi.org/10.1016/j.jamcollsurg.2007.07.022

Helgeson, V. S., Novak, S. A., Lepore, S. J., & Eton, D. T. (2004). Spouse social control efforts: Relations to health behavior and well-being among men with prostate cancer. *Journal of Social and Personal Relationships, 21,* 53–68. https://doi.org/10.1177/0265407504039840

Hendrick, S. S. & Hendrick, C. (2006). Measuring respect in close relationships. *Journal of Social and Personal Relationships, 23,* 881–899. https://doi.org/10.1177/0265407506070471

Hesse, C. & Floyd, K. (2008). Affectionate experience mediates the effects of alexithymia on mental health and interpersonal relationships. *Journal of Social and Personal Relationships, 25,* 793–810. https://doi.org/10.1177/0265407508096696

Hinde, R. A. (1979). *Towards understanding relationships.* London, England: Academic Press.

Hobfoll, S. E. & Schröder, K. E. E. (2001). Distinguishing between passive and active prosocial coping: Bridging inner-city women's mental health and AIDS risk behavior. *Journal of Social and Personal Relationships, 18,* 201–217. https://doi.org/10.1177/0265407501182003

Holmes, J. G. (2002). Interpersonal expectations as the building blocks of social cognition: An interdependence theory perspective. *Personal Relationships, 9,* 1–26. https://doi.org/10.1111/1475–6811.00001

(2004). The benefits of abstract functional analysis in theory construction: The case of interdependence theory. *Personality and Social Psychology Review, 8*, 146–155. https://doi.org/10.1207/s15327957pspr0802_8

Holmes, J. G. & Rempel, J. K. (1989). Trust in close relationships. In C. Hendrick (Ed.), *Close relationships: Review of personality and social psychology* (pp. 187–220). Thousand Oaks, CA: Sage Publications.

Holt-Lunstad, J., Birmingham, W. C., & Light, K. C. (2015). Relationship quality and oxytocin: Influence of stable and modifiable aspects of relationships. *Journal of Social and Personal Relationships, 32*, 472–490. https://doi.org/10.1177/0265407514536294

Holt-Lunstad, J., Smith, T. B., & Layton, J. B. (2010). Social relationships and mortality risk: A meta-analytic review. *PLOS Medicine, 7*(7), e1000316. https://doi.org/10.1371/journal.pmed.1000316

Holt-Lunstad, J., & Uchino, B. N. (2015). Social support and health. In K. Glanz, B. K. Rimer, & K. Viswanath (Eds.), *Health behavior: Theory, research and practice* (5th ed., pp. 183–204). San Francisco, CA: Jossey-Bass.

Holt-Lunstad, J., Uchino, B. N., Smith, T. W., & Hicks, A. (2007). On the importance of relationship quality: The impact of ambivalence in friendships on cardiovascular functioning. *Annals of Behavioral Medicine, 33*, 278–290. https://doi.org/10.1007/BF02879910

Holt-Lunstad, J., Uchino, B. N., Smith, T. W., Olson-Cerny, C., & Nealey-Moore, J. B. (2003). Social relationships and ambulatory blood pressure: Structural and qualitative predictors of cardiovascular function during everyday social interactions. *Health Psychology, 22*, 388–397. https://doi.org/10.1037/0278-6133.22.4.388

House, J. S., Landis, K. R., & Umberson, D. (1988). Social relationships and health. *Science, 241*(4865), 540–545. https://doi.org/10.1126/science.3399889

Huber, M. (2011). Health: How should we define it? *British Medical Journal, 343* (7817), 235–237. https://doi.org/10.1136/bmj.d4163

Iezzoni, L. I. (2006). Make no assumptions: Communication between persons with disabilities and clinicians. *Assistive Technology, 18*, 212–219. https://doi.org/10.1080/10400435.2006.10131920

Impett, E. A., Kogan, A., English, T., John, O., Oveis, C., Gordon, A. M., & Keltner, D. (2012). Suppression sours sacrifice: Emotional and relational costs of suppressing emotions in romantic relationships. *Personality and Social Psychology Bulletin, 38*, 707–720. https://doi.org/1177/0146167212437249

Independent Living Institute. (2005). Independent living empowers people with disabilities. Retrieved March 1, 2017 from www.independentliving.org/docs7/ratzka200507.html

Institute of Medicine. (2001). *Crossing the quality chasm: A new health system for the 21st century*. Washington, DC: National Academy Press.

(2003). *Unequal treatment: Confronting racial and ethnic disparities in health care*. Washington, DC: The National Academies Press.

Jin, S. A. (2012). "To disclose or not to disclose, that is the question": A structural equation modeling approach to communication privacy management in e-health. *Computers in Human Behavior, 28*, 69–77. https://doi.org/10.1016/j.chb.2011.08.012

Kalmijn, M. (2003). Shared friendship networks and the life course: An analysis of survey data on married and cohabiting couples. *Social Networks, 25*, 231–249. https://doi.org/10.1016/S0378–8733(03)00010–8

Kaplan, R. M. (2009). Health psychology: Where are we and where do we go from here? *Mens Sana Monograph, 7*, 3–9. https://doi.org/10.4103/0973–1229.43584

Kellas, J. K., Trees, A. R., Schrodt, P., LeClair-Underberg, C., & Willer, E. K. (2010). Exploring links between well-being and interactional sense-making in married couples' jointly told stories of stress. *Journal of Family Communication, 10*, 174–193. https://doi.org/10.1080/15267431.2010.489217

Kelley, H. H. (1979). *Personal relationships: Their structures and processes*. Hillsdale, NJ: Erlbaum.

(1983). Love and commitment. In H. H. Kelley, E. Berscheid, A. Christensen, J. H. Harvey, T. L. Huston, G. Levinger, … D. R. Peterson (Eds.), *Close relationships* (pp. 265–314). New York, NY: W. H. Freeman.

Kelley, H. H., Berscheid, E., Christensen, A., Harvey, J. H., Huston, T. L., Levinger, G., … Peterson, D. R. (1983a). *Close relationships*. New York, NY: W. H. Freeman.

(1983b). *Close relationships*. New York, NY: Freeman.

Kelley, H. H., Holmes, J. G., Kerr, N. L., Reis, H. T., Rusbult, C. E., & Van Lange, P. A. M. (2003). *An atlas of interpersonal situations*. New York, NY: Cambridge University Press. https://doi.org/10.1017/CBO9780511499845

Kelley, H. H., & Thibaut, J. W. (1978). *Interpersonal relations: A theory of interdependence*. New York, NY: Wiley-Interscience.

Kenny, D. A., & Kashy, D. A. (2011). Dyadic data analysis using multilevel modeling. In J. J. Hox & J. K. Roberts (Eds.), *Handbook for advanced multilevel analysis* (pp. 335–370). New York, NY: Routledge.

Kiecolt-Glaser, J. K., Loving, T. J., Stowell, J. R., Malarkey, W. B., Lemeshow, S., Dickinson, S. L., & Glaser, R. (2005). Hostile marital interactions, proinflammatory cytokine production, and wound healing. *Archives of General Psychiatry, 62*, 1377–1384. https://doi.org/10.1001/archpsyc.62.12.1377

Kilov, A. M., Togher, L., & Grant, S. (2009). Problem solving with friends: Discourse participation and performance of individuals with and without traumatic brain injury. *Aphasiology*, 23, 584–605. https://doi.org/10.1080/02687030701855382

Kivowitz, B. & Weisman, R. (2013). *In sickness as in health: Helping couples cope with the complexities of illness*. Petaluma, CA: Roundtree Press.

Klein, R. (2004). Sickening relationships: Gender-based violence, women's health, and the role of informal third parties. *Journal of Social and Personal Relationships*, 21, 149–165. https://doi.org/10.1177/0265407504039842

Kluwer, E. S. & Karremans, J. (2009). Unforgiving motivations following infidelity: Should we make peace with our past? *Journal of Social and Clinical Psychology*, 28, 1298–1325. https://doi.org/10.1521/jscp.2009.28.10.1298

Knee, C. R., Canevello, A., Bush, A. L., & Cook, A. (2008). Relationship-contingent self-esteem and the ups and downs of romantic relationships. *Journal of Personality and Social Psychology*, 95, 608–627. https://doi.org/10.1037/0022-3514.95.3.608

Knobloch, L. K. (2007). Perceptions of turmoil within courtship: Associations with intimacy, relational uncertainty, and interference from partners. *Journal of Social and Personal Relationships*, 24, 363–384. https://doi.org/10.1177/0265407507077227

Knobloch, L. K. & Delaney, A. L. (2012). Themes of relational uncertainty and interference from partners in depression. *Health Communication*, 27, 750–765. https://doi.org/10.1080/10410236.2011.639293

Knobloch, L. K. & Knobloch-Fedders, L. M. (2010). The role of relational uncertainty in depressive symptoms and relationship quality: An actor – partner interdependence model. *Journal of Social and Personal Relationships*, 27, 137–159. https://doi.org/10.1177/0265407509348809

Knobloch, L. K., Miller, L. E., & Carpenter, K. E. (2007). Using the relational turbulence model to understand negative emotion within courtship. *Personal Relationships*, 14, 91–112. https://doi.org/10.1111/j.1475-6811.2006.00143.x

Knobloch, L. K. & Solomon, D. H. (1999). Measuring the sources and content of relational uncertainty. *Communication Studies*, 50, 261–278. https://doi.org/10.1080/10510979909388499

(2004). Interference and facilitation from partners in the development of interdependence within romantic relationships. *Personal Relationships*, 11, 115–130. https://doi.org/10.1111/j.1475-6811.2004.00074.x

Krause, N. & Shaw, B. A. (2002). Negative interaction and changes in functional disability during late life. *Journal of Social and Personal Relationships*, 19, 339–359. https://doi.org/10.1177/0265407502193003

Kutob, R. M., Yuan, N. P., Wertheim, B. C., Sbarra, D. A., Loucks, E. B., Nassir, R., ... Thomson, C. A. (2017). Relationship between marital transitions, health behaviors, and health indicators of postmenopausal women: Results from the women's health initiative. *Journal of Women's Health, 26,* 313–320. https://doi.org/10.1089/jwh.2016.5925

Lakey, B., Cooper, C., Cronin, A., & Whitaker, T. (2014). Symbolic providers help people regulate affect relationally: Implications for perceived support. *Personal Relationships, 21,* 404–419. https://doi.org/10.1111/pere.12038

Lakey, B. & Orehek, E. (2011). Relational regulation theory: A new approach to explain the link between perceived social support and mental health. *Psychological Review, 118,* 482–495. https://doi.org/10.1037/a0023477

Lang, F., Floyd, M. R., & Beine, K. L. (2000). Clues to patients' explanations and concerns about their illnesses. A call for active listening. *Archives of Family Medicine, 9,* 222–227. https://doi.org/10.1001/archfami.9.3.222

Lawler-Row, K. A., Hyatt-Edwards, L., Wuensch, K. L., & Karremans, J. C. (2011). Forgiveness and health: The role of attachment. *Personal Relationships, 18,* 170–183. https://doi.org/10.1111/j.1475–6811.2010.01327.x

Lazarus, R. S. & Folkman, S. (1984). *Stress, appraisal, and coping.* New York, NY: Springer.

Le, B. M. & Impett, E. A. (2013). When holding back helps: Suppressing negative emotions during sacrifice feels authentic and is beneficial for highly interdependent people. *Psychological Science, 24,* 1809–1815. https://doi.org/10.1177/0956797613475365

Lehmiller, J. J. (2012). Perceived marginalization and its association with physical and psychological health. *Journal of Social and Personal Relationships, 29,* 451–469. https://doi.org/10.1177/0265407511431187

Lehmiller, J. J. & Agnew, C. R. (2007). Perceived marginalization and the prediction of romantic relationship stability. *Journal of Marriage and Family, 69,* 1036–1049. https://doi.org/10.1111/j.1741–3737.2007.00429.x

Lemay, E. P., Jr. & Clark, M. S. (2008). "Walking on eggshells": How expressing relationship insecurities perpetuates them. *Journal of Personality and Social Psychology, 95,* 420–441. https://doi.org/10.1037/0022–3514.95.2.420

Leslie, M. B., Stein, J. A., & Rotheram-Borus, M. J. (2002). The impact of coping strategies, personal relationships, and emotional distress on health-related outcomes of parents living with HIV or AIDS. *Journal of Social and Personal Relationships, 19,* 45–66. https://doi.org/10.1177/0265407502191003

Lewis, M. A. & Butterfield, R. M. (2005). Antecedents and reactions to health-related social control. *Personality and Social Psychology Bulletin, 31,* 416–427. https://doi.org/10.1177/0146167204271600

Lewis, M. A., Butterfield, R. M., Darbes, L. A., & Johnston-Brooks, C. (2004). The conceptualization and assessment of health-related social control. *Journal of Social and Personal Relationships, 21*, 669–687. https://doi.org/10.1177/0265407504045893

Lewis, M. A., McBride, C. M., Pollak, K. I., Puleo, E., Butterfield, R. M., & Emmons, K. M. (2006). Understanding health behavior change among couples: An interdependence and communal coping approach. *Social Science & Medicine, 62*, 1369–1380. https://doi.org/10.1016/j.socscimed.2005.08.006

Lind, C., Hickson, L., & Erber, N. P. (2006). Conversation repair and adult cochlear implantation: A qualitative case study. *Cochlear Implants International, 7*, 33–48. https://doi.org/10.1179/cim.2006.7.1.33

Loving, T. J. & Campbell, L. (2011). Mind–body connections in personal relationships: What close relationships researchers have to offer. *Personal Relationships, 18*, 165–169. https://doi.org/10.1111/j.1475–6811.2011.01361.x

Loving, T. J., Crockett, E. E., & Paxson, A. A. (2009). Passionate love and relationship thinkers: Experimental evidence for acute cortisol elevations in women. *Psychoneuroendocrinology, 34*, 939–946. https://doi.org/10.1016/j.psyneuen.2009.01.010

Loving, T. J. & Sbarra, D. A. (2015). Relationships and health. In M. Mikulincer, P. R. Shaver, J. A. Simpson, & J. F. Dovidio (Eds.), *APA handbook of personality and social psychology, volume 3: Interpersonal relations* (pp. 151–176). Washington, DC: American Psychological Association. https://doi.org/10.1037/14344–006

Luecken, L. J., Roubinov, D. S., & Tanaka, R. (2013). Childhood family environment, social competence, and health across the lifespan. *Journal of Social and Personal Relationships, 30*, 171–178. https://doi.org/10.1177/0265407512454272

Luescher, K. & Pillemer, K. (1998). Intergenerational ambivalence: A new approach to the study of parent–child relations in later life. *Journal of Marriage and the Family, 60*, 413–425. https://doi.org/10.2307/353858

Mack, J. W., Paulk, E., Viswanath, K., & Prigerson, H. G. (2010). Racial disparities in the effects of communication on medical care received near death. *Archives of Internal Medicine, 170*, 1533–1540. https://doi.org/10.1001/archinternmed.2010.322

Mackinnon, S. P., Sherry, S. B., Antony, M. M., Stewart, S. H., Sherry, D. L., & Hartling, N. (2012). Caught in a bad romance: Perfectionism, conflict, and depression in romantic relationships. *Journal of Family Psychology, 26*, 215–225. https://doi.org/10.1037/a0027402

Mann, K., Gordon, J., & MacLeod, A. (2009). Reflection and reflective practice in health professions education: A systematic review. *Advances in Health Sciences Education, 14*, 595–621. https://doi.org/10.1007/s10459-007-9090-2

Manning, J. (2014). A constitutive approach to interpersonal communication studies. *Communication Studies, 65*, 432–440. https://doi.org/10.1080/10510 974.2014.927294

Manning, J. & Kunkel, A. (2014). Making meaning of meaning-making research: Using qualitative research for studies of social and personal relationships. *Journal of Social and Personal Relationships, 31*, 433–441. https://doi.org/10 .1177/0265407514525890

Marks, N. F. & Song, J. (2009). Compassionate motivation and compassionate acts across the adult life course: Evidence from US national studies. In B. Fehr, S. Sprecher, & L. G. Underwood (Eds.), *The science of compassionate love: Theory, research, and applications* (pp. 121–158). Oxford, England: Wiley-Blackwell. http://dx.doi.org.proxy.bc.edu/10.1002/9781444303070.ch5

Martire, L. M. (2013). Couple-oriented interventions for chronic illness: Where do we go from here? *Journal of Social and Personal Relationships, 30*, 207–214. https://doi.org/10.1177/0265407512453786

McLaren, R. M., Solomon, D. H., & Priem, J. S. (2011). Explaining variation in contemporaneous responses to hurt in premarital romantic relationships: A relational turbulence model perspective. *Communication Research, 38*, 543–564. https://doi.org/10.1177/0093650210377896

Merleau-Ponty, M. (1964). In Edie J. (Ed.), *The primacy of perception* (W. Cobb Trans.). Evanston, IL: Northwestern University Press.

Mikulincer, M. (1998). Attachment working models and the sense of trust: An exploration of interaction goals and affect regulation. *Journal of Personality and Social Psychology, 74*, 1209–1224. https://doi.org/10.1037/ 0022-3514.74.5.1209

Mikulincer, M. & Shaver, P. R. (2007). Reflections on security dynamics: Core constructs, psychological mechanisms, relational contexts, and the need for an integrative theory. *Psychological Inquiry, 18*, 197–209. https://doi.org/10 .1080/10478400701512893

Mikulincer, M., Shaver, P. R., Bar-On, N., & Ein-Dor, T. (2010). The pushes and pulls of close relationships: Attachment insecurities and relational ambivalence. *Journal of Personality and Social Psychology, 98*, 450–468. https ://doi.org/10.1037/a0017366

Milardo, R. M. (1987). Changes in social networks of women and men following divorce. *Journal of Family Issues, 8*, 78–96. https://doi.org/10.1177 /019251387008001004

Miller, D. T. (2001). Disrespect and the experience of injustice. *Annual Review of Psychology, 52,* 527–553. https://doi.org/10.1146/annurev.psych.52.1.527

Miller, L. E. & Caughlin, J. P. (2013). "We're going to be survivors": Couples' identity challenges during and after cancer treatment. *Communication Monographs, 80*(1), 63–82. https://doi.org/10.1080/03637751.2012.739703

Miller-Day, M. & Dodd, A. H. (2004). Toward a descriptive model of parent–offspring communication about alcohol and other drugs. *Journal of Social and Personal Relationships, 21,* 69–91. https://doi.org/10.1177/0265407504039846

Mokros, H. & Deetz, S. (1996). What counts as real? A constitutive view of communication and the disenfranchised in the context of health. In E. B. Ray (Ed.), *Communication and disenfranchisement: Social health issues and implications* (pp. 29–44). Mahwah, NJ: Lawrence Erlbaum.

Muraco, A. & Fredriksen-Goldsen, K. (2011). "That's what friends do": Informal caregiving for chronically ill midlife and older lesbian, gay, and bisexual adults. *Journal of Social and Personal Relationships, 28,* 1073–1092. https://doi.org/10.1177/0265407511402419

Murray, S. L. & Holmes, J. G. (2009). The architecture of interdependent minds: A motivation-management theory of mutual responsiveness. *Psychological Review, 116,* 908–928. https://doi.org/10.1037/a0017015

Murray, S. L., Holmes, J. G., & Collins, N. L. (2006). Optimizing assurance: The risk regulation system in relationships. *Psychological Bulletin, 132,* 641–666. https://doi.org/10.1037/0033–2909.132.5.641

Murray, S. L., Holmes, J. G., & Griffin, D. W. (2000). Self-esteem and the quest for felt security: How perceived regard regulates attachment processes. *Journal of Personality and Social Psychology, 78,* 478–498. https://doi.org/10.1037/0022–3514.78.3.478

Napier, A. D., Ancarno, C., Butler, B., Calabrese, J., Chater, A., Chatterjee, H., ... Woolf, K. (2014). Culture and health. *The Lancet, 384*(9954), 1607–1639. https://doi.org/10.1016/S0140–6736(14)61603–2

National Center for Health Statistics. (2015). *Summary health statistics tables for the U.S. population: National health interview survey, 2015, table P-1c.* Hyattsville, MD: US Government Printing Office.

National Coalition for Cancer Survivorship. (2018). Cancer policy matters: A resource for cancer policy analysis and commentary. Retrieved from www.canceradvocacy.org

Neff, L. A. & Karney, B. R. (2009). Compassionate love in early marriage. In B. Fehr, S. Sprecher, & L. G. Underwood (Eds.), *The science of compassionate love:*

Theory, research, and applications (pp. 201–221). Oxford, England: Wiley-Blackwell. http://dx.doi.org.proxy.bc.edu/10.1002/9781444303070.ch7

Newsom, J. T., Nishishiba, M., Morgan, D. L., & Rook, K. S. (2003). The relative importance of three domains of positive and negative social exchanges: A longitudinal model with comparable measures. *Psychology and Aging, 18,* 746–754. https://doi.org/10.1037/0882–7974.18.4.746

Newsom, J. T., Rook, K. S., Nishishiba, M., Sorkin, D. H., & Mahan, T. L. (2005). Understanding the relative importance of positive and negative social exchanges: Examining specific domains and appraisals. *The Journals of Gerontology: Psychological Sciences, 60B,* P304–P312. https://doi.org/10 .1093/geronb/60.6.P304

Ngula, K. W. & Miller, A. N. (2010). Self-disclosure of HIV seropositivity in Kenya by HIV-positive Kamba men and their families. *Southern Communication Journal, 75,* 328–348. https://doi.org/10.1080/1041794x.2010.504443

Novak, S. A. & Webster, G. D. (2011). Spousal social control during a weight loss attempt: A daily diary study. *Personal Relationships, 18,* 224–241. https://doi .org/10.1111/j.1475–6811.2011.01358.x

Nunez-Smith, M., Ciarleglio, M., Sandoval-Minero, T., Elumn, J., Castillo-Page, L., Peduzzi, P., & Bradley, E. (2012). Medical school faculty promotion in the United States: Is there institutional variation by race/ethnicity? *American Journal of Public Health, 102,* 852–858. https://doi.org/10.2105/AJPH.2011 .300552

O'Connor, A. (February 14, 2018). Using art to tackle diabetes in youth. *The New York Times.*

Orbuch, T. L. & Eyster, S. L. (1997). Division of household labor among black couples and white couples. *Social Forces, 76,* 301–332. https://doi.org/10 .2307/2580327

Orbuch, T. L., Veroff, J., Hassan, H., & Horrocks, J. (2002). Who will divorce: A 14-year longitudinal study of black couples and white couples. *Journal of Social and Personal Relationships, 19*(2), 179–202. https://doi.org/10.1177 /0265407502192002

O'Rourke, M. (August 26, 2013). What's wrong with me? I had an autoimmune disease. Then the disease had me. *The New Yorker.*

Orth-Gomér, K. (2009). Are social relations less health protective in women than in men? Social relations, gender, and cardiovascular health. *Journal of Social and Personal Relationships, 26,* 63–71. https://doi.org/10.1177/0265407509105522

Ott, C. H., Sanders, S., & Kelber, S. T. (2007). Grief and personal growth experience of spouses and adult-child caregivers of individuals with Alzheimer's disease

and related dementias. *The Gerontologist, 47*, 798–809. https://doi.org/10
.1093/geront/47.6.798

Ottenstein, S. (2015). The mind-body connection on love. Retrieved April 1, 2018
from www.dreame.me/diaries/the-mind-body-connection-in-love/

Overall, N. C. & Fletcher, G. J. O. (2010). Perceiving regulation from intimate
partners: Reflected appraisal and self-regulation processes in close
relationships. *Personal Relationships, 17*, 433–456. https://doi.org/10.1111/j
.1475–6811.2010.01286.x

Park, C. L., Zlateva, I., & Blank, T. O. (2009). Self-identity after cancer: "Survivor,"
"victim," "patient," and "person with cancer." *Journal of General Internal
Medicine, 24*, S430–S435. https://doi.org/10.1007/s11606-009-0993-x

Parrott, R. L., Silk, K. J., & Condit, C. (2003). Diversity in lay perceptions of the
sources of human traits: Genes, environments, and personal behaviors. *Social
Science & Medicine, 56*, 1099–1109. https://doi.org/10.1016/S0277–9536(02)
00106–5

Paulsen, S. L. & Lanius, U. F. (2014). Introduction: The ubiquity of dissociation.
In U. F. Lanius, S. L. Paulsen, & F. M. Corrigan (Eds.), *Neurobiology and
treatment of traumatic dissociation: Toward an embodied self* (pp. xix–
xxvi). New York, NY: Springer Publishing Company.

Penner, L. A., Albrecht, T. L., Orom, H., Coleman, D. K., & Underwood III, W.
(2010). Health and health care disparities. In J. F. Dovidio, M. Hewstone,
P. Glick, & V. M. Esses (Eds.), *The SAGE handbook of prejudice,
stereotyping and discrimination* (pp. 472–490). London, UK: SAGE
Publications Ltd. https://doi.org/10.4135/9781446200919.n29

Penner, L. A., Hagiwara, N., Eggly, S., Gaertner, S. L., Albrecht, T. L., &
Dovidio, J. F. (2013). Racial healthcare disparities: A social psychological
analysis. *European Review of Social Psychology, 24*, 70–122. https://doi.org/10
.1080/10463283.2013.840973

Penninx, B. W. J. H., van Tilburg, T., Kriegsman, D. M. W., Boeke, A. J. P.,
Deeg, D. J. H., & van Eijk, J. T. M. (1999). Social network, social support, and
loneliness in older persons with different chronic diseases. *Journal of Aging
and Health, 11*(2), 151–168. https://doi.org/10.1177/089826439901100202

Perissinotto, C. M., Stijacic, C. I., & Covinsky, K. E. (2012). Loneliness in older
persons: A predictor of functional decline and death. *Archives of Internal
Medicine, 172*, 1078–1083. https://doi.org/10.1001/archinternmed.2012.1993

Perlman, D., & Sanchez-Aragon, R. (2008). Compassionate love: Concluding
reflections. In B. Fehr, S. Sprecher, & L. G. Underwood (Eds.), *The science of
compassionate love: Theory, research, and applications* (pp. 433–452).
New York, NY: Wiley-Blackwell.

Perry, B. L. (2014). Symptoms, stigma, or secondary social disruption: Three mechanisms of network dynamics in severe mental illness. *Journal of Social and Personal Relationships, 31*, 32–53. https://doi.org/10.1177/0265407513484632

Peterson, L. T., Orbuch, T. L., & Brown, E. (2014). Perceived admiration and transition to parenthood for black and white married couples. *Journal of Family Social Work, 17*, 301–323. https://doi.org/10.1080/10522158.2014.928659

Petronio, S. (2002). *Boundaries of privacy: Dialectics of disclosure.* Albany, NY: State University of New York.

(2004). Road to developing communication privacy management theory: Narrative in progress, please stand by. *Journal of Family Communication, 4*, 193–207. https://doi.org/10.1080/15267431.2004.9670131

(2006). Impact of medical mistakes: Navigating work-family boundaries for physicians and their families. *Communication Monographs, 73*, 462–467. https://doi.org/10.1080/03637750601061174

(2007). Translational research endeavors and the practices of communication privacy management. *Journal of Applied Communication Research, 35*, 218–222. https://doi.org/10.1080/00909880701422443

(2010). Communication privacy management theory: What do we know about family privacy regulation? *Journal of Family Theory & Review, 2*, 175–196. https://doi.org/10.1111/j.1756–2589.2010.00052.x

(2013). Brief status report on communication privacy management theory. *Journal of Family Communication, 13*, 6–14. https://doi.org/10.1080/1526743 1.2013.743426

Petronio, S., DiCorcia, M. J., & Duggan, A. (2012). Navigating ethics of physician-patient confidentiality: A communication privacy management analysis. *The Permanente Journal, 16*(4), 41–45. https://doi.org/10.7812/TPP/12–042

Petronio, S. & Reierson, J. (2009). Regulating the privacy of confidentiality: Grasping the complexities through communication privacy management theory. In T. D. Afifi & W. A. Afifi (Eds.), *Uncertainty, information management, and disclosure decisions: Theories and applications* (pp. 365–383). New York, NY: Routledge.

Petronio, S. & Sargent, J. (2011). Disclosure predicaments arising during the course of patient care: Nurses' privacy management. *Health Communication, 26*, 255–266. https://doi.org/10.1080/10410236.2010.549812

Petronio, S., Sargent, J., Andea, L., Reganis, P., & Cichocki, D. (2004). Family and friends as healthcare advocates: Dilemmas of confidentiality and privacy.

Journal of Social and Personal Relationships, 21, 33–52. https://doi.org/10 .1177/0265407504039838

Petronio, S., Torke, A., Bosslet, G., Isenberg, S., Wocial, L., & Helft, P. R. (2013). Disclosing medical mistakes: A communication management plan for physicians. *The Permanente Journal, 17*(2), 73–79. https://doi.org/10.7812/TP P/12–106

Pinquart, M. & Duberstein, P. R. (2010). Associations of social networks with cancer mortality: A meta-analysis. *Critical Reviews in Oncology Hematology, 75*, 122–137. https://doi.org/10.1016/j.critrevonc.2009.06.003

Planalp, S. & Fitness, J. (1999). Thinking/feeling about social and personal relationships. *Journal of Social and Personal Relationships, 16*, 731–750. https://doi.org/10.1177/0265407599166004

Planalp, S., & Rosenberg, J. (2014). Emotion in interpersonal communication. In C. R. Berger (Ed.), *Interpersonal communication* (pp. 273–296). Berlin, Germany: De Gruyter Mouton.

Power, R., McManus, V., & Fourie, R. (2009). Hardship, dedication and investment: An exploration of Irish mothers commitment to communicating with their children with cerebral palsy. *Journal of Psychiatric and Mental Health Nursing, 16*, 531–538. https://doi.org/10.1111/j.1365–2850.2009.01410.x

Prager, K. J. (1995). *The psychology of intimacy.* New York, NY: Guilford Press. (2014). *The dilemmas of intimacy: Conceptualization, assessment, and treatment.* New York, NY: Routledge.

Quarmby, K. (March 11, 2015). Disabled and fighting for a sex life. *The Atlantic.*

Rauer, A. J., Sabey, A., & Jensen, J. F. (2014). Growing old together: Compassionate love and health in older adulthood. *Journal of Social and Personal Relationships, 31*, 677–696. https://doi.org/10.1177/0265407513503596

Reblin, M., Uchino, B. N., & Smith, T. W. (2010). Provider and recipient factors that may moderate the effectiveness of received support: Examining the effects of relationship quality and expectations for support on behavioral and cardiovascular reactions. *Journal of Behavioral Medicine, 33*, 423–431. https:// doi.org/10.1007/s10865-010–9270–z

Reinhardt, J. P., Boerner, K., & Horowitz, A. (2006). Good to have but not to use: Differential impact of perceived and received support on well-being. *Journal of Social and Personal Relationships, 23*, 117–129. https://doi.org/10.1177 /0265407506060182

Reis, H. T. (2008). Reinvigorating the concept of situation in social psychology. *Personality and Social Psychology Review, 12*, 311–329. https://doi.org/10 .1177/1088868308321721

Reis, H. T. & Arriaga, X. B. (2015). Interdependence theory and related theories. In B. Gawronski & G. Bodenhausen (Eds.), *Theory and explanation in social psychology* (pp. 205–327). New York, NY: New York Guilford Press.

Reis, H. T., Clark, M. S., & Holmes, J. G. (2004). Perceived partner responsiveness as an organizing construct in the study of intimacy and closeness. In D. J. Mashek & A. P. Aron (Eds.), *Handbook of closeness and intimacy* (pp. 201–225). Mahwah, NJ, US: Lawrence Erlbaum Associates Publishers.

Reis, H. T., Collins, W. A., & Berscheid, E. (2000). The relationship context of human behavior and development. *Psychological Bulletin, 126,* 844–872. https://doi.org/10.1037/0033-2909.126.6.844

Reis, H. T. & Shaver, P. (1988). Intimacy as an interpersonal process. In S. Duck, D. F. Hay, S. E. Hobfoll, W. Ickes, & B. M. Montgomery (Eds.), *Handbook of personal relationships: Theory, research and interventions* (pp. 367–389). Oxford, England: John Wiley & Sons.

Rempel, J. K., Holmes, J. G., & Zanna, M. P. (1985). Trust in close relationships. *Journal of Personality and Social Psychology, 49,* 95–112. https://doi.org/10.1037/0022-3514.49.1.95

Roberts, L. J., Wise, M., & DuBenske, L. L. (2009). Compassionate family caregiving in the light and shadow of death. In B. Fehr, S. Sprecher, & L. G. Underwood (Eds.), *The science of compassionate love: Theory, research, and applications* (pp. 311–344). Oxford, England: Wiley-Blackwell. https://doi.org/10.1002/9781444303070.ch11

Robles, T. F., Reynolds, B. M., Repetti, R. L., & Chung, P. J. (2013). Using daily diaries to study family settings, emotions, and health in everyday life. *Journal of Social and Personal Relationships, 30,* 179–188. https://doi.org/10.1177/0265407512457102

Rodriguez, L. M., Knee, C. R., & Neighbors, C. (2014). Relationships can drive some to drink: Relationship-contingent self-esteem and drinking problems. *Journal of Social and Personal Relationships, 31,* 270–290. https://doi.org/10.1177/0265407513494037

Rook, K. S., August, K. J., Stephens, M. A. P., & Franks, M. M. (2011). When does spousal social control provoke negative reactions in the context of chronic illness? The pivotal role of patients' expectations. *Journal of Social and Personal Relationships, 28,* 772–789. https://doi.org/10.1177/0265407510391335

Rusbult, C. E. (1983). A longitudinal test of the investment model: The development (and deterioration) of satisfaction and commitment in heterosexual involvements. *Journal of Personality and Social Psychology, 45,* 101–117. https://doi.org/10.1037//0022-3514.45.1.101

Rusbult, C. E., Agnew, C. R., & Arriaga, X. B. (2011). The investment model of commitment processes. In P. A. M. Van Lange, A. W. Kruglanski, & E. T. Higgins (Eds.), *Handbook of theories of social psychology* (pp. 218–231). London, England: SAGE Publications.

Rusbult, C. E. & Buunk, B. P. (1993). Commitment processes in close relationships: An interdependence analysis. *Journal of Social and Personal Relationships, 10,* 175–204. https://doi.org/10.1177/026540759301000202

Rusbult, C. E., Kumashiro, M., Coolsen, M. K., & Kirchner, J. L. (2004). Interdependence, closeness, and relationships. In D. J. Mashek & A. P. Aron (Eds.), *Handbook of closeness and intimacy* (pp. 137–161). Mahwah, NJ: Lawrence Erlbaum Associates Publishers.

Rusbult, C. E. & Van Lange, P. A. M. (2003). Interdependence, interaction and relationships. *Annual Review of Psychology, 54,* 351–375. https://doi.org/10.1146/annurev.psych.54.101601.145059

Saketkoo, L., Anderson, D., Rice, J., Rogan, A., & Lazarus, C. J. (2004). Effects of a disability awareness and skills training workshop on senior medical students as assessed with self ratings and performance on a standardized patient case. *Teaching and Learning in Medicine, 16,* 345–354. https://doi.org/10.1207/s15328015tlm1604_7

Sandars, J. (2009). The use of reflection in medical education: AMEE guide no. 44. *Medical Teacher, 31,* 685–695. https://doi.org/10.1080/01421590903050374

Sartorius, N. (2006). The meanings of health and its promotion. *Croatian Medical Journal, 47,* 662–664. Retrieved from www.ncbi.nlm.nih.gov/pmc/articles/PMC2080455/

Schillinger, D. & Huey, N. (2018). Messengers of truth and Health – Young artists of color raise their voices to prevent diabetes. *Journal of the American Medical Association,* https://doi.org/10.1001/jama.2018.0986

Schillinger, D., Ling, P. M., Fine, S., Boyer, C. B., Rogers, E., Vargas, R. A., . . . Chou, W. S. (2017). Reducing cancer and cancer disparities: Lessons from a youth-generated diabetes prevention campaign. *American Journal of Preventive Medicine, 53*(3, Suppl. 1), S103–S113. https://doi.org/10.1016/j.amepre.2017.05.024

Schneider, I. K., Konijn, E. A., Righetti, F., & Rusbult, C. E. (2011). A healthy dose of trust: The relationship between interpersonal trust and health. *Personal Relationships, 18,* 668–676. https://doi.org/10.1111/j.1475–6811.2010.01338.x

Schofield, P. E., Butow, P. N., Thompson, J. F., Tattersall, M. H. N., Beeney, L. J., & Dunn, S. M. (2003). Psychological responses of patients receiving a diagnosis of cancer. *Annals of Oncology, 14,* 48–56. https://doi.org/10.1093/annonc/mdg010

Schootman, M. & Jeffe, D. B. (2003). Identifying factors associated with disability-related differences in breast cancer screening. *Cancer Causes & Control, 14*, 97–107.

Schwarzer, R. & Leppin, A. (1991). Social support and health: A theoretical and empirical overview. *Journal of Social and Personal Relationships, 8*, 99–127. https://doi.org/10.1177/0265407591081005

Scott, J. G. (2013). Complexities of the consultation. In J. P. Sturmberg & C. M. Martin (Eds.), *Handbook of systems and complexity in health* (pp. 257–278).

Scully, J. L. (2013). Body alienation and the moral sense of self. *Narrative Inquiry in Bioethics, 3*, 26–28. https://doi.org/10.1353/nib.2013.0013

Segrin, C. (2000). Interpersonal relationships and mental health problems. In K. Dindia & S. Duck (Eds.), *Communication and personal relationships* (pp. 95–111). New York, NY: John Wiley & Sons Ltd.

Segrin, C., Burke, T. J., & Dunivan, M. (2012). Loneliness and poor health within families. *Journal of Social and Personal Relationships, 29*, 597–611. https://doi.org/10.1177/0265407512443434

Sharabi, L. L., Delaney, A. L., & Knobloch, L. K. (2016). In their own words: How clinical depression affects romantic relationships. *Journal of Social and Personal Relationships, 33*, 421–448. https://doi.org/10.1177/0265407515578820

Sharf, B. F., Harter, L. M., Yamasaki, J., & Haidet, P. (2011). Narrative turns epic: Continuing developments in health narrative scholarship. In J. Nussbaum, R. L. Parrott, & T. Thompson (Eds.), *Handbook of health communication* (2nd ed., pp. 36–51). New York, NY: Routledge.

Sharf, B. F. & Vanderford, M. L. (2003). Illness narratives and the social construction of health. In T. L. Thompson, A. M. Dorsey, K. I. Miller, & R. Parrott (Eds.), *Handbook of health communication* (pp. 9–34). Mahwah, NJ: Lawrence Erlbaum Associates Publishers.

Shaughnessy, A., Allen, L., & Duggan, A. (2017). Attention without intention: Explicit processing and implicit goal-setting in family medicine in residents' written reflections. *Education for Primary Care, 28*(3), 150–156. https://doi.org/10.1080/14739879.2016.1278562

Shaughnessy, A. F. & Duggan, A. P. (2013). Family medicine residents' reactions to introducing a reflective exercise into training. *Education for Health, 26*(3), 141–146. https://doi.org/10.4103/1357-6283.125987

Shavers, V. L., Fagan, P., Jones, D., Klein, W. M., Boyington, J., Moten, C., & Rorie, E. (2012). The state of research on racial/ethnic discrimination in the receipt of health care. *American Journal of Public Health, 102,* 953–966. https://doi.org/10.2105/AJPH.2012.300773

Shepler, S., Duggan, A., Kosberg, R., Rosenthal, R., Willets, N., Mattina, A., ... Meadows, M. (2013). Friendships and social support in coping with illness diagnosis: The story of Sherry and the Martha's Vineyard Communication Association. In S. Faulkner (Ed.), *Inside relationships: A creative casebook in relational communication* (pp. 123–133). Walnut Creek, CA: Left Coast Press.

Shilton, T., Sparks, M., McQueen, D., Lamarre, M., & Jackson, S. (2011). Proposal for new definition. *British Medical Journal, 343*(7821), 435. Retrieved from www.jstor.org/stable/23051978

Sillars, A. L. & Canary, D. J. (2013). Conflict and relational quality in families. In A. L. Vangelisti (Ed.), *The Routledge handbook of family communication* (2nd ed., pp. 338–357). New York, NY: Routledge.

Simpson, J. L. & Seibold, D. R. (2008). Practical engagements and co-created research. *Journal of Applied Communication Research, 36,* 266–280. https://doi.org/10.1080/00909880802172285

Slatcher, R. B. (2010). Marital functioning and physical health: Implications for social and personality psychology. *Social and Personality Psychology Compass, 4,* 455–469. https://doi.org/10.1111/j.1751-9004.2010.00273.x

Smith, R. A. (2007). Language of the lost: An explication of stigma communication. *Communication Theory, 17,* 462–485. https://doi.org/10.1111/j.1468-2885.2007.00307.x

(2011). Stigma communication and health. In T. L. Thompson, R. L. Parrott, & J. Nussbaum (Eds.), *Handbook of health communication* (2nd ed., pp. 455–468). New York, NY: Taylor & Francis.

Smith, T. W., Cribbet, M. R., Nealey-Moore, J. B., Uchino, B. N., Williams, P. G., MacKenzie, J., & Thayer, J. F. (2011). Matters of the variable heart: Respiratory sinus arrhythmia response to marital interaction and associations with marital quality. *Journal of Personality and Social Psychology, 100,* 103–119. https://doi.org/10.1037/a0021136

Solomon, D. H. (2016). Relational turbulence model. In C. R. Berger & M. E. Roloff (Eds.), *The international encyclopedia of interpersonal communication* (1st ed., pp. 1–9) https://doi-org.proxy.bc.edu/10.1002/9781118540190.wbeic174

Solomon, D. H. & Knobloch, L. K. (2001). Relationship uncertainty, partner interference, and intimacy within dating relationships. *Journal of Social and Personal Relationships, 18,* 804–820. https://doi.org/10.1177/0265407501186004

(2004). A model of relational turbulence: The role of intimacy, relational uncertainty, and interference from partners in appraisals of irritations.

Journal of Social and Personal Relationships, 21, 795–816. https://doi.org/10 .1177/0265407504047838

Solomon, D. H., Knobloch, L. K., Theiss, J. A., & McLaren, R. M. (2016). Relational turbulence theory: Explaining variation in subjective experiences and communication within romantic relationships. *Human Communication Research, 42,* 507–532. https://doi.org/10.1111/hcre.12091

Solomon, D. H. & Theiss, J. A. (2008). A longitudinal test of the relational turbulence model of romantic relationship development. *Personal Relationships, 15,* 339–357. https://doi.org/10.1111/j.1475–6811.2008.00202.x (2011). Relational turbulence: What doesn't kill us makes us stronger. In W. R. Cupach & B. H. Spitzberg (Eds.), *The dark side of close relationships II* (pp. 197–216). New York, NY: Routledge.

Solomon, D. H., Weber, K. M., & Steuber, K. R. (2010). *Turbulence in relational transitions.* Thousand Oaks, CA: Sage Publications. https://doi.org/10.4135/9 781483349619.n6

Spain, S. M., Jackson, J. J., & Edmonds, G. W. (2012). Extending the actor–partner interdependence model for binary outcomes: A multilevel logistic approach. *Personal Relationships, 19,* 431–444. https://doi.org/10.1111/j.1475–6811 .2011.01371.x

Spiegel, D. (2009). Coming apart: Trauma and the fragmentation of the self. In D. Gordon (Ed.), *Cerebrum 2009: Emerging ideas in brain science* (pp. 1–11). Washington, DC: Dana Press.

Sprecher, S. & Fehr, B. (2005). Compassionate love for close others and humanity. *Journal of Social and Personal Relationships, 22,* 629–651. https://doi.org/10 .1177/0265407505056439 (2006). Enhancement of mood and self-esteem as a result of giving and receiving compassionate love. *Current Research in Social Psychology, 11,* 227–242.

Steuber, K. R. & Solomon, D. H. (2008). Relational uncertainty, partner interference, and infertility: A qualitative study of discourse within online forums. *Journal of Social and Personal Relationships, 25,* 831–855. https://doi .org/10.1177/0265407508096698 (2011). Factors that predict married partners' disclosures about infertility to social network members. *Journal of Applied Communication Research, 39,* 250–270. https://doi.org/10.1080/00909882.2011.585401 (2012). Relational uncertainty, partner interference, and privacy boundary turbulence: Explaining spousal discrepancies in infertility disclosures. *Journal of Social and Personal Relationships, 29,* 3–27. https://doi.org/10 .1177/0265407511406896

Sturmberg, J. P. (2009). The personal nature of health. *Journal of Evaluation in Clinical Practice, 15*, 766–769. https://doi.org/10.1111/j.1365-2753.2009.01225.x

Sturmberg, J. P. & Martin, C. M. (2013). Complexity in health: An introduction. In J. P. Sturmberg & C. M. Martin (Eds.), *Handbook of systems and complexity in health* (pp. 1–17).

Suchman, A. L. (2006). A new theoretical foundation for relationship-centered care: Complex responsive processes of relating. *Journal of General Internal Medicine, 21*, S40–S44. https://doi.org/10.1111/j.1525-1497.2006.00308.x

Tajfel, H. & Turner, J. C. (1979). An integrative theory of intergroup conflict. In W. G. Austin & S. Worchel (Eds.), *The social psychology of intergroup relations* (pp. 33–47). Monterey, CA: Brooks/Cole.

Theiss, J. A. (2018). *The experience and expression of uncertainty in close relationships.* Cambridge, UK: Cambridge University Press.

Theiss, J. A. & Knobloch, L. K. (2013). A relational turbulence model of military service members' relational communication during reintegration. *Journal of Communication, 63*, 1109–1129. https://doi.org/10.1111/jcom.12059

Thibaut, J. W. & Kelley, H. H. (1959). *The social psychology of groups.* Oxford, England: John Wiley.

Thomas, A., Palmer, J. K., Coker-Juneau, C. J., & Williams, D. J. (2003). Factor structure and construct validity of the interaction with disabled persons scale. *Educational and Psychological Measurement, 63*, 465–483. https://doi.org/10.1177/0013164403063003008

Thomas, D. C. (1999). Primary care for people with disabilities. *Mount Sinai Journal of Medicine, 66*, 188–191.

Thompson, J., Petronio, S., & Braithwaite, D. O. (2012). An examination of privacy rules for academic advisors and college student-athletes: A communication privacy management perspective. *Communication Studies, 63*, 54–76. https://doi.org/10.1080/10510974.2011.616569

Thompson, S. C., Galbraith, M., Thomas, C., Swan, J., & Vrungos, S. (2002). Caregivers of stroke patient family members: Behavioral and attitudinal indicators of overprotective care. *Psychology & Health, 17*, 297–312. https://doi.org/10.1080/08870440290029557

Twombly, R. (2004). What's in a name: Who is a cancer survivor? *Journal of the National Cancer Institute, 96*, 1414–1415. https://doi.org/10.1093/jnci/96.19.1414

U.S. Census Bureau. (2001). *Americans with disabilities: Household economic status.* Washington, DC: U.S. Government Printing Office.

U.S. Department of Health and Human Services. (2000). *Healthy people 2010: Understanding and improving health* (2nd ed.). Washington, DC: U.S. Government Printing Office.

Uchino, B. N. (2004). *Social support and physical health: Understanding the health consequences of our relationships.* New Haven, CT: Yale University Press.

(2006). Social support and health: A review of physiological processes potentially underlying links to disease outcomes. *Journal of Behavioral Medicine, 29,* 377–387. https://doi.org/10.1007/s10865-006-9056-5

(2009). Understanding the links between social support and physical health: A life-span perspective with emphasis on the separability of perceived and received support. *Perspectives on Psychological Science, 4,* 236–255. https://doi.org/10.1111/j.1745–6924.2009.01122.x

(2013). Understanding the links between social ties and health: On building stronger bridges with relationship science. *Journal of Social and Personal Relationships, 30,* 155–162. https://doi.org/10.1177/0265407512458659

Uchino, B. N., Bowen, K., Carlisle, M., & Birmingham, W. (2012). Psychological pathways linking social support to health outcomes: A visit with the "ghosts" of research past, present, and future. *Social Science & Medicine, 74,* 949–957. https://doi.org/10.1016/j.socscimed.2011.11.023

Uchino, B. N., Cacioppo, J. T., & Kiecolt-Glaser, J. K. (1996). The relationship between social support and physiological processes: A review with emphasis on underlying mechanisms and implications for health. *Psychological Bulletin, 119,* 488–531. https://doi.org/10.1037/0033–2909.119.3.488

Uchino, B. N., Cacioppo, J. T., Malarkey, W., Glaser, R., & Kiecolt-Glaser, J. K. (1995). Appraisal support predicts age-related differences in cardiovascular function in women. *Health Psychology, 14,* 556–562. https://doi.org/10.1037/0278–6133.14.6.556

Uchino, B. N. & Garvey, T. S. (1997). The availability of social support reduces cardiovascular reactivity to acute psychological stress. *Journal of Behavioral Medicine, 20,* 15–27. https://doi.org/10.1023/A:1025583012283

Uchino, B. N., Holt-Lunstad, J., Uno, D., Betancourt, R., & Garvey, T. S. (1999). Social support and age-related differences in cardiovascular function: An examination of potential mediators. *Annals of Behavioral Medicine, 21,* 135–142. https://doi.org/10.1007/BF02908294

Uchino, B. N., Holt-Lunstad, J., Uno, D., & Flinders, J. B. (2001). Heterogeneity in the social networks of young and older adults: Prediction of mental health and cardiovascular reactivity during acute stress. *Journal of Behavioral Medicine, 24,* 361–382. https://doi.org/10.1023/A:1010634902498

Uchino, B. N., Kiecolt-Glaser, J. K., & Cacioppo, J. T. (1992). Age-related changes in cardiovascular response as a function of a chronic stressor and social support. *Journal of Personality and Social Psychology, 63*, 839–846. https://doi.org/10.1037/0022-3514.63.5.839

Uchino, B. N., & Reblin, M. (2009). Health and relationships. In H. Reis & S. Sprecher (Eds.), *Encyclopedia of human relationships* (pp. 792–797). New York, NY: Sage.

Uchino, B. N., Ruiz, J. M., Smith, T. W., Smyth, J. M., Taylor, D. J., Allison, M., & Ahn, C. (2016). Ethnic/racial differences in the association between social support and levels of C-reactive proteins in the North Texas Heart Study. *Psychophysiology, 53*, 64–70. https://doi.org/10.1111/psyp.12499

Uchino, B. N., Smith, T. W., & Berg, C. A. (2014). Spousal relationship quality and cardiovascular risk: Dyadic perceptions of relationship ambivalence are associated with coronary-artery calcification. *Psychological Science, 25*, 1037–1042. https://doi.org/10.1177/0956797613520015

Uchino, B. N., Smith, T. W., Carlisle, M., Birmingham, W. C., & Light, K. C. (2013). The quality of spouses' social networks contributes to each other's cardiovascular risk. *PLOS One, 8*(8), e71881. https://doi.org/10.1371/journal.pone.0071881

Ugazio, V. (2013). *Semantic polarities and psychopathologies in the family: Permitted and forbidden stories.* New York, NY: Routledge.

Umberson, D. (1987). Family status and health behaviors: Social control as a dimension of social integration. *Journal of Health and Social Behavior, 28*, 306–319. https://doi.org/10.2307/2136848

Umberson, D., Williams, K., Powers, D. A., Liu, H., & Needham, B. (2006). You make me sick: Marital quality and health over the life course. *Journal of Health and Social Behavior, 47*, 1–16. https://doi.org/10.1177/002214650604700101

Underwood, L. G. (2002). The human experience of compassionate love: Conceptual mapping and data from selected studies. In S. G. Post, L. G. Underwood, J. P. Schloss, & W. B. Hurlbut (Eds.), *Altruism & altruistic love: Science, philosophy, & religion in dialogue* (pp. 72–88). New York, NY: Oxford University Press. https://doi.org/10.1093/acprof:oso/9780195143584.003.0009

(2009). Compassionate love: A framework for research. In B. Fehr, S. Sprecher, & L. G. Underwood (Eds.), *The science of compassionate love: Theory, research, and applications* (pp. 3–25). Oxford, England: Wiley-Blackwell. https://doi.org/10.1002/9781444303070.ch1

Valente, T. W. (2015). Social networks and health behavior. In K. Glanz, B. K. Rimer, & K. Viswanath (Eds.), *Health behavior: Theory, research and practice* (5th ed., pp. 205–222). San Francisco, CA: Jossey-Bass.

van der Kolk, B. A. (2014). *The body keeps the score: Brain, mind, and body in the healing of trauma*. New York, NY: Viking.

Van Lange, P. A. M. & Balliet, D. (2015). Interdependence theory. In J. A. Simpson & J. F. Dovidio (Eds.), *APA handbook of personality and social psychology* (pp. 65–92). New York, NY: APA Books.

Van Lange, P. A. M. & Joireman, J. A. (2008). How we can promote behavior that serves all of us in the future. *Social Issues and Policy Review, 2*, 127–157. https://doi.org/10.1111/j.1751–2409.2008.00013.x

Van Lange, P. A. M., Rusbult, C. E., Drigotas, S. M., Arriaga, X. B., Witcher, B. S., & Cox, C. L. (1997). Willingness to sacrifice in close relationships. *Journal of Personality and Social Psychology, 72*, 1373–1395. https://doi.org/10.1037/0022–3514.72.6.1373

Vangelisti, A. L. (2015). Communication in personal relationships. In M. Mikulincer, P. R. Shaver, J. A. Simpson, & J. F. Dovidio (Eds.), *The APA handbook of personality and social psychology: Interpersonal relations and group processes: Vol. 2* (pp. 371–392). Washington, DC: American Psychological Association.

Verheijden, M. W., Bakx, J. C., van Weel, C., Koelen, M. A., & van Staveren, W. A. (2005). Role of social support in lifestyle-focused weight management interventions. *European Journal of Clinical Nutrition, 59*(Suppl. 1), S179–S186. https://doi.org/10.1038/sj.ejcn.1602194

Vicini, A., Shaughnessy, A., & Duggan, A. (2017a). Cultivating the inner life of a physician through written reflection. *Annals of Family Medicine, 15*(4), 379–381. https://doi.org/10.1370/afm.2091

(2017b). On the inner life of physicians: Analysis of family medicine residents' written reflections. *Journal of Religion and Health, 56*(4), 1191–1200. https://doi.org/10.1007/s10943-017–0394-0

Walen, H. R. & Lachman, M. E. (2000). Social support and strain from partner, family, and friends: Costs and benefits for men and women in adulthood. *Journal of Social and Personal Relationships, 17*, 5–30. https://doi.org/10.1177/0265407500171001

Walker, K. L. & Dickson, F. C. (2004). An exploration of illness-related narratives in marriage: The identification of illness-identity scripts. *Journal of Social and Personal Relationships, 21*, 527–544. https://doi.org/10.1177/0265407504044846

Watson, B. & Gallois, C. (1998). Nurturing communication by health professionals toward patients: A communication accommodation theory approach. *Health Communication, 10*, 343–355. https://doi.org/10.1207/s15327027hc1004_3

(2002). Patients' interactions with health providers: A linguistic category model approach. *Journal of Language and Social Psychology, 21*(1), 32–52. https://doi.org/10.1177/0261927x02021001003

Wear, D., Zarconi, J., Garden, R., & Jones, T. (2012). Reflection in/and writing: Pedagogy and practice in medical education. *Academic Medicine, 87*, 603–609. https://doi.org/10.1097/ACM.0b013e31824d22e9

Weber, K., Johnson, A., & Corrigan, M. (2004). Communicating emotional support and its relationship to feelings of being understood, trust, and self-disclosure. *Communication Research Reports, 21*, 316–323. https://doi.org/10.1080/08824090409359994

Weber, K. M. & Solomon, D. H. (2008). Locating relationship and communication issues among stressors associated with breast cancer. *Health Communication, 23*, 548–559. https://doi.org/10.1080/10410230802465233

Weber, K. M., Solomon, D. H., & Meyer, B. J. F. (2013). A qualitative study of breast cancer treatment decisions: Evidence for five decision-making styles. *Health Communication, 28*, 408–421. https://doi.org/10.1080/10410236.2012.713775

Williams, A. (1999). Communication accommodation theory and miscommunication: Issues of awareness and communication dilemmas. *International Journal of Applied Linguistics, 9*, 151–165. https://doi.org/10.1111/j.1473-4192.1999.tb00169.x

World Health Organization. (1986). The Ottawa Charter for Health Promotion. Retrieved from www.who.int/healthpromotion/conferences/previous/ottawa/en/

World Health Organization. (2003). In R. Wilkinson & M. Marmot (Eds.), *Social determinants of health: The solid facts* (2nd ed.). Copenhagen, Denmark: World Health Organization Regional Office for Europe.

World Health Organization. (2008). Closing the gap in a generation: Health equity through action on the social determinants of health. Final report of the Commission on Social Determinants of Health. Geneva, Switzerland: World Health Organization Press.

World Health Organization. (2014). *Basic documents* (48th ed.) Retrieved from http://apps.who.int/gb/bd/

World Health Organization. (2015a). *Beyond bias: Exploring the cultural contexts of health and well-being measurement.* (No. 1). Copenhagen, Denmark: World Health Organization Regional Office for Europe.

World Health Organization. (2015b). *Core health indicators in the WHO European region 2015. Special focus: Human resources for health.* Retrieved from www.euro.who.int/en/data-and-evidence/evidence-resources/core-health-ind icators-in-the-who-european-region/core-health-indicators-n-the-who-eur opean-region-2015.-special-focus-human-resources-for-health

Yamasaki, J., Geist-Martin, P., & Sharf, B. F. (2017). *Storied health and illness: Communicating personal, cultural, & political complexities.* Long Grove, IL: Waveland Press.

Index

Arriaga, Ximena, 222, 224–235
Attachment theory and relational
    ambivalence, 83

Biological systems, 170–172
Biomedical model, 43, 51, 52, 53, 292, 293
Bodily defense responses, 215–218
Bodily doubt, 201
Body alienation, 205
Body as disconnected from
    psychoemotional, 210
Body as objectively measured, 209

Caughlin, John, 89, 113
Changing expectations, 112
Close relationship processes, 64–66
Co-constructing communication, 277–282
Co-generativity through reflection, 294–296
Communication
    Communication accommodation and
        health disparities, 188
    Communication influence processes,
        95–107
    Communication privacy management
        theory, 236–245
    Communication processes and close
        relationships, 87–92
    Communicative process and everyday
        conversation, 150
Compassionate love, 142–145. *See also* Love
Competing demands in close
    relationships, 107
Complexities in definitions as emergent,
    309–318
Complexity theory, 272
Conceptualizing close relationships and
    health and illness, 59
Constitutive communication, 274–277
Constitutive communication in close
    relationships, 282
Coping, 130
Cultural context of health and illness, 39–42

Dark side of close relationships,
    97
Dilemmas of intimacy. *See* Emergence in
    dilemmas of intimacy
Disability, 278–282
Disability communication, 277–282
Disability salience in close relationships,
    187
Disclosure. *See* Communication privacy
    management theory
Disease, 21
Disparities, overall 10, 8, 30, 34, 36, 167, 312,
    318, 319
Disparities in health and illness,
    176–187
Duality between biological and lived
    body, 208
Duggan, Ashley, 55–58, 97–107
Dyadic theories, 222

Embodiment conceptualized,
    197
Emergence, theoretical conceptualization
    Emergence co-generativity in theory,
        323
    Emergence and language, 285
    Emergence in close relationships,
        287–289
    Emergence in dilemmas of intimacy,
        301–304
    Emergence through reflection,
        294–296
Emotional bonds, 75–81
Emotional suppression, 80
Emotions and illness challenges,
    124
Engaged theorizing, 263
Expression-based authenticity doubts model,
    92–95

Fehr, Beverly, 79, 80, 142, 143,
    144,

Finkel, Eli, 62, 63, 70, 71, 73

Gaines, Stanley, 81–83

Health and illness
    Context for relationship research, 58
    Initial definition, 20–30
Health promotion, 27
Human development, 66

Identity and illness progression, 119
Illness
    As lived experience, 198–202
    Sensations in the body, 202
Illness identity, 123, 190
Inconsistent nurturing as control theory,
    98–107
Individual differences, 81
Inequalities, 8, 29, 30, 31, 37, 177, 273, *See
    also* Disparities
Interaction design, 289
Interdependence theory, 224–235
Interdisciplinary, 308
Inter-group
    Communication and disability, 186
    Racial orientation, 183
    Perspective identified, 188

Knobloch, Leanne
    Depression, 137
    Relational turbulence, 246–259
    Uncertainty, 115–117

Labyrinth, 268
Language and body alienation, 211
Language limitations and construction of
    meaning, 290
Lemay, Edward, 92, 93, 94, 95
Life-span implications, 325
Loneliness, 127
Love, 79

Meaning-making in the body, 200
Medical procedures as trauma, 218
Mental health, 8, 25, 172
Mind–body knowing, 319
Multiple lenses as noticing complexities,
    272–274
Multiple-level processes in health-care
    disparities, 181

Narrative research, 44–50
Nonlinearity, 286
Nonverbal behavior, 271

Orbuch, Terri, 79, 165, 166
Ottawa Charter, 27

Perception and use of time, 138
Personality and close relationship
    processes, 81
Petronio, Sandra, 148, 223, 236–245, 257, 258
Physical body in personal relationships, 195
Physical body wisdom, 319
Prager, Karen, 302, 303, 304
Privacy issues, 244
Productive tensions in theory, 284

Questions of lived experience, 199

Reflection as emergence, 299–301
Reflection on health-care communication,
    296–299
Reflective practice, 296–300
Reis, Harry, 62, 66, 95, 222, 224–230, 302, 340
Relational commitment and stability, 67
Relational identity and illness
    challenges, 121
Relational regulation theory, 150
Relational turbulence model. *See* Relational
    turbulence theory
Relational turbulence theory, 246–259
Relationship insecurities, 92–95
Relationship instability, 221
Relationship integration, 70
Relationship science, conceptual, 61
Relationship theories, 56, 70, 321
Relationship theories as part of the system, 321
Relationship-centered health care, 21, 33,
    50–56, 291
    Applications, 54
    Defined, 53
    For theory development, 291
    Versus close relationship processes, 55–58
Relationship-contingent self-esteem, 122
Respect, 80

Scripts and limits for emerging
    understanding, 292
Shared goals, 70–75
Shared health pursuits, 73

Social and economic constructs, 165–169
Social and economic conditions, 42
Social construction of health and illness, 42–44
Social control and influence, 139
Social determinants of health and illness, 33–38. *See also* Social gradient of health and illness
Social gradient of health and illness, 37
Social networks, 117, 159–165
Social production of health, 30–33
Social strain, 134
Social support, 117
  As behavioral pathway, 172–176
  Conceptualized, 219
Societal conditions of health and illness, 155–159
Solomon, Denise, 223, 235, 246–257
Sprecher, 79, 80, 142, 143, 144, 167, 332, 340
Stigma, 135–138
Systematic theorizing, 284–287
Systematic understanding, 266

Theiss, Jennifer, 114, 115, 116, 248, 250, 252
Theoretical foundations, 195, 290
Theoretical attributes of close relationships in healthcare, 111
Theoretical generativity, images, 267
Theories as embedded within social structures, 318
Theory as co-created, 265
Theory of resilience and relational load, 151
Time and space of illness, 203
Transactive goal dynamics theory, 70–75
Trauma and body alienation, 214
Trust and forgiveness, 145

Uncertainty, 114

Vangelisti, Anita, 88, 89, 90, 91

World Health Organization definition of health, 22–30. *See also* Health and Illness, initial definition